FallProof!

Second Edition

A Comprehensive Balance and Mobility Training Program

Debra J. Rose, PhD

California State University, Fullerton

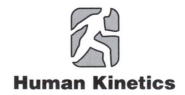

Human Kinetics

Library of Congress Cataloging-in-Publication Data

Rose, Debra J.
  Fallproof! : a comprehensive balance and mobility training program / Debra J. Rose. --
2nd ed.
    p. ; cm.
  Includes bibliographical references and index.
  ISBN-13: 978-0-7360-6747-8 (hard cover)
  ISBN-10: 0-7360-6747-7 (hard cover)
  1. Falls (Accidents) in old age--Prevention. I. Title. II. Title: Compehensive balance and
mobility training program.
  [DNLM: 1. Accidental Falls--prevention & control. 2. Aged. 3. Motor Skills. 4.
Movement. 5. Postural Balance. 6. Safety Management.
WT 104 R7953f 2010]
  RC952.5.R6657 2010
  613'.0438--dc22
                                          2009028325

ISBN-10: 0-7360-6747-7
ISBN-13: 978-0-7360-6747-8

Acquisitions Editor: Judy Patterson Wright, PhD; **Developmental Editors:** Maggie Schwarzentraub and
Kevin Matz; **Assistant Editors:** Katherine Maurer, Nicole Gleeson, and Casey A. Gentis; **Copyeditor:**
Jocelyn Engman; **Indexer:** Dan Connolly; **Permission Manager:** Dalene Reeder; **Graphic Designer:** Joe
Buck; **Graphic Artist:** Yvonne Griffith; **Cover Designer:** Keith Blomberg; **Photographer (cover):** Titan
Communications; **Photographer (interior):** Titan Communications, except as noted. **Photo Asset Manager:**
Laura Fitch; **Visual Production Assistant:** Joyce Brumfield; **Photo Production Manager:** Jason Allen; **Art
Manager:** Kelly Hendren; **Associate Art Manager:** Alan L. Wilborn; **Illustrators:** Accurate Art and Alan L.
Wilborn; **Printer:** Sheridan Books

Printed in the United States of America   10 9 8 7 6 5 4 3 2 1

The paper in this book is certified under a sustainable forestry program.

Human Kinetics
Web site: www.HumanKinetics.com

United States: Human Kinetics
P.O. Box 5076
Champaign, IL 61825-5076
800-747-4457
e-mail: humank@hkusa.com

Canada: Human Kinetics
475 Devonshire Road Unit 100
Windsor, ON N8Y 2L5
800-465-7301 (in Canada only)
e-mail: info@hkcanada.com

Europe: Human Kinetics
107 Bradford Road
Stanningley
Leeds LS28 6AT, United Kingdom
+44 (0) 113 255 5665
e-mail: hk@hkeurope.com

Australia: Human Kinetics
57A Price Avenue
Lower Mitcham, South Australia 5062
08 8372 0999
e-mail: info@hkaustralia.com

New Zealand: Human Kinetics
P.O. Box 80
Torrens Park, South Australia 5062
0800 222 062
e-mail: info@hknewzealand.com

With thanks and gratitude to all the older adults who have touched my life and inspired me to create this program.

Contents

Preface

Maintaining balance and mobility is essential to aging successfully. In addition to making it possible to perform basic activities of daily living, such as rising from a chair or climbing a flight of stairs, good balance forms the foundation on which a healthy and active lifestyle is built. Impairments in any of the multiple systems that contribute to postural stability not only limit the extent and type of physical activities we pursue as we grow older but also may result in falls, leading to further restrictions in activity and profound psychological consequences. The strong association between impaired balance and mobility and greater risk of falling suggests the need for activity-based programs that specifically *and* systematically focus on improving the multiple dimensions of the balance system, particularly among older adults.

The second edition of *FallProof! A Comprehensive Balance and Mobility Training Program* not only builds on the knowledge presented in the first edition but also provides a structured approach to the design and implementation of a balance and mobility program that reduces many of the risk factors that contribute to falling. This program remains the first published balance and mobility program to provide the reader with the fundamental theoretical concepts and practical skills needed to assess and design effective activity programs for older adults with balance and mobility disorders as well as a comprehensive set of progressive balance activities that address the important dimensions of balance and mobility. The program in this guide is based on sound, theoretical research, and a group-based version of the program has been field-tested extensively by many physical activity instructors and rehabilitation specialists working with older adults across a broad continuum of functional abilities. The innovative balance and mobility program described in this book was developed at the Center for Successful Aging at California State University at Fullerton and is currently being implemented in numerous community-based and residential care settings with considerable success. Physical activity professionals who embrace this unique multidimensional programming approach to treating balance and mobility disorders can expect to achieve the same success.

The second edition of *FallProof! A Comprehensive Balance and Mobility Training Program* is divided into three parts. Part I, The Theory Behind the Program, provides the reader with in-depth knowledge about the various body systems that contribute to balance and mobility and the common age-related changes that occur in each of these systems. The external and internal risk factors known to be strongly associated with falls among the older adult population are also discussed, as are the common medical conditions and medications known to adversely affect balance and mobility.

Part II begins by describing a concise set of balance and mobility assessments used to evaluate every client entering the FallProof™ program both before and at regular intervals throughout the program. These assessments measure the multiple dimensions of balance and mobility and provide the instructor with the information needed to determine where each participant should start in each of the six major components of the FallProof program. These components, described in the remainder of part II, include (1) center-of-gravity control training, (2) multisensory training, (3) postural strategy training, (4) gait pattern enhancement and variation training, (5) strength and endurance training, and (6) flexibility training. In addition to describing a set of progressive exercises for each component of the FallProof program, each chapter provides ideas for increasing the challenge associated with each balance activity. Advanced progressions are based on manipulating the task demands and the environmental constraints to progressively challenge the individual capabilities of the participants. At-a-glance summary tables are also provided in chapters 5, 6, 8, and 9 to further guide the instructor.

Part III of the book describes how to implement a balance and mobility program. The first chapter in this part describes contemporary principles of motor learning that will enable instructors to foster optimal learning, develop effective lesson plans, organize the classroom environment to maximize safety and efficiency, and provide meaningful feedback to program participants. The second and final chapter describes the leadership and class management skills needed to be a successful balance and mobility instructor. It covers the important activities that must be completed (a) following the initial assessment of program participants and before the start of the program, (b) before the start of each class session, (c) during each class session, (d) between class sessions, and (e) after each follow-up assessment. It also describes how to communicate effectively with program participants.

This instructor guide will be an invaluable resource for experienced health care professionals and physical activity instructors who want to acquire the specialized knowledge and practical skills needed to develop and implement programs that improve the balance and mobility of older adults. The wide range of exercise progressions described and the ideas for manipulating the challenge associated with each exercise make *FallProof! A Comprehensive Balance and Mobility Training Program* a versatile guide in programming for older adults who come from a broad range of functional levels. Although physical activity instructors who have not yet completed the academic and practical skills training needed to work with at-risk older adults can also use this instructor guide to learn how to incorporate more balance and mobility exercises into their senior fitness programs, they should not develop a specialty balance and mobility program for at-risk older adults until they have completed additional training in the area.

FallProof! A Comprehensive Balance and Mobility Training Program is the first systematic effort to develop a structured and progressive program of activities specifically designed to address the multiple dimensions that contribute to balance and mobility.

This instructor guide serves as the core text for the balance and mobility instructor specialist certification program, which began operating at California State University at Fullerton in 2001. Readers interested in developing their knowledge and practical skills in balance and mobility training so they can become certified to implement the FallProof program should consider enrolling in this certification program. The program is staffed by an outstanding group of experienced kinesiologists and physical therapists with expertise in geriatric assessment and rehabilitation. Information about the certification program and an online application can be obtained by logging onto the Center for Successful Aging Web site at http://hhd.fullerton.edu/csa.

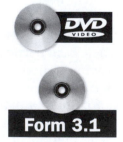

New to the second edition is a supplementary DVD that includes video clips and the forms you will need to assess your clients and monitor their progress throughout the program. Icons (such as the two on this page) appear throughout the text, alerting you to the contents of the DVD. You will find the instructional videos for the Fullerton Advanced Balance (FAB) scale and the 30-foot walk test particularly helpful in preparing you to administer these tests. You can also test your readiness to administer and score the FAB scale by watching the case study video and scoring each test item of the FAB scale after it is administered. Finally, the DVD contains short video clips highlighting different exercise progressions related to each core component of the program and a 30-minute FallProof class with Harriet and Ben, two of my wonderful clients from the Center for Successful Aging.

Acknowledgments

I would first like to extend my heartfelt thanks to the wonderful colleagues I have the pleasure of working with in the balance and mobility instructor specialist certification program at California State University at Fullerton: Dr. Courtney Hall, PhD, PT; Dr. Peggy Trueblood, PhD, PT; Grace Amaya, MS; Judy Aprile, MS; Sue Grant, BS; Danielle Hernandez, MS; and Karen Russell, PTA. In addition, I would like to thank the more than 400 instructors who have been certified to teach the FallProof program over the past several years for providing me with invaluable feedback on the first edition of this book and on the program itself as they implemented it in their communities. Also, thanks to the wonderful group of older adults who served as models for the second edition of this book: Rodolfo Amaya, David Armstrong, Lou Arnwine, John and Myrtle Brothers, Hilda Corral, Ramon Corral, Stanley Dashew, Harriet Dolgin, Carlos Estrada, Ann and Gregory Foster, Ann Gardner, Ted Gibson, Danielle Hernandez, Margaret Low, Bill McGarvey, Mio Sakai, Ralph Scheffer, Ann Siebert, Donna Spradlin, Fritz von Coelln, Andy Washington, and Mildred Kiyo Young.

Many thanks are also extended to the Archstone Foundation of California for providing the generous funding necessary to test the efficacy of this program in a large number of community-based centers serving the needs of older adults. The Archstone Foundation has also provided the Center for Successful Aging at California State University at Fullerton with additional funding for an instructor certification program designed to provide health care professionals with the specialized knowledge needed to implement the FallProof program in their immediate communities. Thanks also to the Retirement Research Foundation for providing additional funding to examine the long-term efficacy of the program in residential care facilities throughout southern California.

Part I

The Theory Behind the Program

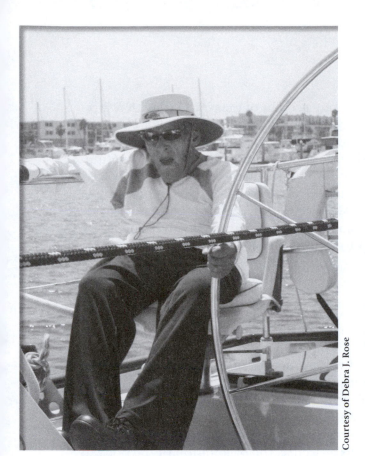

Courtesy of Debra J. Rose

Chapter **1**

Understanding Balance and Mobility

Objectives

After completing this chapter, you will be able to

- describe terminology used in the study of balance and mobility,
- identify the multiple systems that contribute to postural stability, and
- describe the major age-related changes that occur in balance and mobility.

The control of balance depends on a series of complex processes that are triggered by either a conscious or an unconscious decision to act. Our decision to act may be a response to an internal desire to perform a certain task, a reaction to sensory events occurring in the environment, or a combination of the two. Although many of the decisions we make during the day are made at a conscious level, such as rising from a chair to answer the door or walk to the neighborhood store to purchase groceries, others are made at a subconscious level. Subconscious responses are most often associated with well-learned skills that require little or no conscious attention or with the need to respond rapidly to an unexpected threat to our stability. Whether the decision to act is conscious or subconscious, multiple systems within the body are involved.

WHAT IS BALANCE?

center of mass (COM)—In terms of the forces that act on the body and the body's motion, the COM is the point at which all the mass of the body is concentrated. The COM is also referred to as the *center of gravity* (COG) because the gravitational force due to the weight of the body also acts through this point.

balance—The process by which we control the body's COM with respect to the base of support, whether we are stationary or moving.

posture—The biomechanical alignment of the individual body parts as well as the orientation of the body to the environment.

anticipatory postural control—Actions that are planned in advance.

reactive postural control—Actions that cannot be planned in advance due to the unexpected nature of an event.

Balance is the process of controlling the body's **center of mass (COM)** with respect to its base of support, whether the body is stationary or moving. For example, when we are standing upright, our primary goal is to maintain the COM within the confines of the base of support, whereas when we are walking, we are continuously moving the COM beyond the base of support and reestablishing a new base of support with each step taken. Although we often consider upright standing to be a static balance task and leaning or walking to be a dynamic balance task, we must remember that maintaining a stable upright position involves the active contraction of various muscle groups to control the position of the COM against the destabilizing force of gravity.

TERMINOLOGY

Inevitably, when we are introduced to a new area of study, we are overwhelmed by many new and unfamiliar terms. As you read each of the chapters in this instructor guide, you too will be confronted by many new terms that are specific to the study of balance and mobility. In addition to understanding what is meant by the term **balance**, you will need to be able to define the terms *posture, anticipatory and reactive postural control, stability limits, the sway envelope,* and *mobility.*

Good **posture** is critical to good balance, and the term refers to the biomechanical alignment of each of our body parts as well as the orientation of the body to the environment (Shumway-Cook & Woollacott, 2005). When we are standing quietly, our goal is to align each of the body parts vertically and thereby expend the least amount of internal energy necessary to maintain an upright and stable position relative to gravity. To counteract the forces of gravity, a number of muscles are active during quiet standing (see figure 1.1). These include the soleus and gastrocnemius, the tibialis anterior (when the body sways backward), the gluteus medius and tensor fasciae latae, the iliopsoas, the erector spinae in the thoracic region of the trunk, and the abdominal muscles, somewhat more intermittently (Basmajian & De Luca, 1985).

Although many of our balance- and mobility-related activities allow us to plan our actions in advance, there are times when an unexpected event forces us to respond more subconsciously or automatically. **Anticipatory postural control** is the term used to describe those actions that can be planned in advance, whereas **reactive postural control** is the term used to describe the more automatically generated actions that occur when our movements cannot be planned in advance of the required action. Anticipatory postural control helps us avoid obstacles in our path as we walk to the store or run through the forest. It also assists us in adapting our gait pattern as we move from one type of surface to the next (e.g., from firm to compliant or moving surfaces, from wide to narrow surfaces). In contrast, reactive postural control becomes necessary when we have to respond quickly to an event

Figure 1.1 *(a)* Good postural alignment minimizes the amount of muscle activity required to maintain an upright stance. *(b)* Even when we stand quietly, a number of muscles throughout the body are activated.

we did not expect (e.g., stepping in an unseen hole, being bumped in a crowd). Many of the activities described in chapters 4 and 5 will help your older clients improve both of these dimensions of balance.

How far we are willing or able to lean in any direction without having to change our base of support constitutes our **stability limits.** People who are able to align their COM directly above their base of support during quiet standing can sway as much as 12 degrees in a forward–backward direction (8 degrees forward and 4 degrees backward) and 16 degrees laterally before they must take a step because their stability limits have been exceeded (Nashner, 1989). Of course, this **sway envelope,** as it is called, often is much smaller among older adults who are beginning to experience balance problems. Reduced or asymmetric limits of stability may result from musculoskeletal abnormalities caused by weak ankle muscles or reduced range of motion about the ankles, neurological trauma (i.e., stroke, Parkinson's disease, multiple sclerosis) that has resulted in muscle weakness that affects movement in a particular direction, or a fear of falling.

stability limit—The maximum distance an individual is able or willing to lean in any direction without changing the base of support.

sway envelope—The path of the body's movement during quiet standing.

Although stability limits vary according to the individual's inherent biomechanical limitations, the task being performed, or the constraints of the environment, a significant reduction in those limits, particularly in the lateral and backward directions, will place the older adult at a heightened risk for falling. Any small disruption to standing balance quickly moves these individuals beyond their limits of stability and requires them to reach for nearby support or take one or more steps to prevent a fall.

Finally, the term **mobility** has been defined as a person's ability to move independently and safely from one place to another (Shumway-Cook & Woollacott, 2005). Adequate mobility is required for many different types of activities performed in daily life. These may include transfers (e.g., rising from a chair, climbing or descending stairs), walking or running, and other types of recreational activities (e.g., gardening, sports, dancing).

mobility—The ability to move independently and safely from one place to another.

POSTURAL CONTROL STRATEGIES FOR CONTROLLING BALANCE

Studies conducted over the years have discovered at least three distinct postural control strategies that control the amount of body sway. These strategies are referred to as the *ankle, hip,* and *step strategies* (see figure 1.2 on page 6). In the ankle strategy, the body moves as a single entity about the ankle joints as force is exerted against the ground surface. What you see when you watch a person using an **ankle strategy** is the upper and lower body moving in the same direction, or moving in phase. Because the amount of force that can be generated by the muscles surrounding the ankle joint is relatively small, we generally use this strategy to control sway when we are standing upright or swaying slowly through a very small range of motion. The ankle strategy is also used at a subconscious level to restore balance following a small nudge or push.

ankle strategy—The postural control strategy in which the body moves as a single entity about the ankle joints (i.e., the upper and lower body sway in the same direction).

In contrast to the ankle strategy, the **hip strategy** involves activation of the larger hip muscles and is used when the COM must be moved back over the base of support more quickly. When you watch a person using a hip strategy, you will see the upper and lower body move in opposite directions (i.e., move out of phase). The hip strategy becomes increasingly important as the distance and speed of sway increase or when we are standing on a surface that is narrower

hip strategy—The postural control strategy in which the upper and lower body move in opposite directions as a result of the hip muscles being activated to control balance.

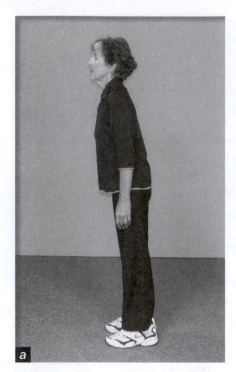
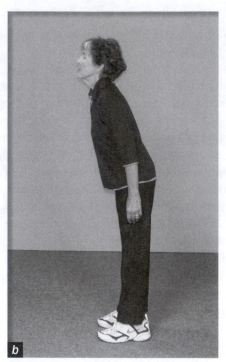
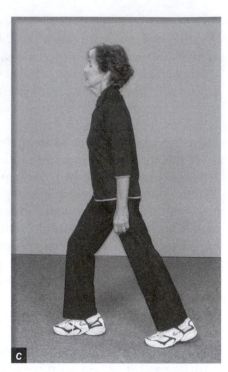

Figure 1.2 Three postural control strategies are used by adults to control balance in a standing position: *(a)* ankle, *(b)* hip, and *(c)* step.

than the length of our feet (e.g., when standing sideways on a narrow beam). In these surface conditions, we can no longer use the ankle strategy because there is not enough surface against which the feet can push in order to generate sufficient force to restore balance using the smaller ankle muscles.

The final postural control strategy used to control balance is the **step strategy**. This strategy comes into play when our COM is displaced beyond our maximum limits of stability or our speed of sway is so fast that a hip strategy is insufficient to maintain the COM within the stability limits. In this situation, we must establish a new base of support if we are to prevent a fall. When executing a step strategy, a person takes one or more steps in the direction of the loss of balance. Although each of the postural control strategies presented in this section are described as distinct movement patterns, various combinations of these strategies are used to control forward and backward sway in a standing position (Horak & Nashner, 1986; Jensen et al., 1996). Moreover, recent research suggests that in many situations stepping or reaching responses may occur even before the COM moves outside of the limits of stability (Brown, Shumway-Cook, & Woollacott, 1999).

What factors are likely to limit our ability to use each of these three movement strategies? In the case of the ankle strategy, adequate range of motion and strength within the muscles surrounding the ankle joint are needed. The surface beneath the feet must also be firm and broad, and the individual must have adequate sensation in the feet to be able to feel the surface. Older adults experiencing a significant decline in sensation in the feet or ankles will find it particularly difficult to employ this strategy.

step strategy—The postural control strategy used when the COM is displaced beyond the maximal stability limits or sway is too great to use a hip strategy effectively. It requires a new base of support to be established.

Key Point

An effective ankle strategy requires
- adequate range of motion and strength in the ankle joints;
- a firm, broad surface below the feet; and
- adequate sensation in the feet and ankles.

Our ability to use a hip strategy to control postural sway is determined more by the amount of muscle strength and range of motion we have in the hip as opposed to the ankle. Although the use of a hip strategy is confined to forward and backward movement, sway in the lateral direction is also controlled by the larger hip muscles, particularly the adductor and abductor muscle groups. Any weakness in these muscles adversely affects lateral stability, a requirement for walking.

As mentioned earlier, the stepping strategy is most likely to be used when the boundaries of stability are exceeded. The ability to use this particular movement strategy is greatly affected by lower-limb strength and muscle power. Also, slowed central processing adversely affects an older adult's ability to use the step strategy effectively. In addition, reduced range of motion at the hip joint is a factor in determining the length of step taken following a loss of balance.

The postural strategy training component of the FallProof program (see chapter 6) contains many progressive exercises that are designed to improve the participants' ability to use each of the three movement strategies just described. This component of the program helps participants learn to select the appropriate postural control strategy and scale it in a way that best matches the demands of the task they are being asked to perform and the environment in which they are working.

MULTIPLE SYSTEMS CONTRIBUTE TO BALANCE AND MOBILITY

Multiple systems contribute to our ability to maintain balance in standing and moving environments. First, the various sensory systems (vision, somatosensory, and vestibular) provide us with information arising from the surrounding environment and from our own actions. This information is critical for successful goal-directed action planning as well as for subconscious or automatic adjustments needed to maintain a given position in space or respond rapidly to a change in task or environmental demands. We use the information from our sensory systems to plan actions, anticipate changes that will affect current or future actions, and respond to changes that have already occurred.

The many structures within the nervous system that make up the motor system are also critical for action. The motor system acts on the sensory information available in the external environment as well as the other sensory areas within the nervous system. Action is accomplished as a result of the nervous system constraining groups of muscles throughout the body to act together. These are referred to as **muscle response synergies** and are responsible for the many coordinated actions we produce in our daily lives. Finally, the cognitive system plays a role in helping us interpret the incoming sensations and plan the ensuing motor responses. This

> **Key Point**
>
> An effective hip strategy requires adequate range of motion and strength in the hip.

> **Key Point**
>
> An effective step strategy requires
> - adequate lower-body muscle strength, power, and range of motion;
> - adequate central processing speed; and
> - the ability to move the limb rapidly during step initiation.

> **Key Point**
>
> Our sensory systems are used to anticipate changes that will affect current and future actions as well as to respond to changes that have already occurred.

muscle response synergies—Groups of muscles constrained to act together.

> ## Key Point
>
> The motor system acts on internally and externally provided sensory information.

system, which encompasses attention, memory storage, and intelligence, provides us with the collective ability to anticipate or adapt our actions in response to changing task demands and environment.

As indicated earlier, three sensory systems are particularly important for good postural control and largely determine how well we perceive what needs to be done based on the information presented to us. These are the visual, somatosensory, and vestibular systems. No individual system provides us with all the sensory information we need to determine our position in space; each system contributes its unique information about body position and movement to the central nervous system (CNS). Each system also responds to different types of incoming information. Whereas vision responds to light, the somatosensory system is sensitive to touch, vibration, and pain and the vestibular system is activated when the head moves.

We depend most heavily on the visual system for information about our movements and our position in space. This system not only provides us with a visual layout of the surrounding environment but also provides us with critical information about our spatial location relative to objects within that environment. Once we begin moving through space, vision also helps us to navigate safely, anticipate changes in surfaces we encounter, and avoid obstacles in our path. It is therefore an important source of mobility information.

> ## Key Point
>
> The somatosensory system provides us with information about our spatial location and the movement of the body relative to the support surface.

In contrast to the visual system, the somatosensory system provides information about the spatial location and movement of our bodies relative to the support surface beneath us. It also informs us about the position and movement of body segments relative to one another. This latter information is provided by proprioceptors located in the muscles and joints (e.g., muscle spindles, joint receptors). In the absence of vision, the somatosensory system becomes our primary source of sensory information for maintaining upright balance and moving about in dark environments.

> ## Key Point
>
> The vestibular system, in conjunction with the visual system, helps us determine whether the world or our body is moving.

The final sensory system that contributes balance information is the vestibular system. This delicate balance mechanism is housed in the inner ear and is activated when we move our head. It works in conjunction with the visual system to help us determine whether the world or our body is moving when we turn quickly in space. It becomes particularly important for maintaining upright balance when sensory information usually received by the visual and somatosensory systems is no longer available, is distorted, or is inaccurate.

Once the information derived from each of the three sensory systems has been organized and integrated by the CNS and we have determined where we are in space and what we wish to do, the motor system generates the appropriate action plan. As we begin to act, the sensory systems continue to receive additional information from the environment and our own movement response so we can quickly modify our current plan of action, change to an alternative plan, or begin planning the next action. This intricate and continuous interplay between the sensory and motor systems is often referred to as the perception–action cycle. Whereas the sensory systems give rise to a perception that is used to guide our initial action, the results of that initial action generated by the motor system are then used to alter or confirm the accuracy of the original perception.

The dynamic equilibrium model was developed by Nashner (1989) as a means of describing each of the processes occurring in the peripheral and central components of the sensory and motor systems that characterize the perception–action cycle (figure 1.3). The visual, somatosensory, and vestibular receptors constitute the peripheral component of the sensory system, and the transmission pathways and specialized areas within the CNS constitute the central components of the sensory system. It is in this central component that the information received from the environment via our visual, somatosensory, and vestibular receptors is compared, selected, and combined so that we can perceive where our body is in space.

Once we have perceived where we are in space, we begin the process of determining what we are going to do, if anything, on the basis of the information received. This action-planning process begins within the central component of the motor system with the selection of the various muscle groups needed to carry out the plan of action and the specific muscle contractile patterns required to accomplish the intended movement. That movement may be as simple as standing quietly in space or as complicated as running over uneven terrain. The many different groups of muscles throughout the body that make up the peripheral component of the motor system ultimately are responsible for generating the desired movement.

Both the speed and the accuracy of the movement generated in response to incoming sensory information are influenced by how well we are able to remember what we are supposed to do in a given situation and our ability to allocate

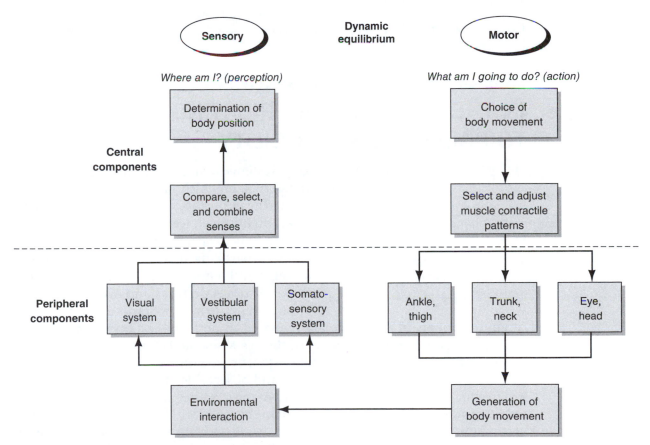

Figure 1.3 The dynamic equilibrium model.
Adapted, by permission, from NeuroCom International.

our attentional resources, particularly when we are required to perform more than one task at a time. Any impairments in cognition or attention will severely compromise our ability to perceive what type of response is needed and then implement the response, or responses, once selected (Dickin & Rose, 2004). It has been well documented that older adults with cognitive impairment not only experience a more rapid decline in function following an acute illness or hospitalization but also experience many more falls than their peers without cognitive impairment experience (Leape, 2000; van Dijk, Meulenberg, van de Sande, & Habbema, 1993).

Several research studies have demonstrated that older adults must allocate more attention to the task of balancing, particularly when less sensory information is available (Shumway-Cook & Woollacott, 2000). Distributing attention between two cognitive tasks has also been found to be increasingly difficult for older adults, especially for older adults with identified balance impairments or a history of falls (Shumway-Cook, Baldwin, Polissar, & Gruber, 1997; Brauer, Woollacott, & Shumway-Cook, 2002).

As a balance and mobility instructor, you need to understand which body systems contribute to postural stability as well as how each system works in collaboration with other systems to solve the many balance problems we face on a daily basis. This knowledge is fundamental to your understanding of the six components of the FallProof program. Not only do the six program components address the dimensions of balance and mobility just described, but the progression of exercises from easier to more challenging will accommodate the heterogeneous capabilities of participants in each program component.

> **Key Point**
>
> Older adults must allocate more attention to the task of balancing.

AGE-ASSOCIATED CHANGES IN THE SYSTEMS CONTRIBUTING TO BALANCE AND MOBILITY

Unfortunately, changes in the body systems that contribute to balance and mobility are an inevitable consequence of aging. Although some of the changes occurring in these systems have no observable effect on how well we perform balance-related tasks across a variety of environments, other changes, particularly those that affect multiple systems, influence the type of strategy we use to perform certain tasks and even whether we choose to perform those tasks at all. The types of environments in which we are prepared to perform certain tasks may also change depending on the severity of the age-associated changes we experience.

> **Key Point**
>
> Changes in the body systems that contribute to balance and mobility are an inevitable consequence of aging.

The structural and functional changes that occur within the CNS with advancing age appear to have the most profound and observable effect on motor function. When older adults are compared with younger adults across a variety of motor tasks, significant differences are evident in the speed with which older adults initiate and execute movements, particularly when the number of available responses and the complexity of the movement to be performed increase (Spirduso, Francis, & MacRae, 2005). Qualitative differences in the strategy used to accomplish the goal of the movement are also evident in some cases.

Despite the many age-associated structural and functional changes occurring within the central and peripheral nervous systems, not all changes occurring within specific regions necessarily result in observable or adverse effects on behavior. That is because optimal motor function is achieved through the interaction of multiple systems both within and external to the CNS. When multiple systems become impaired, however, the quality of the interactions among the impaired systems declines and results in observable motor dysfunction. For example, although adverse changes occurring in the visual system make it more difficult to use visual information for balance, usually information from the somatosensory and vestibular systems can be used to compensate for the impaired visual system. Impairment in one or both of the two remaining sensory systems, however, severely affects the ability to organize and integrate sensory information. Not only does our perception of the surrounding environment and our position in space become inadequate or inaccurate, but our ability to respond appropriately is also compromised.

At a behavioral level, cumulative changes in the aging nervous system manifest themselves in a reduced ability to perform a variety of complex movements that require speed and accuracy, balance, strength, or coordination. Let's now describe the age-related changes occurring in the peripheral and central components of the sensory and motor systems illustrated in Nashner's dynamic equilibrium model (see figure 1.3 on page 9).

> ### Key Point
>
> Optimal motor function is achieved through the interaction of multiple systems that are internal and external to the CNS.

Changes in the Peripheral and Central Components of the Sensory System

Age-related changes in the peripheral and central components of the visual, somatosensory, and vestibular systems can be expected to affect our balance and mobility most adversely because of the interdependency that exists among the processing of incoming sensory information, the selection of an appropriate motor response, and the subsequent control of the motor response. As illustrated in figure 1.3, the peripheral receptors associated with each sensory system are responsible for the initial reception and transmission of sensory information that arises from our interaction with the environment, whereas the sensory areas constituting the central component of the sensory system are responsible for comparing, selecting, and combining the incoming sensory information from each system so that we can determine where we are in space and what we need to do, if anything, in response to it. This sensory information, once organized and integrated within the central sensory areas of the brain, is then used to guide the selection of the ensuing motor response.

Age-Related Changes in Vision

Common age-related changes in the peripheral component of the visual system include reduced acuity, depth perception, and contrast sensitivity as well as narrowing of the visual field, particularly in the peripheral region. These changes alter the quality of the information received within the central component of the system and result in slower processing of the incoming sensory feedback, poorer integration of sensory inputs, and an altered perception of the body's position in space.

At a behavioral level, these age-related changes occurring within the visual system adversely affect the older adult's ability to perceive or anticipate any changes in normal surface conditions and any hazards in the environment. As a result, the ability to avoid obstacles, negotiate curbs and stairs, and move about in conditions of low or changing light is hindered (Lord, Clark, & Webster, 1991). Decrements within the visual system, particularly within the peripheral visual field, are also associated with an increased risk of falling among older adults.

The increasing prevalence of eye diseases such as cataract, glaucoma, and macular degeneration among older adults is associated with increasing fall rates (Ivers, Cumming, Mitchell, & Attabo, 1998; Lord, McLean, & Stathers, 1992). When combined with normal age-related changes occurring within the visual system, these eye diseases further compromise the quality of an older adult's vision. Examples of the ways in which eye diseases affect what an older adult is able to see are illustrated in figure 1.4.

> ### Key Point
>
> Age-related changes in the visual system adversely affect an older adult's ability to perceive or anticipate any changes in surface conditions or any hazards in the environment.

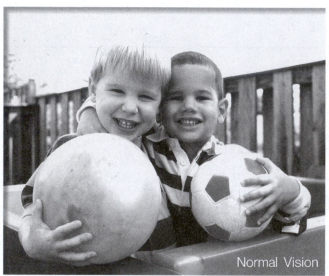

Normal Vision

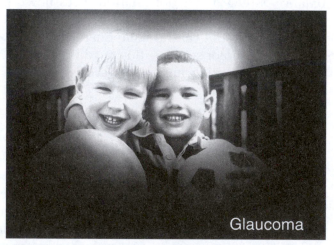

Glaucoma

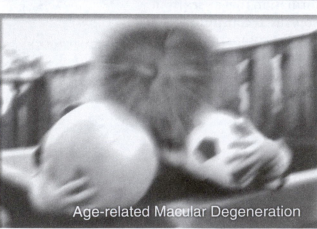

Age-related Macular Degeneration

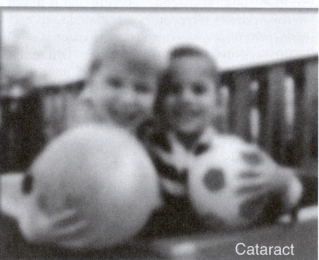

Cataract

Figure 1.4 Normal vision may be adversely affected by diseases such as glaucoma, age-related macular degeneration, and cataract.

Courtesy of the National Eye Institute, National Institutes of Health.

Age-Related Changes in Somatosensation

Age-related changes within the peripheral component of the somatosensory system directly affect postural stability and the ability to restore upright control following a loss of balance. A 2- to 10-fold increase in **vibration threshold,** indicating a reduced ability to feel the contact between the feet and the ground, has been well documented among older adults (Kenshalo, 1986; Perret & Reglis, 1970). Age-related changes in joint position sense have also been shown to adversely influence postural control (Blaszczyk, Hansen, & Lowe, 1993; Thelen, Brockmiller, Ashton-Miller, Schultz, & Alexander, 1998). As mentioned earlier, proprioceptors found within the muscles and joints provide us with information on the static and changing positions of our joints in space and are therefore important for optimal balance and mobility.

> **vibration threshold**—The level at which the somatosensory receptor begins to fire in response to the application of a vibratory stimulus.

Age-Related Changes in the Vestibular System

A gradually decreasing density of hair cells within the vestibular system begins as early as age 30 and progresses through older adulthood. These **hair cells** serve as biological sensors of head motion. Therefore, any significant decline in their number reduces our sensitivity to head movements and results in increased sway, particularly when vision is no longer available and information from the somatosensory system is distorted. A moderate reduction in the gain of the **vestibulo-ocular reflex (VOR)** has also been noted with age. Because this reflex helps us stabilize our vision when we move our heads rapidly, any impairment in the VOR affects our ability to determine whether it is the world or our body that is moving in certain situations.

> **hair cells**—Biological sensors within the vestibular system that are mechanically deformed (bent) when the head moves, causing neural impulses to be generated.
>
> **vestibulo-ocular reflex (VOR)**—The reflex responsible for rotating the eyes in a direction that is equal and opposite to the direction of head movement.

In addition to helping us align our head and body with respect to gravity, the vestibular system becomes critical for balance when sensory information from the visual and somatosensory systems is absent, distorted, or in conflict. For example, we rely heavily on our vestibular system for balance when we are moving around in the dark or on a compliant or unstable surface. The vestibular system also helps resolve the conflict that often arises among the sensory systems when we find ourselves in complex visual environments (e.g., crowded malls, freeway traffic). For example, how often have you found yourself depressing the brake in your stationary car because you erroneously thought that your car was rolling backward? What happened was that the car next to you began moving forward and tricked your visual system into thinking that you were the one moving, even though your somatosensory and vestibular systems were signaling that you were not moving.

> **Key Point**
>
> The vestibular system becomes critical for balance when the sensory information from the visual system is absent or when information from the visual and somatosensory systems is distorted or in conflict.

Older adults who are experiencing balance problems may often comment on how much they dislike going into crowded malls or grocery stores because they feel increasingly unsteady due to people constantly moving in and out of their visual field. Many older adults compensate for this unsteadiness by pushing a shopping cart through the store for better stabilization, whereas others simply avoid these types of sensory environments. These adults are experiencing difficulty in resolving the conflict among the three sensory systems

> **Key Point**
>
> Sensory conflict occurs when information provided by one or more sensory systems is not in agreement with information from one or both of the other sensory systems.

because they are no longer able to identify and then quickly ignore the conflicting input from the visual and somatosensory systems. Older adults with dysfunctional vestibular systems may also report that they are experiencing visual problems, are feeling dizzy or unsteady, or are experiencing unusual sensory illusions when confronted with a conflicting sensory environment (Wolfson, 1997).

Changes in the Central and Peripheral Components of the Motor System

Age-related changes in the central component of the motor system have been well documented. Chronometric measures (i.e., reaction time, movement time, and response time) used to quantify the time required to plan and execute actions have revealed that the most significant age-related decline occurs in the action-planning phase (the time when incoming sensory information is processed and an appropriate motor response is formulated; Spirduso et al., 2005). Many older adults also experience difficulty in selecting the appropriate movement strategy to use in a given situation. Inappropriate scaling of the response strategy is also observed among older adults; that is, older adults tend to over- or underrespond, particularly when they are perturbed. They might overrespond by taking a step, even though the loss of balance was small, or they might underrespond to a larger perturbation by not stepping at all.

perturbation—A disturbance to a system. The disturbance may be external or internal.

Electromyographic (EMG) studies have revealed significant age-related differences in the temporal sequencing of muscle activation patterns in response to unexpected **perturbations.** Unlike their younger counterparts, who demonstrate stereotypical and symmetrical responses, healthy older adults exhibit considerably more variable activation patterns and a reduced ability to inhibit inappropriate responses (Stelmach, Phillips, DiFabio, & Teasdale, 1989). Inappropriate postural responses are most evident when the functional base of support is reduced, the support surface is compliant or unstable, or the visual input is altered (Alexander, 1994).

> ### Key Point
>
> The inappropriate scaling of response strategies is common among older adults.

Finally, as adults age they appear to lose their ability to anticipate changes in the environment or the demands associated with a task. This loss of anticipatory postural control is no doubt a result of declining processing speeds within both the peripheral and central components of the sensory system and the central component of the motor system. This age-associated change is most evident when older adults are asked to start or stop quickly, transition between different surfaces (e.g., move from a firm to compliant surface), or negotiate obstacles in their environment. Instead of using a smooth and continuous stepping action, older adults are more likely to demonstrate a marked slowing in gait speed as they approach an obstacle and a brief pause before initiating the stepping action. Be sure to watch for this changing behavior during your initial assessment of the older adult so you can better match the difficulty of the selected exercises to the individual's capabilities.

muscle strength—The amount of force that an individual muscle or group of muscles can produce with a single maximal contraction.

Age-associated changes in the musculoskeletal component of the motor system also result in longer movement execution times. Decreases in **muscle strength,** particularly in the lower body, have been well documented. Between age 50 and age 70, muscle strength declines as much as 30 percent, and even larger decreases are noted after age 80 (Lindle et al., 1997). This decline is thought to be due to a decrease in both the size and the number of muscle fibers. Physical inactivity also contributes to the loss of muscle strength, particularly in the antigravity or postural muscles required for good upright posture. **Muscle endurance** also decreases with age. This decrease results in an earlier onset of fatigue that places an older adult at a heightened risk for a loss of balance or a fall. Finally, **muscle power** also decreases significantly with age. It is estimated that absolute power declines 6 to 11 percent per decade and is lost at a rate that is 10 percent greater than the rate at which muscle strength is lost, even though the declines in both strength and power begin at a similar age (Metter, Conwitt, Tobin, & Fozard, 1997). This age-related change in muscle probably has the greatest consequences for performing basic activities such as walking, climbing stairs, or rising from a chair because all of these activities require muscle power for their successful completion. Certainly a decline in muscle power is a contributing factor to an older adult's inability to respond quickly and effectively to an unexpected loss of balance.

muscle endurance—A muscle's ability to contract continuously at a submaximal level.

muscle power—A muscle's ability to contract forcefully in a very short time.

> ## Key Point
> Between age 50 and age 70, muscle strength declines by as much as 30 percent.

A selective loss of fast-twitch **motor units** has also been observed; this loss adversely affects the older adult's ability to execute movements quickly. Several studies have shown that age-related changes in the firing behavior of motor units are evident (Erim, Beg, Burke, & De Luca, 1999; Luff, 1998; Roubenoff, 2001). This change in the neuromuscular component of the motor system, coupled with the loss of anticipatory postural control abilities due to slower central processing speeds, places the older adult at greater risk for falling when balance is unexpectedly perturbed.

motor unit—A motor neuron and all the muscle fibers it innervates.

The loss of muscle strength, combined with age-related structural changes occurring within the joints, leads to a reduction in overall flexibility that can adversely affect postural alignment as well as the quality of an older adult's movement. Specific diseases in the joint such as osteoarthritis and rheumatoid arthritis further influence the joint's integrity and have been strongly associated with impaired balance and mobility. The pain associated with each of these conditions also contributes to restrictions in the functional range of motion. Both of these medical conditions are discussed in greater depth in chapter 2.

Changes in the Cognitive System

Whereas age-related declines in the sensory and motor systems adversely affect the older adult's balance and mobility, so too do age-associated changes in the cognitive system. In fact, at least 10 percent of all people older than 65 and 50 percent of those older than 80 have some form of cognitive impairment, ranging from mild deficits to dementia (Yaffe, Barnes, Nevitt, Lui, & Covinski, 2001). Adverse changes occurring in attention, memory, and intelligence are most likely to affect the older adult's ability to anticipate and adapt to changes occurring in the environment.

Older adults find it particularly difficult to store and manipulate information in working memory when a second task that also demands cognition is presented. This requirement to divide attention between tasks, particularly when one of the tasks involves balance, is more problematic for healthy

> ## Key Point
> At least 10 percent of all people older than 65 and 50 percent of those older than 80 have some form of cognitive impairment.

crystallized intelligence— Verbal, numerical, and spatial abilities.

fluid intelligence—The ability to reason, solve problems, and form relationships among abstract concepts.

older adults than it is for their younger counterparts (Shumway-Cook, Woollacott, Baldwin, & Kerns, 1997; Brown et al., 1999). Decrements in performance are even more evident when older adults with known balance impairments are compared with healthy younger and older adults (Shumway-Cook et al., 1997; Brauer et al., 2002).

Intelligence comprises two components: **crystallized intelligence** and **fluid intelligence.** Crystallized intelligence involves the verbal, numerical, and spatial abilities, whereas fluid intelligence involves the ability to reason, solve problems, or form relationships among abstract concepts. Although aging does not appear to affect crystallized intelligence, it does have an adverse effect on fluid intelligence. At a practical level, the changes in fluid intelligence are most likely to affect your older clients' abilities to quickly find solutions to movement problems that are novel or are presented in a new way to them.

> ## Key Point
>
> Age-related changes in fluid intelligence are most likely to affect the ability to quickly find solutions to new movement problems.

Can Age-Associated Changes in Balance and Mobility Be Reversed?

Despite the many age-related changes occurring in the multiple systems that contribute to good balance and mobility, growing evidence suggests that we can reverse, or at least slow, the rate of decline occurring in some or all of these systems. Several intervention studies that include exercise as a stand-alone strategy or as a core component of a multifactorial approach have been conducted among both healthy older adults and adults with existing balance problems and have demonstrated moderate to large improvements in balance and mobility and a reduction in fall risk or fall incidence (Chang et al., 2004; Clemson et al., 2004; Lord et al., 2003). Interventions that target the sources of balance-related problems and repeatedly expose older adults to changing task demands and environmental constraints have been particularly effective (Buchner et al., 1997; Rose & Clark, 2000; Shumway-Cook, Gruber, Baldwin, & Liao, 1997; Wolfson et al., 1996). The FallProof program targets the sources of underlying impairments contributing to postural instability as a result of its comprehensive screening and assessment protocol and its multidimensional programming approach.

> ## Key Point
>
> Interventions that target the sources of balance-related problems and repeatedly expose older adults to changing task demands and environmental constraints are particularly effective in improving balance and preventing falls.

CASE STUDIES

One of the best ways to apply the theoretical information presented in this book is to relate it to an actual person. To help you make the critical connection between theory and practice and to help you develop your problem-solving skills along the way, two case studies are introduced in this section and expanded on in subsequent chapters. Each case study describes an older adult experiencing the types of balance and mobility problems you can expect to encounter in many of the older adults enrolling in a community-based balance and mobility program. This chapter provides a general description of their current status and summarizes the information each client provided on the health and activity questionnaire completed before the start of the program. Health and activity information is presented for case study 1 on pages 18 to 23 and for case study 2 on pages 25 to 30. Both case studies are based on actual people who have participated in the FallProof program at California State University at Fullerton. In addition to the health history provided in this chapter, a complete set of assessment results for each case study is provided in chapter 3. It will be important to review these results carefully and use the interpretation tables provided in chapter 3 to identify the possible underlying impairments that are contributing to the changes in balance and mobility indicated by the test results.

Case Study 1: Phoebe

Current Status

Phoebe is a 74-year-old female who heard about the FallProof program from her primary care physician, who had been treating her for a number of medical conditions over the years. On her first visit to our center, she described how poor her balance and mobility had become since experiencing the latest of several heart attacks in February 2006. Although she had already found it difficult to engage in physical activity because of chronic asthma that she has experienced her entire adult life, complications from recent heart surgery (i.e., theophylline toxicity) have significantly affected her ability to maintain balance and walk confidently.

Health and Activity History

A review of Phoebe's completed health and activity questionnaire (pages 18-23) reveals that in addition to being diagnosed with congestive heart failure and asthma, Phoebe was diagnosed with peripheral neuropathy in both feet in 2002 as well as osteoarthritis in both hips and the right knee that same year. She also reported experiencing a severe bout of vertigo in 1993 that significantly affected her balance. Despite her poor balance and level of conditioning, Phoebe was highly motivated to improve her balance and mobility. She described her health as good despite her physical limitations and reported no depression in the previous month. She rated her quality of life as moderately low because of her inability to perform a number of basic and intermediate daily activities (e.g., making the bed, vacuuming, carrying groceries) without assistance and to be as involved socially as she had been in past years. She also indicated that she experiences quite a bit of pain when performing daily activities. Phoebe is currently taking seven prescription medications for her various medical conditions and two over-the-counter medications. The exact medications are listed under question 9 on Phoebe's completed questionnaire on page 20.

Fall History

Phoebe's fall history indicated that she had fallen twice in the previous six months. Both falls occurred outside the home, the first when she was walking across her front lawn at night and the second when she tripped over an obstacle she did not see in her path. She was very fortunate not to break any bones, but she did sustain severe bruising in the first fall and lacerations to the arms and legs in the second fall. It is not surprising, then, that she indicated she was extremely concerned about falling in response to question 13 on her health and activity questionnaire.

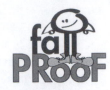

FallProof Health and Activity Questionnaire

Name _Phoebe_____ Date _____

Address _____

City _____ State _____ Zip _____

Home phone # (_____) _____ Gender: Male ❏ Female ☑

Date of birth _6/17/1935_____ Height_5' 6"_____ Weight _200 lbs._____

Person to contact in a case of emergency _____ Phone # (____) _____

Name of your physician _____ Phone # (____) _____

1. Have you ever been diagnosed as having any of the following conditions?

If yes, year of diagnoses

Heart attack	☑ Yes	❏ No	_Feb. 2006_____
Transient ischemic attack	❏ Yes	☑ No	
Angina (chest pain)	❏ Yes	☑ No	
High blood pressure	❏ Yes	☑ No	
Stroke	❏ Yes	☑ No	
Peripheral vascular disease	❏ Yes	☑ No	
Diabetes	❏ Yes	☑ No	
Neuropathies (problems with sensations)	☑ Yes	❏ No	_Both feet 2002_____
Respiratory disease	☑ Yes	❏ No	_Asthma_____
Parkinson's disease	❏ Yes	☑ No	
Multiple sclerosis	❏ Yes	☑ No	
Polio/post-polio syndrome	❏ Yes	☑ No	
Epilepsy/seizures	❏ Yes	☑ No	
Other neurological conditions	❏ Yes	☑ No	
Osteoporosis	❏ Yes	☑ No	
Rheumatoid arthritis	❏ Yes	☑ No	
Other arthritic conditions	☑ Yes	☑ No	_Osteoarthritis—hips/knees 2002_
Visual/depth perception problems	☑ Yes	❏ No	_Vertigo 1993_____
Inner ear problems/recurrent ear infections	❏ Yes	☑ No	
Cerebellar problems (ataxia)	❏ Yes	☑ No	
Other movement disorders	❏ Yes	☑ No	
Chemical dependency (alcohol or drugs)	☑ Yes	❏ No	
Depression	❏ Yes	❏ No	

2. Have you ever been diagnosed as having any of the following conditions?

Cancer ☐ Yes ☑ No

If yes, describe what kind: _____

_____

Joint replacement ☐ Yes ☑ No

If yes, how many times? _____ ☐ Right hip

☐ Left hip

☐ Right knee

☐ Left knee

Cognitive disorder ☐ Yes ☑ No

If yes, describe condition: _____

_____

Uncorrected visual problems ☐ Yes ☑ No

If yes, describe type: _____

_____

Any other type of health problem? ☐ Yes ☑ No

If yes, describe conditions: _____

_____

3. Do you currently experience any of the following symptoms in your legs or feet?

Numbness ☑ Yes ☐ No

Tingling ☑ Yes ☐ No

Arthritis ☑ Yes ☐ No

Swelling ☑ Yes ☐ No

4. Do you currently have any medical conditions for which you see a physician regularly?

☑ Yes ☐ No

If yes, describe conditions: _Heart condition_ _____

_____

_____

(continued)

5. Do you require eyeglasses?   ❑ Yes ☑ No

   If yes, what type of glasses do you wear?
- ❑ Bifocals
- ❑ Graded lenses
- ❑ Magnification only
- ❑ Trifocals

6. Do you have your eyesight checked at least once a year?

                                         ☑ Yes ❑ No

7. Do you require hearing aids?   ☑ Yes ❑ No

   If yes, which ear?   ❑ Left ❑ Right ❑ Both

8. Do you use an assistive device for walking?   ❑ Yes ☑ No   ❑ Sometimes

   If yes or sometimes, what type of assistive device do you use?

- ❑ Single-point cane
- ❑ Three-point cane
- ❑ Quad cane
- ❑ Rolling stand walker
- ❑ Three-wheel walker with seat

9. List all medications that you currently take (including all over-the-counter and alternative medicines)

Type of Medication	For what condition?
Albuterol	Asthma
Azmacort	Asthma
K-Dur (3 × day—10 mg)	Congestive heart failure
Lasix (3 × day—20 mg)	Congestive heart failure
Synthroid (1 × day—0.175 mg)	Hyperthyroidism
Oyster shell calcium (3 × day—500 mg)	Bone health
Centrum Silver (1 × day)	Vitamin supplement
Allopurinol (1 × day—300 mg)	Gout
Glucosamine (3 × day—500 mg)	Osteoarthritis

10. Have you required emergency medical care or hospitalization in the last year?

                                        ❑ Yes ☑ No

   If yes, please list when this occurred and briefly explain why. *But I did in 2006 because of theophylline toxicity.*

11. Have you ever had any condition or experienced any injury that has affected your balance or ability to walk without assistance? ☑ Yes ☐ No

If yes, please list when this occurred and briefly explain condition or injury.

Vertigo 1993 and theophylline toxicity from recent heart surgery.

12. How many times have you fallen *within the past 6 months*? _2_

If you have fallen in the past 6 months, please give a detailed description of the incident.

   a. Date: _October 14_

   b. Location (i.e., indoors, outdoors): _outdoors_

   c. Reason for fall (i.e., uneven surface, going down stairs): _Walking across front lawn at night and fell._

   d. Did you require medical treatment? ☑ Yes ☐ No

   e. Please provide some details for any additional fall you had in the past 6 months:
   I was outdoors walking when I tripped over a tree root in my path.

13. How concerned are you about falling?

☐ 1	☐ 2	☐ 3	☐ 4	☐ 5	☐ 6	☑ 7
Not at all		A little		Moderately		Very		Extremely

14. As a result of this concern, have you stopped doing some of the things you used to do or liked to do?

☑ Yes ☐ No

15. How would you describe your overall health?

☐ Excellent ☐ Very good ☑ Good ☐ Fair ☐ Poor

16. In general, how would you rate the quality of your life?

☐ 1	☐ 2	☑ 3	☐ 4	☐ 5	☐ 6	☐ 7
Very low		Low		Moderate		High		Very high

(continued)

17. Please indicate your ability to do each of the following. (Place a ✔ in the most appropriate box.)

	Can do	Can do with difficulty or with help	Cannot do
a. Take care of own personal needs (e.g., dressing yourself)	☑ 2	☐ 1	☐ 0
b. Bathe yourself, using tub or shower	☑ 2	☐ 1	☐ 0
c. Climb up and down a flight of stairs (e.g, second story)	☑ 2	☐ 1	☐ 0
d. Do light household activities (e.g., cooking, dusting, washing dishes, sweeping a walkway)	☑ 2	☐ 1	☐ 0
e. Do heavy household activities (e.g., scrubbing floors, vacuuming, raking leaves)	☐ 2	☐ 1	☑ 0
f. Do own shopping for groceries or clothes	☐ 2	☑ 1	☐ 0
g. Walk outside (one or two blocks)	☑ 2	☐ 1	☐ 0
h. Walk 1/2 mile (0.8 km, 6-7 blocks)	☐ 2	☑ 1	☐ 0
i. Walk 1 mile (1.6 km, 12-14 blocks)	☐ 2	☐ 1	☑ 0
j. Lift and carry 10 pounds (4.5 kg, e.g., a full bag of groceries)	☐ 2	☑ 1	☐ 0
k. Lift and carry 25 pounds (11 kg, e.g, medium to large suitcase)	☐ 2	☐ 1	☑ 0
l. Do strenuous activities (e.g., hiking, calisthenics, moving heavy objects, bicycling, aerobic dance activities, strenuous digging in garden)	☐ 2	☐ 1	☑ 0

18. In general, do you currently require household or nursing assistance to carry out daily activities?

☑ Yes   ☐ No

If yes, please check the reasons.

☐ Health problems
☑ Chronic pain
☑ Lack of strength or endurance
☑ Lack of flexibility or balance
☐ Other reasons: _____

_____

_____

19. In a typical week, how often do you leave your house (to run errands, go to work, go to meetings, classes, church, social functions, etc.)?

❏ less than once   ☑ 3-4 times

❏ 1-2 times   ❏ almost every day

20. Do you *currently* participate in regular physical exercise (such as walking, sports, exercise classes, housework, or yard work) that is strenuous enough to cause a noticeable increase in breathing, heart rate, or perspiration?

                                          ❏ Yes   ☑ No

If yes, how many days per week?

❏ One   ❏ Two   ❏ Three   ❏ Four   ❏ Five   ❏ Six   ❏ Seven

21. When you go for walks (if you do), which of the following best describes your walking pace?

❏ Strolling (easy pace, takes 30 minutes or more to walk a mile)

❏ Average or normal (can walk a mile in 20-30 minutes)

❏ Fairly brisk (fast pace, can walk a mile in 15-20 minutes)

☑ Do not go for walks on a regular basis

22. Did you require assistance in completing this form?

☑ None (or very little)   ❏ Needed quite a bit of help

Reason: _____

_____

_____

From D. Rose, 2010, *Fallproof!* 2nd ed. (Champaign, IL: Human Kinetics). Reprinted by permission, from the Center for Successful Aging at California State University, Fullerton. Question 17 of this form is reprinted, by permission, from R. Rikli and J. Jones, 1998, "The reliability and validity of a 6-minute walk test as a measure of physical endurance in older adults," *Journal of Aging and Physical Activity*, 6: 363-375.

Case Study 2: Larry

Current Status

Larry is a 70-year-old male who resides in the community with his wife of 34 years. Larry enrolled in the FallProof program in 2008 because he was experiencing a steady decline in his balance abilities. Although he was a regular participant in an exercise program that operated 3 days a week at the local senior center, he was looking for a program that specifically focused on improving balance and mobility.

Health and Activity History

Larry reported five medical diagnoses on his completed health and activity questionnaire (see pages 25-30). He sustained a heart attack in 1999 that resulted in triple bypass surgery, followed by a stroke in 2004 that left him with weakness on the right side. He was also diagnosed with type 2 diabetes in 2002 and osteoarthritis in the back and right knee in 2004. He was first diagnosed with high blood pressure in 1996. The condition is currently being controlled with medication. Although he reported swelling in his legs and feet, Larry has not been diagnosed with peripheral neuropathy, a common condition secondary to diabetes. Larry rated his health as good and his quality of life high. He experiences some difficulty performing daily activities, particularly those requiring aerobic endurance and strength.

Larry currently takes seven prescription medications and two over-the-counter medications for his various medical conditions. The exact medications are listed in question 9 on his completed health and activity questionnaire. He wears eyeglasses for reading purposes only, as well as a hearing aid in the right ear. Because of his increasing problems in balance, he uses a single-point cane on occasion, usually when he is planning to be out in the community for a good portion of the day.

Fall History

Larry reported no falls in the previous six months, although he had some near misses, particularly when walking on uneven surfaces. Even though he had not actually fallen in the previous six months, he reported that he was very concerned about falling.

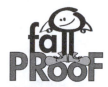

FallProof Health and Activity Questionnaire

Name _Larry_ _____ Date _____

Address _____

City _____ State _____ Zip _____

Home phone # (_____) _____ Gender: Male ☑ Female ☐

Date of birth _1/20/1939_ _____ Height _6'0"_ _____ Weight _220 lbs_ _____

Person to contact in a case of emergency _____ Phone # (_____) _____

Name of your physician _____ Phone # (_____) _____

1. Have you ever been diagnosed as having any of the following conditions?

			If yes, year of diagnoses
Heart attack	☑ Yes	☐ No	Triple bypass 1999
Transient ischemic attack	☐ Yes	☑ No	
Angina (chest pain)	☐ Yes	☑ No	
High blood pressure	☑ Yes	☐ No	1996
Stroke	☑ Yes	☐ No	2004 (right side)
Peripheral vascular disease	☐ Yes	☑ No	
Diabetes	☑ Yes	☐ No	2002
Neuropathies (problems with sensations)	☐ Yes	☑ No	
Respiratory disease	☐ Yes	☑ No	
Parkinson's disease	☐ Yes	☑ No	
Multiple sclerosis	☐ Yes	☑ No	
Polio/post-polio syndrome	☐ Yes	☑ No	
Epilepsy/seizures	☐ Yes	☑ No	
Other neurological conditions	☐ Yes	☑ No	
Osteoporosis	☐ Yes	☑ No	
Rheumatoid arthritis	☐ Yes	☑ No	
Other arthritic conditions	☑ Yes	☐ No	2004 (osteoarthritis)
Visual/depth perception problems	☐ Yes	☑ No	
Inner ear problems/recurrent ear infections	☐ Yes	☑ No	
Cerebellar problems (ataxia)	☐ Yes	☑ No	
Other movement disorders	☐ Yes	☑ No	
Chemical dependency (alcohol or drugs)	☐ Yes	☑ No	
Depression	☑ Yes	☐ No	2006

2. Have you ever been diagnosed as having any of the following conditions?

Cancer   ❑ Yes   ☑ No

If yes, describe what kind: _____

_____

_____

Joint replacement   ❑ Yes   ☑ No

If yes, how many times? _____   ❑ Right hip

                                                           ❑ Left hip

                                                             ❑ Right knee

                                                             ❑ Left knee

Cognitive disorder   ❑ Yes   ☑ No

If yes, describe condition: _____

_____

_____

Uncorrected visual problems   ❑ Yes   ☑ No

If yes, describe type: _____

_____

_____

Any other type of health problem?   ❑ Yes   ☑ No

If yes, describe conditions: _____

_____

_____

3. Do you currently experience any of the following symptoms in your legs or feet?

Numbness   ❑ Yes   ☑ No

Tingling   ❑ Yes   ☑ No

Arthritis   ❑ Yes   ☑ No

Swelling   ☑ Yes   ❑ No

4. Do you currently have any medical conditions for which you see a physician regularly?

                                       ❑ Yes   ☑ No

If yes, describe conditions: _____

_____

_____

5. Do you require eyeglasses?   ☑ Yes   ❑ No

    If yes, what type of glasses do you wear?   ❑ Bifocals

         ❑ Graded lenses

         ☑ Magnification only

         ❑ Trifocals

6. Do you have your eyesight checked at least once a year?

         ☑ Yes   ❑ No

7. Do you require hearing aids?   ☑ Yes   ❑ No

    If yes, which ear?   ❑ Left   ☑ Right   ❑ Both

8. Do you use an assistive device for walking?   ❑ Yes   ❑ No   ☑ Sometimes

    If yes or sometimes, what type of assistive device do you use?

    ☑ Single-point cane   ❑ Rolling stand walker

    ❑ Three-point cane   ❑ Three-wheel walker with seat

    ❑ Quad cane

9. List all medications that you currently take (including all over-the-counter and alternative medicines)

Type of Medication	For what condition?
Lanoxin (0.25 mg)	*Heart medication*
Glucophage (500 mg)	*Diabetes*
Lipitor (20 mg)	*Cholesterol*
Furosemide (40 mg)	*Swelling (water retention)*
Atenolol (50 mg)	*Blood pressure*
Feldene (20 mg)	*Arthritis*
Plendil (5 mg)	*Blood pressure*
Aspirin (81 mg)	*Blood thinner*
Citracal	*Osteoporosis*

10. Have you required emergency medical care or hospitalization in the last year?

         ❑ Yes   ☑ No

    If yes, please list when this occurred and briefly explain why. _____

_____

_____

_____

(continued)

11. Have you ever had any condition or experienced any injury that has affected your balance or ability to walk without assistance?   ☑ Yes   ☐ No

   If yes, please list when this occurred and briefly explain condition or injury.

   Stroke (March 2004). Right side weakness. _____

   _____

   _____

12. How many times have you fallen *within the past 6 months*? _____ 0 _____

   If you have fallen in the past 6 months, please give a detailed description of the incident.

   a. Date:_____

   b. Location (i.e., indoors, outdoors): _____

   c. Reason for fall (i.e., uneven surface, going down stairs): _____

   _____

   _____

   d. Did you require medical treatment?   ☐ Yes   ☐ No

   e. Please provide some details for any additional fall you had in the past 6 months:

   _____

   _____

   _____

13. How concerned are you about falling?

   ☐ 1   ☐ 2   ☐ 3   ☐ 4   ☑ 5   ☐ 6   ☐ 7
   Not at all   A little   Moderately   Very   Extremely

14. As a result of this concern, have you stopped doing some of the things you used to do or liked to do?

   ☐ Yes   ☑ No

15. How would you describe your overall health?
   ☐ Excellent   ☐ Very good   ☑ Good   ☐ Fair   ☐ Poor

16. In general, how would you rate the quality of your life?

   ☐ 1   ☐ 2   ☐ 3   ☐ 4   ☑ 5   ☐ 6   ☐ 7
   Very low   Low   Moderate   High   Very high

17. Please indicate your ability to do each of the following. (Place a ✔ in the most appropriate box.)

	Can do	Can do with difficulty or with help	Cannot do
a. Take care of own personal needs (e.g., dressing yourself	✔ 2	☐ 1	☐ 0
b. Bathe yourself, using tub or shower	✔ 2	☐ 1	☐ 0
c. Climb up and down a flight of stairs (e.g, second story)	☐ 2	✔ 1	☐ 0
d. Do light household activities (e.g., cooking, dusting, washing dishes, sweeping a walkway)	✔ 2	☐ 1	☐ 0
e. Do heavy household activities (e.g., scrubbing floors, vacuuming, raking leaves)	✔ 2	☐ 1	☐ 0
f. Do own shopping for groceries or clothes	✔ 2	☐ 1	☐ 0
g. Walk outside (one or two blocks)	✔ 2	☐ 1	☐ 0
h. Walk 1/2 mile (0.8 km, 6-7 blocks)	✔ 2	☐ 1	☐ 0
i. Walk 1 mile (1.6 km, 12-14 blocks)	☐ 2	✔ 1	☐ 0
j. Lift and carry 10 pounds (4.5 kg, e.g., a full bag of groceries)	✔ 2	☐ 1	☐ 0
k. Lift and carry 25 pounds (11 kg, e.g, medium to large suitcase)	☐ 2	✔ 1	☐ 0
l. Do strenuous activities (e.g., hiking, calisthenics, moving heavy objects, bicycling, aerobic dance activities, strenuous digging in garden)	☐ 2	☐ 1	✔ 0

18. In general, do you currently require household or nursing assistance to carry out daily activities?

☐ Yes ✔ No

If yes, please check the reasons.
☐ Health problems
☐ Chronic pain
☐ Lack of strength or endurance
☐ Lack of flexibility or balance
☐ Other reasons: _____

_____

_____

(continued)

19. In a typical week, how often do you leave your house (to run errands, go to work, go to meetings, classes, church, social functions, etc.)?

   ❑ less than once   ❑ 3-4 times

   ❑ 1-2 times   ☑ almost every day

20. Do you *currently* participate in regular physical exercise (such as walking, sports, exercise classes, housework, or yard work) that is strenuous enough to cause a noticeable increase in breathing, heart rate, or perspiration?

   ☑ Yes   ❑ No

   If yes, how many days per week?

   ❑ One   ❑ Two   ☑ Three   ❑ Four   ❑ Five   ❑ Six   ❑ Seven

21. When you go for walks (if you do), which of the following best describes your walking pace?

   ❑ Strolling (easy pace, takes 30 minutes or more to walk a mile)

   ❑ Average or normal (can walk a mile in 20-30 minutes)

   ❑ Fairly brisk (fast pace, can walk a mile in 15-20 minutes)

   ☑ Do not go for walks on a regular basis

22. Did you require assistance in completing this form?

   ☑ None (or very little)   ❑ Needed quite a bit of help

   Reason: _____

   _____

   _____

   _____

Now that you have been introduced to our two case studies and understand a little more about each individual's current status and health history, examine each of the completed questionnaires to learn more about the two clients. Become familiar with the different medical diagnoses listed on their HAQs, their primary signs and symptoms, and how each condition is likely to affect the clients' ability to perform certain activities in an exercise class. Over the course of the next two chapters you will be asked to complete a number of activities based on the information provided on the health and activity questionnaires in this chapter.

SUMMARY

The purpose of this chapter was to introduce you to the terminology used in the study of balance and mobility as well as provide you with an overview of the multiple body systems that contribute to balance and mobility and the types of movement strategies used to control balance. The major age-related changes you are likely to observe in the clients you serve in a balance and mobility program were also described. As you learned in this chapter, the sensory, motor, and cognitive systems are integral to the development and maintenance of good balance and mobility. Whereas the sensory systems provide us with the information needed to perceive where we are in space, the motor system plans and carries out actions. The cognitive system, which includes memory, attention, and intelligence, plays a critical role in helping older adults anticipate changes occurring in the environment as well as adapt their actions in response to changing task or environmental demands.

Although some changes occurring in certain systems may be small (e.g., slight reduction in visual acuity), others may be so large (e.g., macular degeneration) as to adversely affect an older adult's ability to perform many daily activities that require balance and mobility. The good news is that many of the age-associated changes occurring in the systems that contribute to balance and mobility can be reversed, or at least compensated for, once they are identified. Certainly each of the core exercise components that make up the FallProof program addresses each of the dimensions of balance and mobility that, although altered by the aging process, can be positively influenced by a targeted and multidimensional exercise program.

This chapter also introduced two case studies to help you better apply the theory presented in this book to actual physical activity settings. The case studies are also intended to sharpen your problem-solving abilities in preparation for working with individual clients or leading group-based balance and mobility classes in the future. In order to be a successful individual or group instructor of this program, you must be able to analyze each client's health history thoroughly so you can learn as much about the client as possible even before any baseline tests are administered. Each case study will be further developed during the next two chapters, and practical problems will be presented to you as you begin to acquire the theoretical knowledge needed to design and implement an effective balance and mobility training program.

Test Your Understanding

1. In which of the following situations is anticipatory postural control most likely to be used?
    a. maintaining upright balance
    b. avoiding an obstacle in our path
    c. restoring balance after unexpectedly stepping in a hole
    d. running in the forest at night
    e. sitting on an unstable surface with the eyes closed

2. The boundaries of a person's stability limits are
   a. 12 degrees in the forward, backward, and lateral directions
   b. determined by the task demands
   c. limited by the person's biomechanical limitations
   d. dependent on the constraints of the environment
   e. b, c, and d

3. Muscle response synergies are
   a. groups of muscles that must be inhibited if movement is to occur
   b. groups of muscles constrained to work together to produce movement
   c. any group of muscles in the body
   d. muscles that are involved in reflexive movements only
   e. a group of muscles that are activated together to produce movement

4. Which sensory system provides us with information about our position in space relative to the ground?
   a. the visual system
   b. the somatosensory system
   c. the vestibular system
   d. the visual *and* somatosensory systems
   e. all three sensory systems

5. The hip strategy is most likely to be used when
   a. the surface beneath the feet is narrow or compliant
   b. the sway distance is small
   c. we exceed our limits of stability
   d. the speed of the sway is slow
   e. the step strategy cannot be used

6. Which of the following is *not* a common age-related change that occurs in the visual system?
   a. reduced visual acuity
   b. reduced contrast sensitivity
   c. narrowing of the visual field
   d. glaucoma
   e. decreased depth perception

7. The primary role of the proprioceptors is to inform us about
   a. the position of the head and body in space
   b. the visual layout of the environment
   c. the position and movement of body parts in relation to one another
   d. the changing tension of the muscles as they move
   e. the type of surface below the feet

8. The primary role of the vestibulo-ocular reflex is to
   a. stabilize the head when the eyes are moving
   b. stabilize the body when the head is moving
   c. stabilize the eyes when the head is moving
   d. stabilize the body when the feet are moving
   e. force the head and eyes to move in the same direction

9. A situation of sensory conflict arises when
   a. the visual, somatosensory, and vestibular systems are providing the same information
   b. the information provided by one or more sensory systems is not in agreement with the information provided by the other sensory systems
   c. information provided to the motor system is not in agreement with the information provided to the sensory systems
   d. the cognitive system is not functioning properly
   e. vision is no longer available

10. The loss of anticipatory postural control that accompanies aging is likely due to
   a. a reduction in muscle strength
   b. cognitive impairment
   c. a decline in central processing speed
   d. impaired memory
   e. improved reactive postural control

Practical Problems

This set of age-simulation activities is intended to help you better understand how age-related changes in multiple body systems are likely to affect balance and mobility. You will require the following equipment to complete this set of activities: eyeglasses, petroleum jelly, black tape, athletic tape, gloves, foam-filled shoes, cotton balls or earplugs, and dry macaroni. Although you can perform this activity alone, it is usually best to do it with a partner for safety reasons. After you have made each alteration described in the following directions, attempt to navigate an obstacle course and try to follow a set of visual and verbal instructions delivered by your partner as though you were in a physical activity setting.

1. Smear petroleum jelly on a set of clear eyeglasses so that your vision is blurred. This simulates age-related changes in visual acuity and also simulates diseases such as macular degeneration or cataract.

2. Eliminate the peripheral regions of each eyeglass lens with black tape to simulate visual field loss or glaucoma.

3. Insert cotton balls or earplugs in your ears and try to follow a set of softly delivered verbal instructions from your partner.

4. Put dry macaroni in each shoe to simulate the discomfort associated with arthritis.

5. Use the athletic tape to reduce range of motion in key joints (e.g., ankle, knee, and hip). Perform sit-to-stand, walking, and obstacle negotiation activities.

6. Tie a length of resistance band around the ankles to simulate reduced stride length and a narrow base of support.

7. Put on a pair of foam-filled booties to simulate sensation loss in the feet.

Once you have experienced moving about the room with each of these simulated age-related impairments, combine impairments (e.g., 1 and 3 or 1, 2, and 4) so you can better understand how changes in multiple body systems influence balance and mobility. Record your thoughts on paper when you have finished each of the activities.

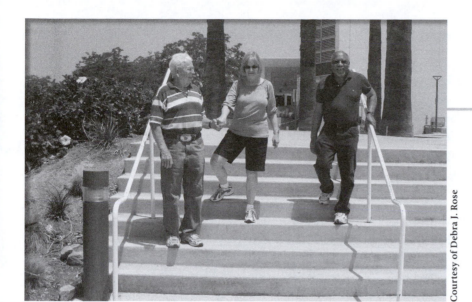

Courtesy of Debra J. Rose

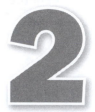

Chapter 2

Why Do Many Older Adults Fall?

Objectives

After completing this chapter, you will be able to

- identify the intrinsic and extrinsic risk factors contributing to falls among older adults,
- describe the signs and symptoms associated with common medical conditions evident among older adults,
- understand the importance of modifying balance and mobility activities that are contraindicated or likely to exacerbate symptoms associated with a medical condition,
- identify categories of medications that produce side effects likely to adversely affect balance and mobility,
- identify areas in and around the home that contribute to heightened fall risk, and
- better understand which biological and behavioral risk factors can be eliminated or reduced through targeted exercise programming.

Falls are all too common among older adults, often leading to physical injury and psychological trauma. In the United States, falls in the population aged 65 and older lead to high rates of morbidity and mortality. In fact, falls are the leading cause of nonfatal injuries requiring medical attention in the United States (Adams, Dey, & Vickerie, 2007). Falls are also very costly. For example, the total cost of fall-related injuries in the United States was $27.3 billion in 1994; this figure is expected to rise to as much as $43.8 billion in 2020. Fall injury rates increase with age and are higher among women than among men. Older adults with certain chronic medical conditions and activity limitations also experience higher rates of fall injuries when compared with older adults without these conditions (Schiller, Kramarow, & Dey, 2007). Many possible causes have been attributed to the higher-than-average incidence of falls among older adults, and a number of fall-related risk factors have been identified over the past decade. Four categories of these risk factors will be identified and discussed in greater detail later in this chapter.

As gloomy as these statistics might appear, the good news is that many falls are potentially preventable. Well-designed physical activity programs, often combined with a comprehensive fall risk assessment, behavioral counseling, and home safety inspections and modifications, have been shown to significantly lower fall risk and fall incidence rates among older adults (Chang et al., 2004; Gillespie et al., 2009).

To better prepare you as a balance and mobility instructor, this chapter discusses the different categories of risk factors that have been shown to be associated with increased fall risk among older adults. The chapter also presents several strategies that you, as an instructor, can employ to help your older adult clients become more aware of the need to engage in safe behaviors while improving their own physical capabilities, particularly in the area of balance and mobility. With this knowledge, you will be better able to identify the risk factors that are most likely to contribute to each individual client's risk of falling. This knowledge will also help you develop an individualized exercise plan that targets the specific risk factors identified.

MULTIPLE FACTORS CAUSE FALLS

Older adults do not all fall for the same reason. In fact, a multitude of factors contribute to the increased fall rates observed among older adults. Four main categories of risk factors are discussed in this section: biological, behavioral, environmental, and socioeconomic (Scott et al., 2001; World Health Organization, 2007). Figure 2.1 presents a model illustrating how these different types of risk factors both individually and interactively contribute to a heightened risk for falls and fall-related injuries.

Biological Risk Factors

A number of biological risk factors contributing to heightened fall risk have been identified in the literature. These include nonmodifiable factors such as age, sex, and race as well as factors that are somewhat more modifiable with targeted interventions (e.g., age-associated physical and cognitive decline, chronic diseases). Biological factors that are moderately to strongly associated with falling include being older than 80 years and female. Difficulty performing a variety of activities of daily living (ADLs) and impaired mobility have also been identified as risk factors for falls (Nevitt, 1997). Poor performance on specific tests of balance and

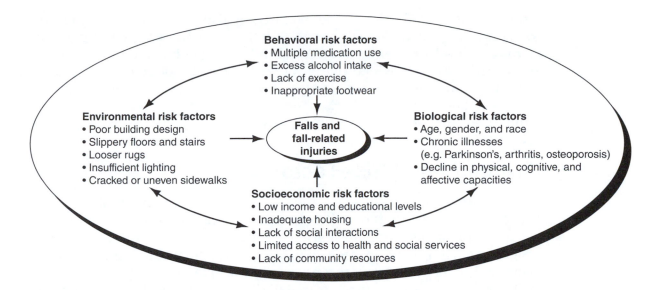

Figure 2.1 Risk factor model for falls occurring among older adults.

Reprinted, by permission, from WHO, 2008. *Global Report on falls prevention in older age* (Geneva, Switzerland: World Health Organization), 5.

gait is also strongly associated with increased fall rates. In addition, age-associated changes in vision contribute to heightened fall risk. The specific types of vision changes associated with increased fall risk are discussed in chapter 1.

Certain chronic medical conditions such as Parkinson's disease, stroke, osteoporosis, arthritis, and dementia have also been shown to be moderately to strongly predictive of increased falls. The increased risk is likely due to the negative effect these diseases have on the various dimensions of balance and mobility as well as cognition. The increased joint pain and reduced range of motion that accompany the various arthritic conditions have also been shown to have a strong association with increased falls among older adults. The common medical conditions observed in the older adult population that adversely affect balance and mobility are described in more detail in the next section of this chapter.

Behavioral Risk Factors

A number of behavioral factors increase the risk for falls and fall-related injuries among older adults. Examples include multiple medication use, excessive intake of alcohol, physical inactivity, poor diet, inappropriate footwear, and risk-taking behaviors. It has been well documented in the literature that older adults who take four or more prescription medications, irrespective of type, are at a significantly greater risk for falls (Campbell, Borrie, & Spears, 1989). Benzodiazepines (e.g., sedatives and hypnotics, antidepressants, anti-anxiolytics) in particular are strongly associated with increased risk of falling among older adults (Leipzig, Cumming, & Tinetti, 1999a). The effect of medication use on balance and mobility specifically, and on falls in general, is discussed in greater detail in a later section of this chapter. Inadequate amounts of physical activity, coupled with a poor diet, certainly exacerbate the age-associated changes that older adults experience while also elevating the risk for falls. Engaging in regular physical activity (30 minutes of activity on most days of the week) not only is important for maintaining muscle strength, aerobic endurance, flexibility, and balance but also is critical for maintaining good cognitive function (Nelson et al., 2007). Similarly, eating a well-balanced diet is integral to a healthy body and mind. Wearing inappropriate footwear also constitutes a behavioral risk factor for falling. Too often older adults pay little attention to what they put on their feet and are prone to slips and trips as a result. Shoes with high heels, shoes with very soft or slippery soles, or ill-fitting shoes that do not provide firm ankle support should be avoided (Lord, Sherrington, Menz, & Close, 2007).

Environmental Risk Factors

Older adults who reside independently within the community face numerous environmental risk factors on a daily basis. These may be hazards in and around the home or in the community itself. Clutter, unsecured floor rugs, poorly designed stairwells, and inadequate lighting in the home are just a few of the many environmental hazards that have been linked to increased fall risk. Poorly maintained sidewalks, varying curb heights, sloping driveways, lack of curb ramps, and generally poor building design also pose risks for older adults moving about the community.

Social and Economic Risk Factors

Although not directly linked to increased fall risk, low income, less education, and a lack of supportive social networks or access to health or social services place older adults at a much greater risk for chronic medical conditions that increase the risk of falling. Being socially, academically, and economically disadvantaged also adversely affects an older adult's physical health, diet, and ability to benefit from educational materials covering a number of health topics as well as falls.

The good news is that many of these risk factors are modifiable. Modest safety changes made to the home environment (e.g., installation of grab bars in the bathroom, placement of night-lights in dark corridors, removal of unnecessary clutter) can significantly reduce an older adult's overall risk for falls (see figure 2.2). Muscle weakness, as well as impaired balance and gait, has also been identified as a biological risk factor for falling that can be significantly improved with a targeted intervention. In fact, many of the balance and mobility activities introduced in part II of this instructor guide target the biological and behavioral risk factors that contribute to falls and fall-related injuries among older adults.

> **Key Point**
>
> Many of the primary causes of falls among community-residing older adults are preventable.

EFFECTS OF COMMON MEDICAL CONDITIONS

A large proportion of the older adults who enroll in your balance and mobility program will already have been diagnosed with one or more chronic medical conditions that influence their ability to perform certain balance and mobility activities. Although the degree to which performance is affected will depend on both the type and the severity of the medical condition, you should become familiar with the signs and symptoms associated with the more common medical conditions so that you can eliminate or adapt any balance and mobility activities that might be contraindicated or harmful to your participants. This section therefore discusses

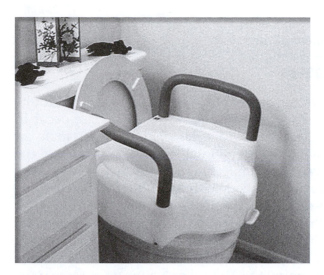 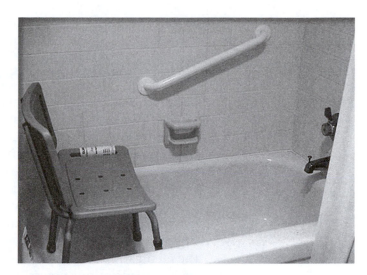

Figure 2.2   Installing devices that *(a)* raise the height of a toilet or *(b)* provide increased safety during bathing can reduce the risk of falling during transfer maneuvers.

selected medical conditions you are likely to observe among your older adult participants. The conditions to be discussed include stroke, cardiovascular disease, arthritis, osteoporosis, Parkinson's disease, diabetes, and vestibular dysfunction. Program considerations related to joint replacement surgery are also discussed.

Stroke

When a person experiences a stroke, also known as a *cerebrovascular accident* (CVA), one of two things happens: A blood vessel in the brain either becomes occluded (blocked) or hemorrhages (a wall has burst). The loss of blood supply that accompanies either of these events causes an **infarction** in the area that was supplied by the blood vessel, causing brain cell death. A less serious medical event, in which the blood supply is reduced (ischemia) but not cut off, is a **transient ischemic attack (TIA).** A person experiencing a TIA may exhibit symptoms such as weakness, temporary paralysis or loss of speech, and confusion.

Given the prevalence of stroke among the older adult population (approximately three-quarters of all strokes occur in adults older than 65 years; Centers for Disease Control and Prevention, 2008), you are likely to encounter a number of older adults in your community-based class who have experienced a stroke or TIA. Older adults who have experienced a stroke often demonstrate weakness or even paralysis that affects one or more limbs on one side of the body. Depending on the location of the stroke, speech, cognition, or memory may also be affected. Individuals with impaired cognition are often impulsive or lack good judgment regarding their abilities. Others experiencing memory loss may find it difficult to complete the health and activity questionnaire without assistance or to follow verbal directions during class. You can expect their progress to be much slower than that of clients without cognitive or memory impairments.

Knowing the exact nature of the deficits each client experiences after a stroke will help you decide which exercise progressions are most appropriate for the client and, more important, which exercises should be eliminated. Having this knowledge can provide a safe practice environment for these clients. You will recall that Larry, the second case study described in chapter 1, experienced a stroke in 2004

infarction—An event in which brain cells die in the area of the brain that is deprived of blood supply following a stroke.

transient ischemic attack (TIA)—The result of a temporary interruption of the blood supply to the brain.

that left him with weakness on the right side. His stroke was due to occlusion of a major artery in the left hemisphere of the brain.

Cardiovascular Disease

Because of the high prevalence of cardiovascular disease among older adults (approximately 84 percent of deaths related to cardiovascular disease occur in people aged 65 years and older; American Heart Association, 2002), many of the clients in your balance and mobility program will check one or more of the boxes related to heart disease when they complete their health and activity questionnaires at the outset of the program. Clients with heart disease may become fatigued or short of breath when exercising, particularly if they have congestive heart failure. If your participants have **hypertension (HTN),** their blood pressure must be medically managed so that they can participate in the program. Check the medications section of the health and activity questionnaire to determine the type of medications prescribed to control their blood pressure. At the same time, look to see if any clients have been prescribed anticoagulant medications, which are designed to prevent blood clots. These clients will be susceptible to excessive bleeding if they sustain a cut, so extra precaution will be needed to ensure their safety during class.

Although the program does not involve high-intensity exercise, you will need to closely monitor clients who have a history of heart disease. Be sure to check with them regularly to find out whether there has been any change in either the type or the dose of medication they have been prescribed. Recall from chapter 1 that Phoebe indicated she has high blood pressure and experienced a severe heart attack in 2006 that seriously compromised her balance and mobility. She was subsequently diagnosed with **congestive heart failure (CHF).** Familiarize yourself with this condition so you can better understand what precautions might be needed when assessing Phoebe prior to entry into a balance and mobility program. Screening for fall risk and assessing balance and mobility will be the focus of chapter 3.

Arthritis

More than 21 percent (46.4 million) of adults in the United States have self-reported doctor-diagnosed arthritis (Helmick et al., 2008). Osteoarthritis affects approximately 50 percent of all adults older than 65 years and 80 percent of those older than 75 years (Brandt & Slemenda, 1993). This form of arthritis typically affects the weight-bearing joints, thereby reducing the joints' ability to transmit or absorb the forces associated with impact. Predisposing factors for osteoarthritis include obesity, hypermobility, trauma, overuse, infection, inflammation, and genetics. The joint pain that accompanies osteoarthritis invariably leads to inactivity and loss of strength, range of motion, and cardiovascular endurance. Although exercise has been shown to be an effective intervention, it does not cure the disease.

Land-based programming consisting of aerobic conditioning, resistance training, and flexibility exercises can moderately improve function, and aquatics exercise programs have also produced moderate improvements in strength and flexibility, particularly among older adults with moderate to severe joint damage (Deyle et al., 2000; Ettinger, Burns, & Messier, 1999). Significant improvements in physical function and pain have also been documented following aquatics programs (Foley, Halbert, Hewitt, & Crotty, 2003; Fransen, Nairn, Winstanley, Lam, & Edmonds,

hypertension (HTN)—A condition diagnosed when systolic blood pressure is greater than 140 mmHg and diastolic pressure is greater than 90 mmHg.

congestive heart failure (CHF)—A condition in which the heart is unable to deliver adequate amounts of oxygen to the metabolizing tissues of the body.

2007). Both Phoebe and Larry have osteoarthritis in multiple joints. Although Larry reported that he does not experience much pain on a daily basis, Phoebe indicated that she experiences quite a bit of pain and therefore requires assistance to complete daily tasks in the home and community.

In contrast to osteoarthritis, rheumatoid arthritis (RA) causes joint deformities that are often more severe and affect the entire joint. Because RA is a systemic inflammatory disease process, it usually affects multiple joints throughout the body. The systemic disease also produces symptoms that include increased fatigue, sleep disorders, and anemia. As with osteoarthritis, exercise is an effective intervention for RA. Moderate gains in aerobic endurance and muscle strength have been reported with no adverse effect on progression of the disease (Van den Ende, Vliet Vlieland, Munneke, & Hazes, 1998; Brady, Kruger, Helmick, Callahan, & Boutaugh, 2003).

The main goal of any exercise program for older adults with arthritis is to minimize the progression of the existing damage in the affected joints. With that in mind, you as an instructor should focus on selecting activities that promote awareness of postural alignment, good body mechanics when performing dynamic activities, and improved strength and flexibility. When conducting any of the strength activities associated with the program, encourage participants with arthritis to perform a higher number of repetitions (to fatigue) with resistance bands or hand weights that offer a lower level of resistance. This is particularly important when using resistance bands because resistance increases as the band is stretched. The greatest resistance is therefore encountered at the end range of the joint's movement, when the exercising muscle has exceeded its range of mechanical advantage.

You should also encourage participants with arthritis to stop performing any exercise that increases their pain. In some cases, you may be able to adapt an exercise, whereas in others, you may have to eliminate an exercise altogether because the required plane of motion irritates the joint. Watch these clients carefully when they perform exercise progressions you suspect might cause pain and ask them regularly during the class whether certain exercises are causing them unnecessary pain. Many older adults may be reluctant to tell you they are experiencing pain during a certain exercise because they want to please you or do not want to be labeled as a complainer. Continually reiterate the mantra "Where there is pain there is *no* gain" to these clients in particular.

> ### Key Point
>
> Encourage your participants with arthritis to stop performing any exercise that increases their pain. Reiterate the mantra "Where there is pain there is *no* gain."

Joint Replacement Surgery

Unfortunately, if conservative nonoperative approaches fail to improve function and quality of life for older adults with osteoarthritis and RA, it is often necessary to replace a joint surgically with a prosthesis. In 1997, approximately 60 percent of the primary hip replacements and 69 percent of the primary knee replacements performed in the United States were for adults aged 65 years and older (Helmick et al., 2008). Other common conditions that may lead to joint replacement include joint deterioration, the loss of articular cartilage, severe joint pain that compromises functional mobility, a significant reduction in joint range of motion, and marked deformity (Kisner & Colby, 1990).

Although participants who have recently undergone successful joint replacement surgery generally are able to perform all of the activities described in this instructor guide, you will need to review the medical release form obtained from the primary care physician to see whether any exercise restrictions have been indicated. An older adult who has delayed the surgery until it was absolutely necessary, spending years living with chronic pain and instability, may exhibit lower self-confidence and a reluctance to trust the new hip or knee during some of the more challenging activities. By starting with easier balance activities that can be performed successfully after only a few attempts, you can foster increased confidence and greater motivation in these participants. As their confidence increases, you can introduce more challenging balance and mobility activities. Emphasizing good postural alignment and symmetry during standing and walking activities is necessary with this group of clients due to their tendency to adopt a misaligned posture (i.e., anterior pelvic tilt, asymmetrical weight bearing) in order to reduce the amount of pain emanating from the involved joint. Many of the standing balance activities described in the chapter on COG control training (chapter 4) that emphasize weight shifting and transfers with the eyes open and closed are particularly beneficial for participants with joint replacements. Transferring on and off benches of different heights and between chairs of different heights also strengthens the muscle groups surrounding the hip and knee joints. Finally, participants with joint replacements should practice the activities described in the gait pattern enhancement and variation chapter (chapter 7).

> **Key Point**
>
> Providing balance activities that foster increased confidence and greater motivation is particularly important for clients who have recently had joint replacement surgery.

Osteoporosis

Osteoporosis is a metabolic bone disease characterized by a progressive loss of bone mass that increases an individual's susceptibility to fractures. It is the major underlying cause of bone fractures in women and older adults. In the United States, an estimated 10 million adults have osteoporosis of the hip (Surgeon General's Report on Bone Health and Osteoporosis, 2004), and approximately 4 in 10 women and 1 in 10 men over the age of 50 will break a hip, spine, or wrist due to poor bone health. Bone mineral density (BMD) is measured to determine whether an individual is within a normal range. Individuals with below-normal BMD may be diagnosed with osteopenia (low bone mass) or osteoporosis. Table 2.1 outlines the classification of osteopenia and osteoporosis (WHO Study Group, 1994).

Individuals with osteoporosis often sustain compression fractures in the thoracic and lumbar spine. These types of fractures lead to increased **kyphosis** (rounding of the upper back) and back pain in many older adults. In advanced cases of osteoporosis, fractures can result from the performance of everyday activities such as bending over, lifting objects, and rising from a chair. Although certain compression fractures cause significant pain, many do not and can be detected only on radiographic examination. The lack of observable symptoms makes it difficult for you as an instructor to select balance and mobility activities that are appropriate for this group of older adults.

Women have a higher risk for osteoporosis than men have because they have lower bone mass in general and experience an accelerated loss of bone mass following menopause. Women who are underweight are at greater risk for the disease, as are Caucasian men and women. In addition to medical treatment, weight-bearing

kyphosis—Increased posterior curvature of the spine.

Table 2.1 The World Health Organization Classification of Osteopenia and Osteoporosis

Condition	Description
Normal	BMD is within 1 SD of that of a normal young adult (T-score greater than –1)
Low bone mass (osteopenia)	BMD is between 1 and 2.5 SD below that of a normal young adult (T-score between –1 and –2.5)
Osteoporosis	BMD is 2.5 SD or more below that of a normal young adult (T-score at or below –2.5)

BMD = bone mineral density; SD = standard deviation. T-scores are derived from measurements provided by dual-energy X-ray absorptiometry (DXA). Values are based on measurements performed on Caucasian women.

Reprinted, by permission, from World Health Organization, 1994, *Report of a WHO study group*, WHO technical report series 843: 1-129.

exercise is strongly recommended as an effective method of preventing further bone loss in individuals diagnosed with osteoporosis. Resistance exercises, both isotonic and isometric, have been shown to be an effective way of strengthening muscle and therefore bone.

In considering which activities are most appropriate for the older adult with osteoporosis, you need to review the health and activity questionnaire or interview the participant to ascertain whether the participant already has a history of compression fractures. Knowing the exact BMD for an individual diagnosed with osteoporosis or osteopenia is particularly helpful, especially when selecting balance, resistance, or flexibility activities for these clients. Although most of the balance and mobility activities described in this text should not place older adults with osteopenia or osteoporosis at undue risk, any activities that require forward flexion of the spine combined with either stooping or spinal rotation (e.g., lifting weighted objects from low levels, toe touching, spine twists) should be avoided. Instead, exercises that require spinal extension (e.g., standing backward bends, isometric spinal extension, prone spinal extension for individuals who can tolerate lying on the floor) should be emphasized. Upper-body resistance exercises are also recommended to induce weight-bearing stress on the spine and wrists. Begin these exercises with a low level of resistance and increase resistance slowly (i.e., begin with one set of 8-12 repetitions and increase to a maximum of three sets). Standing weight-bearing activities are also desirable for this group of older adults. Assigning a set of resistance exercises (isotonic and isometric) as homework is particularly beneficial for these participants.

Because older adults diagnosed with osteoporosis often have a heightened fear of falling, you should select activities that provide sufficient challenge but also a large dose of success. Being able to perform balance activities that are perceived to be challenging leads to elevated self-confidence and a reduced fear of falling over the long term. This improved self-confidence eventually carries over to daily life and leads to increased levels of weight-bearing activity that delay the progression of the disease. Fear of falling is discussed in a later section of this chapter. Although fear of falling is not a medical condition, you will need to identify older adults with this syndrome during the initial assessment so that the program can be individualized to meet their needs.

> **Key Point**
>
> Older adults with osteoporosis should not perform any activities that require forward flexion of the spine combined with stooping or spinal rotation.

Parkinson's Disease

bradykinesia—Extreme slowness of movement.

festinating gait—An abnormal and involuntary increase in gait speed.

Parkinson's disease (PD) is a progressive neurological disease resulting from reduced availability of the vital neurotransmitter dopamine in the substantia nigra of the basal ganglia. You can expect program participants with PD to exhibit one or more of the following symptoms: resting tremor, **bradykinesia** (slow movements), gait and balance abnormalities, and increasing rigidity. Specific problems you are likely to see include difficulty with initiating movements; a slow, shuffling gait pattern with shortened, **festinating** steps (uncontrollable hurrying); reduced arm swing; and a general inability to move the limbs quickly or respond effectively to an unexpected loss of balance.

Since balance and mobility are particularly affected by PD, the risk for falling is extremely high in this group of participants and requires additional safeguards to ensure a safe practice environment. These participants should use additional support in the form of a chair or wall when performing standing balance exercises, and close supervision should be provided during any of the gait pattern enhancement and variation activities. What makes it even more challenging for the instructor to program effectively for the participant with PD is that the symptoms are likely to fluctuate from class to class and even within a class depending on where in the medication cycle the participant happens to be on a given day. Also, careful screening of older adults with PD is necessary to ensure that they are appropriate candidates for a group exercise class of this type. In some cases, older adults with PD may be better suited to a one-to-one environment with a physical therapist (if their balance impairments are severe enough) or a well-educated personal trainer.

Diabetes Mellitus

The number of older adults diagnosed with diabetes has increased considerably during the past decade, and many clients in your program are likely to be affected by this chronic metabolic disease. Two types of diabetes mellitus have been identified: type 1, or insulin-dependent diabetes, and type 2, or non-insulin-dependent diabetes. Type 1 diabetes is the more serious of the two and requires careful medical management. Exercise, combined with a proper diet designed to control blood glucose levels in the body, has been shown to be particularly beneficial for individuals with diabetes mellitus. The benefits include greater glucose tolerance and a lower insulin response to a glucose challenge. Older adults engaged in vigorous exercise programs are also likely to reduce their overall body fat, which may result in the need for lower doses of insulin or oral medications. In addition to his other medical conditions, Larry was diagnosed with type 2 diabetes in 2002.

hypoglycemia—Low blood glucose levels. Hypoglycemia may be caused by too much insulin (or oral medications), too little food intake (relative to medication dose), or too much physical activity (relative to medication dose).

As an instructor of a balance and mobility program, you must understand the side effects associated with diabetes and the signs and symptoms of **hypoglycemia.** Signs and symptoms of hypoglycemia include the following:

Anxiety, uneasiness	Sweating, palpitation
Irritability	Headache
Nausea	Loss of motor coordination
Extreme hunger	Strong, rapid pulse
Confusion	Insomnia
Pale, moist skin	Double vision

Hypoglycemia occurs when the blood glucose level falls below 60 milligrams per deciliter. Experts consider this condition to be much more problematic than **hyperglycemia** (high blood glucose) because it can occur quickly and lead to an insulin reaction as a result of too little blood glucose or too much insulin circulating throughout the body (Rimmer, 2005). In addition to watching for hypoglycemia, you will need to know whether any of your program participants with diabetes is experiencing significant vision loss (diabetic retinopathy) or sensation loss, particularly in the feet. Exercises that involve standing or moving on a compliant surface may be problematic for participants with reduced or absent vision or loss of sensation in the feet, as these participants are no longer able to extract good information from the surface. Participants who have unhealed ulcers on their feet may also need to exercise in a seated position to avoid further complications. Certain exercises coordinating head and eye movements (described in chapter 5) may also be ineffective if severe vision loss is evident.

As a general precaution, always check that participants with diabetes have eaten a light snack before class or have one with them in case any symptoms of hypoglycemia develop during the exercise session. Clients with diabetes should also be encouraged to bring a portable glucometer to class so they can check their glucose levels before and after exercising if warranted. Exercise should *not* be initiated if the blood glucose level is not within a safe range (i.e., is less than 100 or greater than 300 milligrams per deciliter). Although the balance activities presented in this program often tax the mind more than the body, you must monitor your clients with diabetes carefully and ensure that they remain hydrated at all times.

Vestibular Disorders

The final set of medical conditions discussed in this section are those related to disorders of the vestibular system. Although it is often difficult to identify why an older adult is experiencing problems in the inner ear, you must understand how to safeguard a participant who is experiencing dizziness that is not caused by hypertension. In older adults, vestibular dysfunction is caused by specific diseases of the inner ear such as **Ménière's disease** or vascular diseases of the labyrinth, an important area within the vestibular system (Diener & Nutt, 1997). In some cases, a more temporary disturbance in vestibular function is caused by **benign positional vertigo (BPV)**, a condition that develops as a result of small crystals called **otoconia** falling into the semicircular canals and causing dizziness with certain movements of the head. Although BPV can be treated quite easily by a trained physical therapist, it is not uncommon to see older adults who have had the problem for a long time and have not received treatment for it.

Although it is well beyond the scope of your professional boundaries (unless you are a licensed physical therapist) to deduce the cause of any dizziness an older adult may experience during class, you must monitor these adults closely, particularly during activities that require rapid tilting or turning of the head or activities in which vision is absent and the ground surface is compliant or unstable. Older adults with an impaired vestibular system are at a greater risk for losing their balance during these types of activities. A careful review of the results of selected items on the Fullerton Advanced Balance (FAB) scale (e.g., test items 3, 4, 7, and 9), which is described in greater detail in the next chapter, will help you identify individuals who may be experiencing difficulties using the information provided by the vestibular system for balance. Although Phoebe did not list a specific

hyperglycemia—High blood glucose levels.

Ménière's disease—A disorder of the inner ear that causes severe disequilibrium lasting anywhere from 30 minutes to 72 hours during an attack.

benign positional vertigo (BPV)—An inner ear condition that produces dizziness or vertigo (illusion of movement) with a rapid change in head position.

otoconia—Calcium carbonate crystals found in the otolithic membranes of the inner ear.

vestibular diagnosis on her health and activity questionnaire, she did indicate that she experienced a severe bout of vertigo in 1993 that affected her balance and mobility. You should monitor her closely when she is performing item 7 on the FAB scale (stand on foam with eyes closed), as this test item requires the person being tested to rely more on the vestibular system to maintain balance. Test item 9 on the FAB scale may also be challenging for Phoebe, as it involves turning the head from side to side while walking.

When working with clients who experience dizziness, encourage them to sit down and rest if a particular activity is making them dizzy to the point that they are at risk of losing their balance. In some cases, you can encourage clients to pace themselves during an exercise so that the symptoms do not become too severe. Because some types of dizziness can be helped by activities that stimulate the vestibular system, teaching your older adult clients to move a little more slowly during a particular activity rather than stop altogether can be helpful. It is also a good idea to ask your clients to rate their dizziness on a scale from 0 (none at all) to 10 (so dizzy they are about to fall down) so you can get a better sense of how dizzy they are feeling. Generally, clients who report a dizziness level or 5 or higher should sit down and rest. An activity that increases a participant's dizziness with each repetition is also a sign that the exercise should be discontinued immediately. Increasing dizziness might occur during an activity such as rock hopping, in which the participants might be bending down to pick up objects as they move down an imaginary creek. If clients repeatedly experience dizziness as a result of activities performed during the class, you should encourage them to talk with their primary care physician. Excellent educational resources are also available to provide more information about vestibular disorders to your older adult clients. The Vestibular Disorders Association (VEDA) Web site (www. vestibular.org) is just one example of these resources.

> ### Key Point
>
> If any clients repeatedly experience dizziness during class activities, encourage them to consult with their primary care physician.

EFFECT OF MEDICATIONS ON BALANCE AND MOBILITY

In addition to certain medical conditions, both the type and the number of medications prescribed to older adults contribute to heightened fall risk. It has been demonstrated that older adults who are taking more than four prescription medications are four times more likely to sustain a fall when compared with peers who are taking fewer prescription medications (Tinetti, 2003; Neutel, Perry, & Maxwell, 2002). In addition, specific types of medications have been shown to elevate fall risk in older adults (Leipzig et al., 1999a). Side effects such as dizziness, reduced alertness, weakness, fatigue, and postural hypotension that result from taking these medications are all likely contributors to heightened fall risk.

Given that most, if not all, of the clients enrolled in your balance and mobility program will be taking one or more prescription medications, you need to ask prospective program participants to provide you with the names of all their medications and the medical condition for which the drugs were prescribed. Although numerous research studies have identified many individual medications that increase the risk for falling due to their effects on CNS function, little

Table 2.2 Potential Adverse Effects of Medications Contributing to Falls in Older Adults

Adverse drug effects	Medications*
Agitation	Antidepressants, caffeine, neuroleptics, stimulants
Arrhythmias	Antiarrhythmics
Cognitive impairment, confusion	Benzodiazepines, narcotics, neuroleptics, any drug with anticholinergic effects
Dizziness, orthostatic hypotension	Anticonvulsants, antidepressants, antihypertensives, benzodiazepines, narcotics, neuroleptics
Gait abnormalities, extrapyramidal reactions	Antidepressants, metoclopramide, neuroleptics
Increased ambulation	Diuretics
Postural disturbances (e.g., problems with balance)	Anticonvulsants, benzodiazepines, neuroleptics
Sedation, drowsiness	Anticonvulsants, antidepressants, benzodiazepines, narcotics, neuroleptics
Syncope	Beta-blockers, nitrates, vasodilators (e.g., alpha$_1$-adrenergic blockers such as doxazosin)
Visual disturbances (e.g., blurred vision)	Neuroleptics, any drug with anticholinergic effects

*This is not an exhaustive list; many other agents may cause the adverse effects specified.

Reprinted, by permission, from B. Ruddock, 2004, "Medications and falls in the elderly," *Revue Des Pharmacies Du Canada*, July/August 137(6): 17.

is known about how the interactive or additive effects of taking multiple medications might further affect balance and mobility. The classes of medications that are positively associated with increased fall risk include most classes of psychotropic drugs, such as tricyclic antidepressants, neuroleptics, sedatives and hypnotics, and benzodiazepines (both long and short acting). Table 2.2 summarizes adverse effects associated with certain types of medications that are likely to increase the risk for falling.

Antidepressants in particular are associated with an increased risk for falling, and new users of these drugs are at a greater risk for falling than are the individuals who have been taking them for a while. It has also been demonstrated that older adults taking a higher dosage of an antidepressant drug experience a higher fall rate. Little difference in fall rates exists among older adults prescribed different types of antidepressants (Thapa, Gideon, Cost, Milam, & Ray, 1998). Older adults taking more than one psychotropic agent or having other risk factors for falls are at a greater risk of falling (Leipzig et al., 1999a). Cardiac and analgesic medications (e.g., digoxin, type Ia antiarrhythmics, and diuretics) have also been studied but were found to be only weakly associated with heightened fall risk (Leipzig et al., 1999b).

Antidepressant use is higher among older adults living in nursing homes (35.5 percent) or assisted-living facilities (39.8 percent) when compared with older adults dwelling in the community (8 percent; Ray & Griffin, 1990). The loss of perceived

> ### Key Point
>
> Certain classes of prescription medications are associated with a higher fall risk among older adults. These include psychotropics, sedatives and hypnotics, and antidepressants.

independence and control over life no doubt contributes to the higher use of anti-depressants by older adults who are no longer able to live independently within the community. Increased frailty is also often accompanied by increased depression. In addition, the loss of a spouse or family member is likely to precipitate the use of these types of drugs. Although interventions aimed at reducing the number of psychotropic medications taken by older adults have been shown to be very effective in reducing fall rates, the benefits have been short lived. A large percentage of the older adults studied began using the withdrawn medications within 3 months of the study ending (Campbell, Robertson, Gardner, Norton, & Buchner, 1999). The investigators concluded that in order for this type of intervention strategy to be successful, it needs to be combined with a behavioral counseling program.

FEAR OF FALLING

Although fear of falling is not a medical condition, per se, this psychological syndrome has been identified as a risk factor for falls. Previous research on postfall syndrome (Murphy & Isaacs, 1982) indicates that between 35 and 56 percent of community-residing older adults significantly curtail their activities due to being fearful of falling (Howland, Peterson, & Ohayon, 2000). Although heightened fear of falling is common after a fall, even if the fall did not result in injury, it has also been observed among older adults who have not yet fallen. Some of the risk factors associated with developing fear of falling include a history of multiple falls, dizziness, certain medical conditions that affect mobility (e.g., RA, osteoarthritis, PD, stroke), and self-rated poor health (Lach, 2005). As an instructor of a balance and mobility program, you are likely to find that a number of participants are fearful of falling and require specialized attention over the course of the program. In the FallProof program, fear of falling, as well as balance-related self-confidence, is evaluated before the start of the program and at regular intervals after the program has started. Question 13 on the health and activity questionnaire asks older adults how concerned they are about falling. Responses can range from "Not at all" to "Extremely" on a 7-point Likert scale. As you will learn in chapter 3, you can glean even more information about older adults' confidence when performing balance-related tasks by having them complete the Balance Efficacy Scale (BES; Rose, 2003; Gunter et al., 2003). Unlike the general question on the health and activity questionnaire, the BES can help you identify which specific tasks and environments adversely affect the older adult's level of confidence.

Once you know which participants are fearful of falling or lack confidence in their abilities to perform tasks requiring balance, you should structure the practice environment in a manner that will raise their confidence levels. You must select exercise progressions carefully so that your participants experience a high dose of success during each class or training session. Regularly including activities that lower anxiety, such as breathing exercises, relaxation training, and visualization, also constitutes an effective way to treat fear of falling. Cognitive-behavioral intervention techniques have also been successful in reducing fear of falling and increasing physical activity levels among older adults identified with the syndrome. These techniques form the basis of a well-known program, A Matter of Balance, which was designed by researchers at the Roybal Center at Boston University and was demonstrated to be an effective program for increasing self-efficacy among older adults (Tennstedt et al., 1998).

ARE THE RISKS THE SAME FOR ALL OLDER ADULTS?

As mentioned earlier in this chapter, fall risk is not the same for all older adults. It has also been shown to change over time. With advancing age and declining physical function, both the level of risk and the factors contributing to risk change. Older adults who remain physically active as they age and thereby retain good postural competence are at a lower risk for falls than are older adults who severely limit or curtail their levels of physical activity. Sedentary older adults are more likely to experience increased difficulty performing activities that require balance and mobility as their level of conditioning declines. Although their risk of falling may decrease in the short term as a function of their reduced exposure, their long-term risk increases significantly as their physical function and confidence in their ability to engage in certain activities or venture into more challenging environments decline (Tinetti, Mendes de Leon, Doucette, & Baker, 1994).

> ### Key Point
>
> The level of fall risk is not the same for all older adults and changes over time.

The setting in which an older adult resides influences the type of risk factors associated with increased falls. Frail older adults residing in long-term care settings, for example, rarely fall as a result of environmental factors. Intrinsic risk factors (e.g., general weakness, cognitive impairment, adverse drug events, medical conditions) are much more likely to constitute the primary reasons for increased falls in this group of older adults (Lipsitz, Jonsson, Kelley, & Koestner, 1991). In contrast, at least one-third to one-half of all falls sustained by community-residing older adults can be attributed to environmental or extrinsic risk factors (Rubenstein & Josephson, 1992; Tinetti, Speechley, & Ginter, 1988).

Researchers who have analyzed fall patterns in the home have identified several patterns, including collisions with objects in a dark environment, inability to avoid temporary hazards or conditions, experiencing adverse frictional contact with different surface types, and careless negotiation or use of the environment. It has also been demonstrated that older adults who continue to be active within their community though their physical capabilities are declining, take unnecessary personal risks when performing daily activities, or expose themselves to hazardous environments are at especially high risk for falls (Studenski et al., 1994).

PRACTICAL IMPLICATIONS FOR PROGRAM PLANNING

Why should instructors of balance and mobility programs know about the various risk factors that contribute to heightened fall risk? Instructors who know about the risk factors related to increased fall incidence among older adults glean vital clues when they review a client's completed health and physical activity history (e.g., age, sex, diagnoses, medications, self-reported joint pain). These clues help instructors to understand the client's initial level of function and to design a more individualized exercise plan that better addresses the client's balance and mobility problems.

Given that falls are often due to many different factors, the exercises you prescribe for your older adult clients should directly address the biological and behavioral risk factors that are most amenable to change (e.g., muscle strength, balance and gait, fear of falling). For example, an older adult client who demonstrates low muscular strength, particularly at the ankle, knee, and hip, should be provided with resistance exercises, both in class and at home, that specifically strengthen these muscle groups (see chapter 8 for appropriate exercises). Similarly, an older adult who demonstrates poor mobility skills or impaired gait speed should be prescribed progressive activities that target those impairments. Several activities presented in the gait pattern enhancement and variation section of chapter 7, coupled with activities described in the weight shift and transfer sections of chapter 4, should address these problems very well.

Although your primary focus as an instructor is to address the physical risk factors that contribute to increased fall rates among older adults, you may have several opportunities to educate your clients about environmental and behavioral risk factors such as environmental hazards and risk-taking behaviors. Following a review of the client's health history, you can provide the client with educational materials on various topics such as home safety, medication use and abuse, home exercise programs, or community activity resources. It is also a good idea to have your clients complete a home safety checklist and return it to you during the first week of class (see the internet resources related to home safety and modifications listed on page 51). This activity not only increases your clients' awareness of home safety issues but also lets you know if there are hazards in a client's home that are likely to increase the overall fall risk. Depending on the resources available in your community, you may even be able to go a step further by providing your client with a list of local organizations that conduct home safety inspections and repairs. Many hospitals and home health nursing agencies provide this type of service. You might also inquire as to whether your community has a local chapter of Rebuilding Together, a national nonprofit organization that provides a home safety inspection and repair service.

In addition to having clients complete a home safety checklist, consider incorporating role-playing into your classes as a means of helping your clients make good judgments about how to perform daily activities and the types of environments in which they are likely to encounter problems. For example, a client with sensory peripheral neuropathy needs to learn that taking the trash out to the curb at night might not be as prudent as performing the same activity in the morning. The loss of sensation in the feet, coupled with reduced vision at night, places that adult at unnecessary risk for falls when the same activity can be performed much more safely during the day, when vision is better. Be sure to inquire regularly about any changes in your clients' medications or dosages so that you can maintain a current list of the various medications being used. Because many older adults use complementary and alternative medicine (CAM), you need to maintain a list of those medications as well (Eisenberg et al., 1993, 1998). Although little is currently

> ### Key Point
>
> Have your clients complete a home safety checklist during the first week of class. This activity raises your clients' awareness of home safety issues and lets you know if a client has hazards in the home that are likely to increase overall fall risk.

> ### Key Point
>
> In addition to knowing which prescription medications your clients have been prescribed, maintain a list of any complementary and alternative medicine (CAM) being used by your older adult clients.

Internet Resources

There are a number of very good internet resources devoted to various fall prevention topics. I recommend that you take some time to familiarize yourself with the content of the sites identified in this section. They will provide you with up-to-date information on important issues related to fall prevention such as medications, home assessment and modification, and exercise, as well as many excellent educational materials that you can use to further educate your clients about how to avoid falls and maintain an independent lifestyle. The Web site hosted by the Fall Prevention Center of Excellence is one of my favorite fall prevention internet resources. It has sections with information pertinent to older adults, caregivers, professionals, and researchers. The internet can be a wonderful source of information to you as long as you know that the sites you use are hosted by reputable organizations and regularly updated.

Fall Prevention

One of the newest and most rapidly growing Web sites providing fall prevention information and educational resources is available through the Fall Prevention Center of Excellence at the University of Southern California. By logging onto **www.stopfalls.org** you can access the latest and greatest information on preventing falls among older adults. The Web site provides information for older adults and their families, educators, researchers, and health professionals and also provides a number of fact sheets that you can use to educate your clients and their families about preventing falls.

Home Safety and Modifications

One of the most comprehensive Web sites addressing home safety and modification is that of the National Resource Center on Supportive Housing and Home Modification. This nonprofit organization, housed at the University of Southern California, promotes aging in place and independent living for people of all ages and disabilities. The Web address is **www.homemods.org**.

Medications

Information about medications and their known side effects can be obtained by logging onto either of the following Web sites:

- ◆ **www.nlm.nih.gov/medlineplus/druginformation.html**. In addition to providing information on prescription medications, this Web site links to Natural Standard, a Web site that provides information about complementary and alternative medications.
- ◆ **www.rxlist.com**. This Web site is particularly easy for older adults to use to learn more about the medications they have been prescribed as well as the types of side effects that may result from taking them.

known about possible interactions between CAM and prescription medications, it is a good idea to maintain a record of all prescription medications as well as over-the-counter supplements being taken by your class participants.

SUMMARY

Many factors contribute to an older adult's heightened risk for falls. Although it is not possible for you as an instructor to eliminate certain risk factors known to contribute to increased fall rates, such as advancing age or sex, you can positively affect many physical risk factors through careful program planning. Helping your clients understand which activities and environments they should avoid until their balance improves will prove invaluable. Having clients complete a home safety checklist as a homework assignment will also make them more aware of potential hazards in and around the home and perhaps lead them to make some changes to reduce their chances of falling. Of course, your primary goal as an instructor is to improve the balance and mobility of your clients as a means of significantly reducing their overall risk for falls. As their postural competence increases, so too will their self-confidence, hopefully to a level that will motivate them to become more physically active on a daily basis.

Test Your Understanding

1. Which of the following is *not* an example of a biological risk factor for falls?
    a. chronic illness
    b. age
    c. gender
    d. unsecured mats or rugs in the home
    e. cognitive impairment

2. Which of the following is an impairment associated with a stroke?
    a. stooped posture
    b. asymmetrical gait pattern
    c. shortness of breath
    d. anemia
    e. shuffling gait

3. A person is diagnosed with hypertension when
    a. systolic blood pressure is greater than 140 mmHg and diastolic blood pressure is less than 90 mmHg
    b. systolic blood pressure is greater than 100 mmHg and diastolic blood pressure is greater than 140 mmHg
    c. systolic blood pressure is greater than 200 mmHg
    d. diastolic blood pressure is greater than 110 mmHg
    e. diastolic blood pressure is greater than 90 mmHg and systolic blood pressure is greater than 140 mmHg

4. A diagnosis of osteoporosis is made once bone mineral density is
    a. between 1 and 2.5 SDs below that of normal young adults
    b. at least 2.5 SDs above that of normal young adults
    c. within 1 SD of that of normal young adults
    d. a T-score that is at or below −2.5
    e. between 2 and 2.5 SDs below that of young adults

5. Which types of exercises should not be performed by older adults with a diagnosis of osteoporosis?
    a. forward flexion of the spine combined with stooping
    b. lower-body strength exercises
    c. spinal extension
    d. weight-bearing activities
    e. a and c

6. Bradykinesia is a symptom associated with Parkinson's disease that is characterized by
   a. an abnormal and involuntary increase in gait speed
   b. extremely slow movements
   c. an unstable movement pattern
   d. increased rigidity
   e. a shuffling gait pattern

7. The following medications have been positively associated with increased fall risk:
   a. coenzyme Q10
   b. benzodiazepines
   c. ibuprofen
   d. analgesics
   e. gingko biloba

8. Which of the following is *not* a symptom of hypoglycemia?
   a. strong, rapid pulse
   b. insomnia
   c. pale, moist skin
   d. loss of appetite
   e. nausea

9. An observable characteristic of kyphosis is
   a. an increased posterior curvature of the spine
   b. a decreased posterior curvature of the spine
   c. BMD that is lower than normal
   d. BMD that is higher than normal
   e. swelling in joint structures

10. At least one-third to one-half of all falls sustained by community-residing adults can be attributed to
   a. intrinsic risk factors
   b. poor judgment
   c. extrinsic risk factors
   d. a low level of physical activity
   e. muscle weakness

Practical Problems

Review the health and activity questionnaires associated with the two case studies presented in chapter 1. Complete the following tasks:

1. Identify the primary signs and symptoms associated with the medical diagnoses reported by Larry and Phoebe. Indicate whether any special precautions might be necessary when testing either client before the program and designing an exercise program for each of them.

2. Research each of the medications listed in the health and activity questionnaires completed by Larry and Phoebe. List the medical condition that each medication is prescribed for and any side effects likely to adversely affect balance and mobility. Also identify any medications on the list that are associated with a heightened risk for falls. Any of the internet sites listed on page 51 will provide you with additional information about the side effects associated with each medication.

3. Develop a list of the biological and behavioral risk factors for Larry and Phoebe based on your review of their completed health and activity questionnaires.

Part II

The FallProof Program for Improving Balance and Mobility

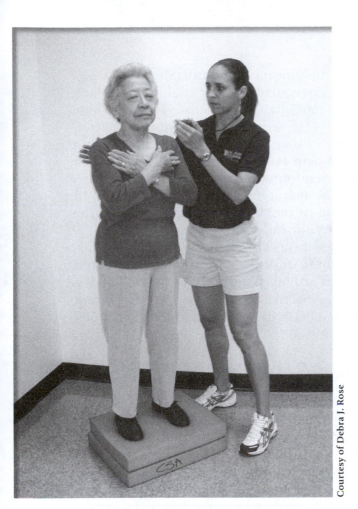

Courtesy of Debra J. Rose

Chapter 3

Screening and Assessment

Objectives

After completing this chapter, you will be able to

- identify several tests used to evaluate balance and mobility in older adults,
- screen and evaluate the multiple dimensions of balance and mobility,
- interpret the test results, and
- identify the possible causes of the impairments identified.

The assessment of multiple dimensions of physical function (in particular, balance and mobility) assists the instructor in many ways. Assessment not only facilitates the early identification of older adults who are beginning to experience significant changes in multiple body systems resulting in observable changes in postural stability and mobility but also helps you, the instructor, develop an appropriate exercise plan that targets the identified impairments. When assessments are readministered on a regular basis, the information obtained can be used to guide the selection or deletion of certain exercises, help participants set appropriate short- and long-term goals, and motivate participants to meet each of those goals. Finally, assessment is a way of documenting the overall effectiveness of the program and your teaching.

Consistent with a systems approach to studying motor control (Shumway-Cook & Woollacott, 2007), any screening and assessment of older adults, particularly those already experiencing balance and mobility impairments, should include tests that assess the multiple body systems (e.g., sensory, motor, musculoskeletal, cognitive) that contribute to balance. Such a multisystem assessment will provide you with in-depth information that can be used to select the most appropriate exercise progressions. In addition to providing information about the multiple dimensions of balance and mobility, the assessment described in this chapter reveals important information about lifestyle and physical activity patterns. It is now well understood that lifestyle factors such as physical inactivity and disuse are as important as pathology in contributing to frailty and disability in the later years (Chandler & Hadley, 1996; Di Pietro, 1996; Rikli & Jones, 1997).

> ### Key Point
>
> Screening and assessment facilitate the early identification of balance impairments in the older adult and help the instructor develop a more tailored exercise plan for the older adult.

HEALTH AND PHYSICAL ACTIVITY PATTERNS

Information about participants' overall health status and physical activity patterns is obtained from the health and activity questionnaire administered before any physical assessment of clients (see form 3.1 on pages 84-89). In addition to providing information about existing medical diagnoses and medications and overall health status, the questionnaire asks participants three questions related to their physical activity and exercise patterns (see questions 19-21 of the questionnaire). For example, participants are asked how often they leave the house during the week. They are also asked whether they participate in regular physical exercise that is strenuous enough to increase their breathing, heart rate, or perspiration, and, if so, how many days they exercise per week. Finally, they are asked to select, from a list of four options, the pace at which they walk (if they walk on a regular basis).

> ### Why Test?
>
> Assessment should be conducted before the start of the program
> - ◆ to help participants understand the specific nature of their balance and mobility impairments,
> - ◆ to help establish a starting point for each participant in each component of the FallProof program, and
> - ◆ to individualize program content based on the identified impairments and functional limitations.
>
> Assessment should be conducted regularly during the program
> - ◆ to determine whether each participant's balance and mobility impairments are being addressed,
> - ◆ to determine the program's effectiveness,
> - ◆ to provide valuable feedback to participants about their progress, and
> - ◆ to motivate participants to continue the program.

Let's review the responses that Phoebe provided on her health and activity questionnaire (chapter 1, pages 18-23) so that we can learn more about her pathology or disease and pattern of physical activity. On the questionnaire, Phoebe indicated that she has been diagnosed with cardiovascular disease, a respiratory disease (i.e., chronic asthma), peripheral neuropathy, arthritis, an inner ear disorder, and depression—a total of six medical conditions. Her prescription medications include Albuterol, Azmacort, Lasix, Synthroid, Allopurinol, K-Dur, and Beconase—a total of seven prescription medications. It would be reasonable to conclude that her overall health status is good based on her responses to question 15. She also rated the overall quality of her life as being only low to moderate (question 16).

Phoebe's responses to questions 19 through 21 indicate that despite her numerous health issues, she remains active socially. She leaves the house 3 to 4 times per week. She does not, however, engage in any regular physical exercise, and she does not go for walks on a regular basis. From her self-report, it is clear that Phoebe is a sedentary person who would benefit from being involved in a regular exercise program of low to moderate intensity. Take a moment now to review the same questions on Larry's completed health and activity questionnaire (chapter 1, pages 25-30) to learn more about his overall health and physical activity patterns.

ASSESSING FUNCTIONAL ABILITY

The health and activity questionnaire in form 3.1 (pages 84-89) also includes the self-report Composite Physical Function (CPF) scale (in question 17), which assesses a wide range of functional abilities, from those associated with basic ADLs (e.g., bathing, dressing) to those associated with instrumental or intermediate ADLs (e.g., housework, shopping) as well as advanced ADLs (e.g., strenuous household activities, sport or recreational activities). The CPF scale is an expanded version of three previously published scales and was developed by Rikli and Jones (1998). It can be used to assess a participant's functional ability not only at the beginning of the program but also at regular intervals during the program. Individuals who indicate that they are able to complete all 12 items independently are considered to be high functioning while individuals who report that they are unable to perform six or fewer of the items (score of 12 or lower) without

> ### Key Point
>
> The CPF scale should be used to assess a participant's perceived level of functional ability at the beginning of the program and at regular intervals (every 3-6 months) during the program.

difficulty are considered to be low functioning (Rikli & Jones, 2001). It is a good idea to ask program participants to complete the CPF scale periodically (every 3-6 months) so you can see whether any improvements you have documented on the physical tests of balance and mobility are positively influencing your participants' perceived abilities to perform basic, intermediate, and advanced ADLs. For your convenience, a short form of the health and activity questionnaire that includes the CPF scale (in question 10) is provided in form 3.2 on pages 90-92.

As you can see by reviewing question 17 on Phoebe's health and activity questionnaire (see page 22), she scored 13 out of a total of 24 points on the CPF scale. This score places her just above the category of low function. A closer look at her individual responses reveals that Phoebe is able to perform the basic ADLs (e.g., dressing and bathing oneself) without assistance but requires assistance to complete most of the intermediate ADLs (e.g., shopping, lifting and carrying 10 lbs) and is unable to do any of the advanced ADLs (e.g., strenuous activities, heavy household chores, lifting and carrying 25 pounds, or 11 kg). Now look at the same question on Larry's completed questionnaire on page 29 and calculate his CPF score. What types of activities does he report having difficulty performing on a daily basis?

ASSESSING FALL RISK

In addition to having participants self-assess their fall risk using a tool such as the Stay Independent Self-Risk Assessment Guide (Centers for Disease Control and Prevention, 2008; see bibliography for more information), you can also administer the 8-foot (2.4 m) up-and-go test (Rikli & Jones, 2001) as a means of physically evaluating an individual's fall risk. Older adults who are unable to complete the timed test in 8.5 seconds or less are at a heightened risk for falling (Rose, Jones, & Lucchese, 2002). A full description of the test and the procedures for administering it are available in the *Senior Fitness Test Manual* developed by Rikli and Jones (2001).

Let's review how Phoebe and Larry fared on the 8-foot (2.4 m) up-and-go test. Phoebe's best score on the two recorded test trials was 11 seconds (see figure 3.2, p. 79), placing her well below the criterion threshold of 8.9 seconds on this SFT test item. According to Rikli and Jones (1999b), people who fall below the established criterion for any of the Senior Fitness Test items may be considered to be at risk for loss of functional mobility. Perhaps more importantly, Phoebe's score places her in the high-risk category for falls. Larry fared a little better than Phoebe did on the 8-foot (2.4 m) up-and-go test, although his best score of 9 seconds is just a little slower than the 8.9-second criterion threshold score and still suggests that he is close to being at risk for loss of functional mobility and also at high risk for falls. You will find an empty report card at the end of this chapter (form 3.3, pp. 93-94) that you can begin filling in as you are provided with more performance scores for Larry in the sections to follow. Completing the report card as you continue reading the next few sections will also prepare you to complete practical problem #2 at the end of this chapter.

ASSESSING THE MULTIPLE DIMENSIONS OF BALANCE AND MOBILITY

Before starting your balance and mobility program, and at regular intervals throughout the program, you should conduct the following tests to assess the multiple dimensions of balance and mobility: the Fullerton Advanced Balance (FAB) scale (Rose, Lucchese, & Wiersma, 2006; Hernandez & Rose, 2008) or Berg Balance Scale (BBS) (Berg, Wood-Dauphinee, Williams, & Maki, 1992), the 30-foot (9 m) walk performed at preferred and maximum speeds (Hernandez, Rose, & Theou, 2008; Theou, French, Hernandez, & Rose, 2006), and the walkie-talkie test (Lundin-Olsson, Nyberg, & Gustafson, 1997). In addition, selected test items from the Senior Fitness Test (Rikli & Jones, 2001) should be administered for the purpose of learning more about the function of the cardiovascular and musculoskeletal systems (e.g., aerobic endurance, strength, and flexibility). Descriptions of how to administer, score, and interpret the results of each of these tests are presented in the following sections of this chapter.

> ### Key Point
>
> There are several available clinical and field tests that provide valid and reliable information, require little or no equipment, and are quick and easy to administer in community-based settings.

Balance

The two tests used to measure balance are the FAB scale (Rose et al., 2006; Hernandez & Rose, 2008) and the BBS (Berg et al., 1992). Both are described in the following sections.

Fullerton Advanced Balance Scale

The FAB scale is a relatively new test designed to measure subtle changes in balance occurring in independently functioning older adults. It is appropriate to use with the independently residing older adults who are most likely to enroll in a community-based balance and mobility program. The FAB scale is composed of 10 items that are scored on an **ordinal scale** ranging from 0 to 4 points. The maximum possible score for the FAB scale is 40 points. The scale includes a combination of static and dynamic balance activities performed in different sensory environments. Items include standing on foam with the eyes closed, walking with head turns, stepping up onto and over an obstacle, and tandem walking. Detailed test administration procedures are provided in the feature that follows, and a scoring form is provided in form 3.4, "Score Sheet for Fullerton Advanced Balance Scale," which is on pages 95-97.

ordinal scale—A numerical ranking of performance from best (4 points on FAB scale) to worst (0 points on FAB scale). The difference between two adjacent scores is not the same throughout the scale.

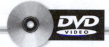

Test Administration Instructions for the Fullerton Advanced Balance Scale

1. Stand with feet together and eyes closed

   Purpose: Assess participant's ability to use somatosensory input (i.e., ground and body position cues) to maintain upright balance while standing on a reduced base of support with vision removed

   Equipment: Stopwatch

   Testing procedure: Demonstrate the correct test position and then instruct the participant to move the feet independently until they are together. If some participants are unable to achieve the correct position due to lower-extremity joint impairments, encourage them to bring their heels together even though the fronts of their feet are not touching. Have participants adopt a position that will ensure their safety as they fold their arms across the chest and prepare to close the eyes. Begin timing as soon as the participant closes the eyes. Instruct participants to open the eyes if they feel so unsteady that a loss of balance is imminent.

   Verbal instructions: Bring your feet together, fold your arms across your chest, close your eyes when you are ready, and remain as steady as possible until I instruct you to open your eyes.

2. Reach forward with outstretched arm to retrieve an object (pencil).

   Purpose: Assess participant's ability to lean forward to retrieve an object without altering the base of support and measure the participant's stability limits in a forward direction

   Equipment: Pencil and 12-inch (30 cm) ruler

   Testing procedure: Instruct the participant to raise the preferred arm to 90 degrees and extend it with the fingers outstretched. Follow with a demonstration of the correct action. Use

(continued)

the ruler to measure a distance of 10 inches (25 cm) from the fingertips of the outstretched arm. Hold the object (a pencil) horizontally and level with the height of the participant's shoulder. Instruct the participant to reach forward, grasp the pencil, and return to the initial starting position without moving the feet, if possible. (It is acceptable to raise the heels as long as the feet do not move.) If the participant is unable to reach the pencil within 2 to 3 seconds of initiating the forward lean, tell the participant that it is OK to move the feet in order to reach the pencil. Record the number of steps the participant takes in order to retrieve the pencil.

Verbal instructions: Try to lean forward, take the pencil from my hand, and return to your starting position without moving your feet from their present position. (Allow 2-3 seconds of lean time.) You can move your feet in order to reach the pencil.

3. Turn in a full circle in right and left directions

Purpose: Assess the participant's ability to turn in a full circle in both directions without losing balance and using a minimum number of steps

Equipment: None

Testing procedure: Verbally explain and then demonstrate the task to be performed, making sure to complete each circle in four steps or less and to pause briefly between turns. Instruct the participant (who is facing you) to turn in a complete circle in one direction, pause, and then turn in a complete circle in the opposite direction. Count the number of steps taken to complete each circle. Stop counting steps as soon as the participant is facing you after completing each turn. Allow for a small correction in foot position before a turn in the opposite direction is initiated.

Verbal instructions: Turn around in a full circle, pause, and then turn around in a full circle in the opposite direction.

4. Step up onto and over a 6-inch (15 cm) bench

Purpose: Assess participant's ability to control COG in dynamic task situations and measure lower-body strength and bilateral motor coordination

Equipment: 6-inch (15 cm) bench with an 14- by 18-inch (36 by 46 cm) stepping surface

Testing procedure: Verbally explain and then demonstrate the step up onto and over the bench in both directions. Instruct the participant to step onto the bench with the right foot, swing the left leg directly up and over the bench, step off the other side, and then repeat the movement in the opposite direction with the left leg leading the action. While the participant performs the test, watch to see that the trailing leg does not make contact with the bench or swing around, as opposed to going directly up and over, the bench.

Verbal instructions: Step up onto the bench with your right leg, swing your left leg directly up and over the bench, and step off the other side. Repeat the movement in the opposite direction with your left leg as the leading leg.

5. Walk with feet in a tandem position

Purpose: Assess participant's ability to dynamically control COM with an altered base of support

Equipment: Masking tape

Testing procedure: Verbally explain and demonstrate how to perform the test correctly before allowing the participant to attempt the test. Instruct the participant to tandem walk (heel to toe) on the line until you say to stop. Allow participants who are unable to achieve a tandem stance within the first two steps to repeat the test *one time*. The participant may elect to step forward with the opposite foot on the second attempt. Score as interruptions any instances where the participant takes one or more steps away from the line when performing the tandem walk or is unable to achieve the correct heel-to-toe position during any step taken along the course. Do not ask the participant to stop until 10 steps have been completed.

Verbal instructions: Walk forward along the line, placing one foot directly in front of the other such that the heel and toe are in contact on each step forward. I will tell you when to stop.

6. Stand on one leg

Purpose: Assess participant's ability to maintain upright balance with a reduced base of support

Equipment: Stopwatch

Testing procedure: Instruct the participant to fold the arms across the chest, lift one leg off the floor, and maintain balance until instructed to return the foot to the floor. Begin timing as soon as the participant lifts the foot from the floor and allow 20 seconds to elapse. Stop timing if the legs touch, the raised leg contacts the floor, or the participant removes the arms from the chest before the 20 seconds are up. Allow participants who are unsure which leg to raise to perform the test once on each leg.

Verbal instructions: Fold your arms across your chest, lift one leg off the floor (without touching your other leg), and stand with your eyes open as long as you can.

7. Stand on foam with eyes closed

Purpose: Assess participant's ability to maintain upright balance while standing on a compliant surface with the eyes closed

Equipment: Stopwatch and two Airex Balance Pads, with a length of nonslip material placed between the two pads and an additional length of nonslip material placed between the floor and the bottom pad if the test is being performed on an uncarpeted surface

Testing procedure: Following a demonstration of the task, instruct the participant to step onto the foam pads without assistance, fold the arms across the chest, and close the eyes when ready. (Be sure to demonstrate the correct standing position on the balance pads.) Make sure the position that you adopt as the test administrator ensures the safety of the participant. Position the foam pads close to a wall in all cases and in a corner of the room if the participant appears unsteady. Begin timing as soon as the eyes close. Stop the trial if the participant (a) opens the eyes before 20 seconds have elapsed, (b) lifts the arms off the chest, or (c) loses balance and requires manual assistance to prevent falling. Be sure to instruct participants to open their eyes if they feel so unsteady that a loss of balance is imminent. Have the participant step forward off the foam at the completion of the test. Provide manual assistance if needed.

Verbal instructions: Step up onto the foam and stand with your feet shoulder-width apart. Fold your arms over your chest, and close your eyes when you are ready. I will tell you when to open your eyes.

8. Jump with both feet for distance

Purpose: Assess participant's upper- and lower-body coordination and lower-body power

Equipment: 36-inch (91 cm) ruler, masking tape

Testing procedure: Do not introduce this test item if the participant cannot perform test item 4 safely, has a diagnosis of osteoporosis, or complains of lower-body joint pain. Score

(continued)

a 0 on the test form and move immediately to test item 9. Otherwise, instruct the participant to perform a jump with both feet (i.e., jump with two feet and land on two feet). Demonstrate the correct movement before having the participant perform the jump. Do not jump much more than twice the length of your own feet when demonstrating the test. Use the ruler to measure the length of the participant's foot and then multiply by 2 to determine the ideal distance to be jumped. Observe whether the participant leaves the floor with both feet and lands with both feet. Be sure to move with the participant during the performance and place your hand on the participant's back to provide stability as soon as the feet contact the ground following the jump.

Verbal instructions: Jump as far but as safely as you can. Try and make sure that both feet leave the floor and land at the same time.

9. Walk while turning head

Purpose: Assess participant's ability to maintain dynamic balance while walking and turning the head

Equipment: Metronome set at 100 beats per minute

Testing procedure: After demonstrating the test item, allow the participant to practice turning the head in time with the metronome while standing in place. Encourage participants to turn the head at least 30 degrees in each direction by instructing them to turn the head to look into each corner of the room. When the participant is finished practicing, instruct the person to walk forward while turning the head from side to side in time with the metronome. Begin counting steps as soon as the participant attempts to turn the head to the beat of the metronome. Observe whether the person deviates from a straight path while walking or is unable to turn the head the required distance (30 degrees) to the timing of the metronome. In most cases, the steps will be synchronized with the head turns, making the counting of 10 steps easier.

Verbal instructions: Walk forward while turning your head from side to side with each beat of the metronome. I will tell you when to stop.

10. Restore balance after backward disturbance

Purpose: Assess participant's ability to restore balance following an unexpected perturbation

Equipment: None

Testing procedure: Instruct the participant to stand with the back turned toward you. Extend your arm, lock your elbow, and place the palm of your hand in the middle of the participant's back. Instruct the participant to lean back slowly against your hand until you say to stop. Quickly flex your elbow to remove your hand from the participant's back as soon as the participant applies a sufficient amount of force against your hand to require a movement of the feet to restore balance once the hand is removed. Try to quickly release your hand while you are still giving the instructions. This release should be unexpected, so do not prepare the participant for the moment of release or allow the participant to lean too far back onto your hand before releasing it.

Verbal instructions: Slowly lean back into my hand until I ask you to stop.

The FAB scale has demonstrated high test–retest and inter- and intrarater reliability (Rose et al., 2006). It can be used to identify people who are at a high risk for falls; a person scoring 25 points or lower on the FAB scale can be considered to be at a heightened risk for falling and in need of immediate intervention (Hernandez & Rose, 2008). The total score on the FAB scale also correlates well with the total score on the BBS ($r = .75$), another measure of balance-related abilities. The FAB scale was developed as an alternative measure of balance because of the tendency of the BBS to produce ceiling effects (i.e., very high scores on repeated tests) when administered to independently functioning older adults with less severe balance impairments. The FAB scale also includes items that identify older adults who may be experiencing increased fall risk as a result of sensory system impairments (Farrar & Rose, 2007), while the BBS has been criticized for its lack of sensitivity in identifying sensory system impairments (Allison & Rose, 1998). An older adult's performance on each of the FAB scale test items can also be evaluated and the possible underlying impairments identified so that exercise progressions can be selected to target those impairments. Table 3.1 lists the possible underlying impairments associated with poor performance on each of the 10 test items and provides a set of recommended exercises to address those impairments.

> ### Key Point
> The FAB scale measures changes in multiple dimensions of balance in independently functioning community-dwelling older adults with less severe balance impairments.

A short form version of the FAB scale (SF-FAB) has been developed recently. It comprises the four test items that have been shown to be the strongest predictors of fall risk (Hernandez & Rose, 2008): 4 (step up onto and over a bench), 5 (tandem walk), 6 (stand on one leg), and 7 (stand on foam with eyes closed). Although the SF-FAB scale does not provide as much information about balance, it is a useful alternative for instructors who do not feel that they have the time to conduct the longer version of the scale. The total score for the SF-FAB scale is 16, and the cutoff value for increased fall risk is 9 points or lower (Hernandez & Rose, 2008).

Table 3.1 Interpretation of the Individual Test Items on the Fullerton Advanced Balance Scale

Item	Possible impairments	Recommended exercises
1. Stand with feet together and eyes closed	1. Weak hip abductors or adductors	Lateral weight shifts against resistance, side leg raises against gravity or resistance
	2. Poor COG control	Seated or standing balance activities emphasizing weight shifts in multiple directions
	3. Poor use of somatosensory cues	Standing balance activities with eyes closed (controlled sway in A-P and lateral directions)
2. Reach forward to retrieve object	1. Reduced limits of stability	Seated or standing COG control activities
	2. Reduced ankle ROM	Ankle circles, heel lifts, and drops from height
	3. Fear of falling	Confidence-building activities that can be performed with a high level of success
	4. LB muscle weakness	Wall sits and LB exercises with resistance

(continued)

Table 3.1 *(continued)*

Item	Possible impairments	Recommended exercises
3. Turn in full circle to right and left	1. Poor dynamic COG control	Standing weight transfers, gait pattern enhancement (turns, directional changes)
	2. Possible vestibular impairment (e.g., dizziness)	Exercises coordinating head and eye movements
	3. LB weakness	LB exercises with resistance that emphasize hip and knee flexion and hip abduction and adduction
4. Step up onto and over a bench	1. Poor dynamic COG control	Seated or standing balance activities emphasizing backward weight shifts
	2. LB weakness	LB exercises with resistance (body weight or resistance band) that emphasize sustained unilateral stance positions
	3. Reduced ROM at ankle, knee, hip	Seated and standing flexibility exercises emphasizing hip, knee, or ankle flexion
5. Walk with feet in tandem position	1. Poor dynamic COG control	Standing or moving COG control activities that emphasize A-P control during weight shifts
	2. Poor use of vision	Activities emphasizing gaze stabilization
	3. Weak hip abductors or adductors	Side leg raise against gravity or resistance, lateral weight shift and lunge activities
6. Stand on one leg	1. Poor COG control	Standing A-P weight shifts and transfers, reduced BOS activities
	2. LB muscle weakness	LB exercises with resistance (body weight or resistance band) that emphasize hip abductors or adductors
	3. Poor use of vision	Activities emphasizing gaze stabilization
7. Stand on foam with eyes closed	1. Poor use of vestibular input for balance	Seated or standing activities performed with reduced or absent vision on altered surfaces
	2. LB muscle weakness	LB exercises with resistance (body weight or resistance band) that emphasize quadriceps, gastrocnemius, and soleus
	3. Heightened fear of falling when vision is absent	Confidence-building activities with progressive reduction in availability of vision
8. Jump with both feet for distance	1. Poor dynamic COG control	Standing or moving COG activities emphasizing leaning away from and back to midline
	2. Poor UB and LB coordination	Selected exercises to improve UB and LB coordination, multiple task activities
	3. LB muscle weakness	LB exercises with resistance (body weight or resistance band) performed at progressively faster speeds
9. Walk while turning head	1. Possible vestibular impairment	Exercises coordinating head and eye movements, gait pattern enhancement (turns, directional changes)
	2. Poor use of vision	Activities emphasizing gaze stabilization
	3. Poor dynamic COG control	Standing or moving activities with head turns that progressively increase in speed and frequency
10. Restore balance after backward disturbance	1. Absent postural strategy (e.g., step strategy)	Activities emphasizing step strategy (e.g., manual perturbations, resistance band release activities)
	2. Poor COG control	Standing COG control activities, volitional stepping activities in multiple directions
	3. LB muscle weakness	LB exercises with resistance that emphasize hip and knee flexion and hip abduction and adduction

A-P = anteroposterior direction; BOS = base of support; COG = center of gravity; LB = lower body; ROM = range of motion; UB = upper body.

Berg Balance Scale

An alternative measure for assessing balance is the BBS, a test that has been shown to be highly reliable and valid when used across a broad continuum of functional levels (Berg et al., 1989; Berg et al., 1992; Berg et al., 1995). The BBS is an effective means of assessing each participant's ability to perform a series of functional tasks that require balance. Many of the tasks presented in this test simulate activities encountered in daily life (e.g., transfers, object retrieval, turning). The procedures for administering and scoring the BBS are provided in the feature that follows. A scoring form is provided in form 3.5, "Score Sheet for Berg Balance Scale," which is on pages 98-101.

As well as providing valuable information about the types of balance activities that are most difficult for participants to perform, the BBS can identify older adults who are appropriate for intervention (Harada, Chiu, Fowler, Lee, & Reuben, 1995). However, many practitioners argue that the BBS is less useful for identifying who will actually fall (Thorbahn & Newton, 1996; Chandler, 1996; Muir, Berg, Chesworth, & Speechley, 2008). It is suggested that older adults who score less than 46 out of the possible 56 points will benefit from immediate intervention. This test, as opposed to the FAB scale, is recommended for assessing older adults with lower functional abilities (i.e., those who score no higher than 12 out of 24 on the CPF scale or who use an assistive device for safe ambulation). The BBS is also more appropriate to use

> ### Key Point
>
> The BBS is recommended when assessing older adults with lower levels of function.

Test Administration Instructions for the Berg Balance Scale

Purpose: Evaluate participant's functional limitations associated with the performance of ADLs requiring balance

Equipment: Stopwatch; two straight-back chairs, one with armrests and one without; 12-inch (30 cm) ruler; slipper; 6-inch (15 cm) bench

Testing procedure: Conduct each test item in the order described on the test form (form 3.5). Demonstrate each test item or read the instructions aloud (as written) to each participant. Performing the scale does not permit the use of assistive devices. In selected questions there may be limited assistance from a person, but that assistance should be at most intermittent physical assistance. No points are awarded if the participant has to be supported or held throughout the activity. Record the score on the test form after the participant completes each test item, recording any additional comments (e.g., tended to look down as she attempted to rise from chair, very unstable immediately after rising from chair) next to each test item. The BBS is not intended to be a test of endurance, so allow participants to rest as needed.

Interpreting the results: The total score possible on the full version of the BBS is 56. A score of 45 or less is associated with a high risk of falling (Thorbahn & Newton, 1996). A more recent study, however, suggests that a cutoff score of 50 improves the test's ability to predict which older adults are more likely to fall (Riddle & Stratford, 1999). Remember that you will learn more about each participant and be able to identify specific limitations in function if you review each of the individual test item scores in addition to the total score.

when evaluating older adults who are homebound or residing in assisted-living facilities.

As with the FAB scale, reviewing the individual test item scores on the BBS will help you identify possible underlying impairments that can be addressed with the exercise progressions described in the FallProof program. An appropriate set of exercises can then be selected to address the identified impairments (see table 3.2).

Table 3.2 Interpretation of the Individual Test Items on the Berg Balance Scale

Item	Possible impairments	Recommended exercises
1. Sit to stand	1. LB or UB weakness	Wall sits, UB and LB exercises with resistance (quadriceps, biceps, triceps, hip abductors, hip adductors)
	2. Poor dynamic COG control	Seated or standing balance activities emphasizing forward weight shifts
	3. Abnormal weight distribution	Standing balance activities with eyes closed (controlled sway in A-P and lateral directions)
2. Stand for 2 minutes	1. Poor gaze stabilization	Gaze fixation and stabilization
	2. LB weakness	Wall sits, LB exercises with resistance
	3. Abnormal weight distribution in standing	COG standing balance activities
3. Sit for 2 minutes	1. Poor trunk stabilization or UB weakness	UB exercises with resistance (body weight), seated balance activities on compliant surfaces
	2. Abnormal perception of true vertical	Standing against wall with eyes closed, somatosensory cues
4. Stand to sit	1. Poor dynamic COG control	Seated or standing balance activities emphasizing backward weight shifts
	2. LB or UB weakness	UB and LB exercises with resistance (body weight or resistance band) that emphasize eccentric component
	3. Poor trunk flexibility	Seated and standing flexibility exercises emphasizing trunk rotation and flexion
5. Transfer (chair to chair)	1. Poor dynamic control of COG	Seated and standing balance activities emphasizing multidirectional weight shifts
	2. LB or UB weakness	UB and LB exercises with resistance
6. Stand with eyes closed	1. Poor use of somatosensory input, visual dependency, or fear of falling	Seated and standing balance activities with eyes closed Use of surface cues
	2. LB weakness	Wall sits, LB exercises with resistance
7. Stand with feet together	1. Poor COG control	Standing balance activities with reduced BOS
	2. Weak hip abductors and adductors	Lateral leg raises, weight shifts against resistance

Item	Possible impairments	Recommended exercises
8. Reach forward with outstretched arm	1. Poor dynamic COG control (reduced limits of stability)	Seated or standing COG activities emphasizing leaning away from and back to midline
	2. LB weakness	LB exercises with resistance (body weight or resistance band) that emphasize dorsiflexors, gastrocnemius, soleus
	3. Reduced ankle ROM	Flexibility exercises that emphasize dorsiflexion
9. Pick up object	1. Poor dynamic COG control	Seated or standing COG activities emphasizing leaning away from and back to midline
	2. Poor UB and LB flexibility	Selected exercises to improve UB and LB flexion
	3. LB weakness	LB exercises with resistance (body weight or resistance band)
	4. Vestibular impairment (dizziness)	Habituation exercises involving head and eye movements
10. Turn to look over shoulders	1. Poor dynamic COG control	Standing weight shifts in lateral direction
	2. Poor neck or trunk flexibility	Selected exercises emphasizing rotation of neck, shoulders, and hips
	3. LB weakness	LB exercises with resistance, ball movement exercises in standing position
11. Turn 360 degrees	1. Poor dynamic COG control	Standing weight transfer activities, gait pattern enhancement (turns, directional changes)
	2. Possible vestibular impairment (e.g., dizziness)	Exercises coordinating head and eye movements
	3. LB weakness	LB exercises with resistance that emphasize hip and knee flexion and hip abduction and adduction
12. Alternate placing left or right foot on bench	1. Poor dynamic COG control	Standing weight shifts in lateral and A-P directions
	2. LB weakness	LB exercises with resistance that emphasize hip and knee flexion and hip abduction and adduction
13. Stand with one foot in front	1. Poor static and dynamic COG control	Standing A-P weight shifts and transfers, reduced BOS activities
	2. LB weakness	LB exercises with resistance (body weight or resistance band) that emphasize hip abductors and adductors
	3. Poor gaze stabilization	Focusing on visual targets in front and at head height during standing and moving activities
14. Stand on one leg	1. Poor static and dynamic COG control	Standing A-P weight shifts and transfers, reduced BOS activities
	2. LB weakness	LB exercises with resistance (body weight or resistance band) that emphasize hip abductors and adductors
	3. Poor gaze stabilization	Focusing on visual targets during standing and moving activities

A-P = anteroposterior direction; BOS = base of support; COG = center of gravity; LB = lower body; ROM = range of motion; UB = upper body.

A shorter version of the BBS (the BBS-3P) has been developed in recent years. In addition to reducing the number of test items to seven, it reduces the scoring levels from 5 to 3 (Chou, Chien, Hsueh, Sheu, Wang, & Hsieh, 2006). Chou and colleagues reduced the number of scoring levels by collapsing the 2nd, 3rd, and 4th scoring levels on the original scale into a single scoring level. The three scoring levels were subsequently renumbered as 0, 2, and 4. The test items included in the BBS-3P are as follows: 1 (sit to stand), 6 (stand unsupported with eyes closed), 8 (reach forward with outstretched arm), 9 (pick up object from the floor from a standing position), 10 (turn to look over left and right shoulders while standing), 13 (stand unsupported with one foot in front), and 14 (stand on one leg).

Despite her medical history, Phoebe was administered the FAB scale before the start of the FallProof program. The decision to administer the FAB scale was based on the fact that Phoebe scored 13 out of 24 on the CPF scale and did not require the use of an assistive device for walking (question 8 on the health and activity questionnaire). She was also still residing in the community and maintained a relatively active social life. Phoebe's total score on the FAB scale was 16 out of 40. This relatively low score indicates that she is at high risk for falls based on the established cutoff score of 25 or less. As you can see by reviewing her test results in table 3.3, Phoebe experienced the greatest difficulties on the following items: turning in a full circle in a right and left direction (2/4), stepping up onto and over a 6-inch (15 cm) bench (0/4), tandem walking (1/4), standing on foam with the eyes closed (0/4), jumping with both feet for distance (0/4), walking while turning head (1/4), and restoring balance after a backward disturbance (1/4). She did not perform test item 8 (jumping with both feet) because she was unable to perform test item 4 (stepping up onto and over a bench) safely. As such, she was given an automatic score of 0 on test item 8 as per the test administration instructions.

As you review the activities performed in each test item and the physical abilities each item requires, a clear pattern of impairment begins to emerge for Phoebe.

Table 3.3 Fullerton Advanced Balance Scores for Phoebe

Item number	Description	Score
1	Stand with feet together and eyes closed	4
2	Reach forward to retrieve object	4
3	Turn in a full circle in right and left directions	2
4	Step up onto and over a 6-inch bench	0
5	Walk with feet in tandem position	1
6	Stand on one leg	3
7	Stand on foam with eyes closed	0
8	Jump with both feet for distance	0
9	Walk while turning head	1
10	Restore balance after a backward disturbance	1

Table 3.4 Fullerton Advanced Balance Scores for Larry

Item number	Description	Score
1	Stand with feet together and eyes closed	4
2	Reach forward to retrieve object	4
3	Turn in full circle in right and left directions	2
4	Step up onto and over a 6-inch bench	4
5	Walk with feet in tandem position	1
6	Stand on one leg	1
7	Stand on foam with eyes closed	4
8	Jump with both feet for distance	2
9	Walk while turning head	1
10	Restore balance after backward disturbance	3

She scored poorly on all items that require good sensory reception and integration skills, strength and flexibility, static and dynamic balance, and the ability to use the compensatory step strategy following an unexpected loss of balance. Take a moment now to review Larry's scores on the FAB scale (see table 3.4) and identify any trends in underlying impairments that might account for the balance difficulties observed on his completed test.

Although usually you administer either the FAB scale or the BBS (not both) to clients before the start of a balance and mobility program, the BBS was administered to Phoebe and Larry in addition to the FAB scale so that the final scores achieved on each scale could be compared. In contrast to her performance on the FAB scale, Phoebe scored 48 out of a possible total score of 56 on the BBS. What is surprising about this score is that it does not categorize Phoebe at a high risk for falls because it is above the cutoff value of 46. Phoebe can improve by only 8 points on the BBS, whereas her score of only 16 out of 40 on the FAB scale leaves her with considerable room for improvement. Her total FAB scale score also indicates that she is at high risk for falls. The scenario is similar for Larry, who scored only 26 out of 40 on the FAB scale but as high as 51 out of 56 on the BBS. His BBS score leaves him with little room for improvement, while his FAB scale score leaves him with considerably more room. Note that his total score on the FAB scale places him just a little above the threshold for high fall risk.

Mobility

In addition to the 8-foot (2.4 m) up-and-go test (a Senior Fitness Test item) described earlier in this chapter, a second test used to identify functional limitations in mobility is the 30-foot (9 m) walk test. Participants are required to walk a total distance of 50 feet (15 m), first at a preferred speed and then at a maximal speed, and the distance between 10 and 40 feet (3 and 12 m) is timed for the purpose of calculating velocity and other useful measures of gait. Counting the number of steps achieved by the participant over the 30-foot (9 m) distance can be used to calculate cadence (i.e., steps per second) and stride length (divide number of steps by 2 to get the number of strides, and then divide 30 if working in feet or 9 if working in meters by the number of strides to get the stride length). A gait stability ratio (GSR) can be calculated from cadence and velocity (GSR = ratio of cadence to velocity expressed in units of steps per foot or meter; Cromwell & Newton, 2004). The GSR is a useful measure of gait stability, with higher values indicating more time spent with the feet in contact with the ground during the gait cycle. Cromwell and Newton (2004, p. 94) stated that "this type of walking pattern is more stable because participants avoid the dynamic components of walking." Instructions for administering this test are provided in the feature on page 75, and scoring procedures are described in form 3.6 on page 102. This test serves as a useful measure of both functional mobility and walking stability. Comparing the times recorded for the preferred and maximum walking speeds can also provide you with information about the participant's ability to adapt walking speed to accommodate a change in task demands (i.e., walk at maximal speed). A participant's gait velocity, cadence, stride length, and GSR can also be compared with the reference values presented in table 3.5 *a-d*. The reference values for preferred and maximal speeds are based on data collected on 399 community-residing adults between ages 65 and 89. The results of the 30-foot (9 m) walk provide the instructor with additional information needed to select the most appropriate gait pattern enhancement and variation activities for each participant.

> ## Key Point
>
> The 30-foot (9 m) walk is a useful measure of functional mobility and walking stability. It can also be used to demonstrate whether older adults are able to adapt their gait speed to changing task demands.

Phoebe was able to complete the 30-foot (9 m) walk test at preferred speed in a time of 13 seconds (30/13 = 2.3 feet per second, or 9/13 = .7 m/sec) and 23 steps, whereas she completed the test at maximal speed in 10 seconds (30/10 = 3.0 feet per second, or 9/10 = .9 m/sec) and 21 steps. Comparing Phoebe's scores with the reference values presented in table 3.5*a* demonstrates that Phoebe is well below average in terms of gait speed for both test conditions. The average preferred speed for females in the 70 to 74 age category is 3.90 feet per second (1.19 m/sec), and the average maximum speed for the same age group is 4.97 feet per second (1.52 m/sec). Including a number of gait pattern enhancement and variation training activities (see chapter 7) will be important if Phoebe is to improve both the speed and the flexibility of her gait pattern. Improving her strength and flexibility will also be important for increasing her stride length as well as her cadence.

Larry was considerably faster than Phoebe at both the preferred and maximum speeds of the 30-foot (9 m) walk test. His preferred speed time was 7.2 seconds (30/7.2 = 4.17 feet per second, or 9/7.2 = 1.25 m/sec) and 14 steps, while his maximum speed time was 6 seconds (30/6 = 5.00 feet per second, or 9/6 = 1.50 m/sec) and 13 steps. Comparing Larry's scores with the reference values in table 3.5*a*, we find that Larry's preferred speed is just below the mean of 4.16 feet per second (1.27 m/sec) for men aged between 65 and 69 years, while his maximum speed is further below the mean of 5.82 feet per second (1.77 m/sec). Using the time taken to complete the 30-foot (9 m) walk as well as the number of steps recorded for each client across the two walking conditions, you should be able to calculate the additional measures of stride length, cadence, GSR, and gait adaptation for both Phoebe and Larry.

Table 3.5a Normative Values for Gait Velocity in Men and Women Between Ages 65 and 89

Age group	Preferred (ft/sec)		Maximum (ft/sec)	
	Men	Women	Men	Women
65-69 (n = 60)	4.16 ± .87	4.08 ± .88	5.82 ± 1.45	5.33 ± 1.17
70-74 (n = 67)	4.46 ± 1.26	3.90 ± .89	6.07 ± 1.95	4.97 ± 1.13
75-79 (n = 98)	3.99 ± .76	3.73 ± .65	5.49 ± 1.39	4.86 ± 1.04
80-84 (n = 101)	3.80 ± .97	3.48 ± .82	5.09 ± 1.37	4.37 ± .99
85-89 (n = 73)	3.51 ± .83	3.25 ± .75	4.65 ± 1.24	3.99 ± .91
Age group	Preferred (m/sec)		Maximum (m/sec)	
	Men	Women	Men	Women
65-69 (n = 60)	1.27 ± .26	1.24 ± .27	1.77 ± .44	1.62 ± .36
70-74 (n = 67)	1.36 ± .38	1.19 ± .27	1.85 ± .59	1.52 ± .34
75-79 (n = 98)	1.22 ± .23	1.14 ± .20	1.67 ± .42	1.48 ± .32
80-84 (n = 101)	1.16 ± .30	1.06 ± .25	1.55 ± .42	1.33 ± .30
85-89 (n = 73)	1.07 ± .25	0.99 ± .23	1.42 ± .38	1.22 ± .28

Table 3.5b Normative Values for Stride Length in Men and Women Between Ages 65 and 89

Age group	Preferred (ft/stride)		Maximum (ft/stride)	
	Men	Women	Men	Women
65-69 (n = 60)	4.31 ± .74	4.10 ± .60	4.96 ± .99	4.58 ± .73
70-74 (n = 67)	4.36 ± .82	3.91 ± .53	5.13 ± 1.05	4.38 ± .61
75-79 (n = 98)	4.29 ± .62	3.77 ± .52	4.93 ± .62	4.22 ± .60
80-84 (n = 101)	4.15 ± .81	3.53 ± .56	4.61 ± .94	3.88 ± .60
85-89 (n = 73)	3.81 ± .73	3.43 ± .60	4.27 ± .76	3.74 ± .62
Age group	Preferred (m/stride)		Maximum (m/stride)	
	Men	Women	Men	Women
65-69 (n = 60)	1.31 ± .23	1.25 ± .18	1.51 ± .30	1.40 ± .22
70-74 (n = 67)	1.33 ± .25	1.19 ± .16	1.56 ± .32	1.33 ± .19
75-79 (n = 98)	1.31 ± .19	1.15 ± .16	1.50 ± .19	1.29 ± .18
80-84 (n = 101)	1.27 ± .25	1.07 ± .17	1.40 ± .29	1.18 ± .18
85-89 (n = 73)	1.16 ± .22	1.04 ± .18	1.30 ± .23	1.14 ± .19

Table 3.5c Normative Values for Cadence in Men and Women Between Ages 65 and 89

Age group	Preferred (steps/sec)		Maximum (steps/sec)	
	Men	Women	Men	Women
65-69 (n = 60)	1.92 ± .14	1.98 ± .23	2.32 ± .21	2.32 ± .36
70-74 (n = 67)	2.02 ± .32	1.97 ± .28	2.32 ± .43	2.25 ± .33
75-79 (n = 98)	1.85 ± .17	1.98 ± .22	2.22 ± .41	2.30 ± .34
80-84 (n = 101)	1.82 ± .23	1.96 ± .26	2.20 ± .30	2.24 ± .30
85-89 (n = 73)	1.84 ± .25	1.87 ± .21	2.16 ± .33	2.13 ± .31

Table 3.5d Normative Values for Gait Stability Ratio in Men and Women Between Ages 65 and 89

Age group	Preferred (steps/ft)		Maximum (steps/ft)	
	Men	Women	Men	Women
65-69 (n = 60)	.48 ± .10	.50 ± .08	.42 ± .10	.45 ± .08
70-74 (n = 67)	.48 ± .11	.52 ± .08	.41 ± .10	.47 ± .07
75-79 (n = 98)	.48 ± .08	.54 ± .08	.41 ± .05	.48 ± .07
80-84 (n = 101)	.50 ± .10	.58 ± .10	.45 ± .10	.53 ± .09
85-89 (n = 73)	.55 ± .12	.60 ± .11	.49 ± .10	.55 ± .10
Age group	Preferred (steps/m)		Maximum (steps/m)	
	Men	Women	Men	Women
65-69 (n = 60)	1.57 ± .34	1.64 ± .27	1.38 ± .32	1.47 ± .26
70-74 (n = 67)	1.57 ± .37	1.71 ± .26	1.34 ± .34	1.53 ± .23
75-79 (n = 98)	1.56 ± .26	1.78 ± .25	1.35 ± .17	1.59 ± .24
80-84 (n = 101)	1.64 ± .34	1.91 ± .32	1.49 ± .32	1.74 ± .29
85-89 (n = 73)	1.79 ± .39	1.98 ± .36	1.59 ± .34	1.80 ± .33

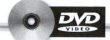

Test Administration Instructions
for the 30-Foot (9 m) Walk
at Preferred and Maximum Speeds

Purpose: Measure participant's gait velocity at preferred and maximum speeds (slow gait velocities are associated with increased risk for falls) and calculate stride length by counting the number of steps taken over the test distance

Equipment: Stopwatch, measuring tape (at least 100 feet, or 30 m), masking tape or chalk

Testing procedure: Measure out 50 feet (15 m) and use the masking tape or chalk to place small marks at 0, 10, 40, and 50 feet (0, 3, 12, and 15 m), as shown in figure 3.1. Instruct the participant to begin walking at a comfortable speed until you say to stop. Start timing the participant as soon as either foot crosses the 10-foot (3 m) mark. Stop timing once either foot crosses the 40-foot (12 m) mark. An additional 10 feet (3 m) are included at the start of the walkway to ensure that the participant has reached a relatively consistent walking velocity after accelerating from a standing position. The additional 10 feet (3 m) at the end of the 30-foot (9 m) walkway are included to ensure that participants do not begin to slow down as they reach the 30-foot (9 m) marker. In addition to starting the stopwatch when the participant's lead leg crosses the 10-foot (3 m) mark, begin counting the number of steps taken between the 10- and 40-foot (3 and 12 m) marks. Each time either foot contacts the ground between the 10- and 40-foot (3 and 12 m) marks constitutes a step.

Make sure that you walk slightly behind and to the side of the person performing the test so as not to influence the walking speed. Have the participant perform the 30-foot (9 m) walk at preferred speed and then at maximum speed to see whether the person is able to change gait speed noticeably on command. Instruct the participant to walk as quickly but as safely as possible. Assistive devices may be used to perform this test. Be sure to indicate on the score sheet what type of device (e.g., cane, walker with wheels) is used so that the same device can be used on subsequent tests.

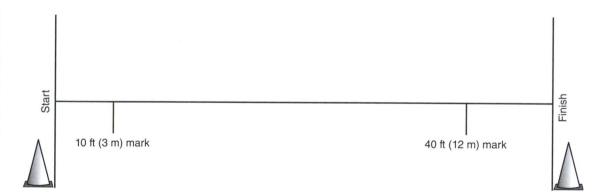

Figure 3.1 Walkway for the 30-foot (9 m) walk.

Ability to Divide Attention

The walkie-talkie test is used to measure an older adult's ability to divide attention between tasks (see the feature that follows for instructions on how to administer the test). You or an assistant can conduct this quick test while walking with the participant to the location where the 30-foot (9 m) walk begins. Initiate a conversation by asking an open-ended question that requires more than a simple *yes* or *no* from the participant. The walkie-talkie test is positive if the participant stops walking in order to respond to the question. Alternatively, if a person is able to continue walking while answering the question, the test is negative. A positive score on this test suggests that the person is unable to divide attention between the tasks of walking and talking (see form 3.7 on page 103). Although the test has been criticized because it lacks the sensitivity needed to discriminate between fallers and nonfallers (Shumway-Cook & Woollacott, 2007), it still provides information about the individual's ability to divide attention between two tasks. Watch for older adults who don't actually stop but do slow down as they respond to your question. This behavior is worthy of noting on your scoring form and does suggest that the participant has difficulty doing two things at once. The results of this test can be used to determine the nature of the task demands that should be introduced during the early stages of the program. For example, an individual who achieves a positive score on this test (or perhaps slows down significantly when responding) is best suited to performing activities with a single goal (e.g., standing quietly on a foam surface while fixating on a point in space), whereas a person who earns a negative score (and doesn't appear to slow down when responding)

> ### Key Point
>
> The walkie-talkie test measures an older adult's ability to divide attention between two tasks.

Test Administration Instructions for the Walkie-Talkie Test

Purpose: Evaluate participant's ability to divide attention between two tasks—in this case, the task of talking and the task of walking

Testing procedure: As you walk to the location where you plan to start the 30-foot (9 m) walk, begin a conversation with the individual you are testing. Stopping walking in order to respond to you is a sign that participants are unable to divide their attention adequately between the tasks of walking and talking. It is important to ask open-ended questions that require more than a *yes* or *no* in response.

Interpreting the results: Record a positive score if the person stops walking in order to respond to your question. Alternatively, if the person is able to continue walking while conversing with you, record a negative score. A positive score on this test suggests that the person needs to direct attention to the task of balancing while walking and will therefore not be ready to perform multiple tasks in the class until better overall balance has been developed.

can engage in tasks with multiple demands (e.g., reaching for or catching objects while standing on a foam surface) much earlier in the program.

Phoebe actually recorded a negative score on the walkie-talkie test, indicating that she is able to divide her attention between two tasks. On the basis of this test, it appears that Phoebe is limited physically more than cognitively. Although it will still be important to have her perform the lower-level exercise progressions in each component of the program, her ability to divide attention between a task that requires balance and a second cognitive task means that you will be able to introduce additional tasks once she can perform the various balance and gait activities correctly. Larry also recorded a negative score on this test.

Physical Function

An excellent test of functional fitness for older adults is the Senior Fitness Test developed by Rikli and Jones (1999a, 1999b). This six-item test battery includes measures of upper- and lower-body strength and flexibility, aerobic endurance, and dynamic balance and agility. When performed in accordance with the administration guidelines, the results derived from each test item can be compared with norm-referenced standards based on a sample of 7,183 community-dwelling older adults ranging in age from 60 to 94 years. The Senior Fitness Test has demonstrated reliability and validity and can be performed successfully by older adults ranging from healthy to physically frail. Although it may be necessary to modify how certain test items are administered for older adults who are frail (e.g., allow use of hands during the chair stand or asymmetrical leg lift or use of external support during the 2-minute step test), the results can still be used to identify each participant's immediate program needs when administered at the beginning of the program and each participant's progress when administered at regular intervals throughout the program. A brief description of each of the six test items is provided in table 3.6. The actual test procedures and norm-referenced tables are provided in the *Senior Fitness Test Manual* (Rikli & Jones, 2001).

> ### Key Point
>
> A client's performance on the Senior Fitness Test can be compared with norm-referenced standards obtained for community-dwelling older adults ranging in age from 60 to 94 years.

Let's review Phoebe's test results on four of the Senior Fitness Test items to see how she fared. As her report card indicates (see figure 3.2 on p. 79), Phoebe was able to complete six arm curls within 30 seconds when using the right arm. A quick review of the national norms for women between 70 and 74 years of age indicates that Phoebe is below the 5th percentile for her age group on this measure of upper-body strength. Her score of 4 on the 30-second chair stand also places her in the lowest 5th percentile for her age group. This score indicates that she has very poor lower-body strength. Phoebe was placed in the lowest 10th percentile based on her performance on the back scratch (–7 inches, or –18 cm), a measure of upper-body flexibility, and below the 5th percentile on the chair sit-and-reach test (–6.5 inches, or –16.5 cm), a measure of lower-body flexibility. As was the case for strength, Phoebe demonstrates very poor flexibility. Finally, Phoebe was able to complete 53 unassisted steps in place on the 2-minute step test. Once again, her performance placed her below the 5th percentile for her age and gender. This indicates that her aerobic endurance is very poor.

Larry scored higher on most of the Senior Fitness Test items when compared with Phoebe. He completed 14 arm curls and 10 chair stands in separate 30-second

Table 3.6 Brief Descriptions of the Six Senior Fitness Test Items

Test item	Purpose	Description
30-second chair stand	To assess lower-body strength needed for numerous tasks such as climbing stairs, walking, and getting out of a chair, tub, or car; also reduces the chance of falling	Number of full stands that can be completed in 30 seconds with arms folded across chest
Arm curl	To assess upper-body strength needed for performing household and other activities involving lifting and carrying things such as groceries, suitcases, and grandchildren	Number of biceps curls that can be completed in 30 seconds holding a hand weight of 5 lb (2.3 kg) for women or 8 lb (3.6 kg) for men
6-minute walk or	To assess aerobic endurance that is important for distance walking, climbing stairs, shopping, and sightseeing while on vacation	Number of yards or meters that can be walked in 6 minutes around a 50 yd (45.7 m) course
2-minute step test	To assess aerobic endurance when space limitations or weather prohibit the 6-minute walk	Number of full steps, raising each knee to a point midway between the patella (kneecap) and the iliac crest (top hip bone) completed in 2 minutes; score is number of times right knee reaches the required height
Chair sit-and-reach test	To assess lower-body flexibility, which is important for good posture, for normal gait patterns, and for various mobility tasks such as getting into and out of a bathtub or car	From a sitting position at the front of the chair with one leg extended and the hands reaching toward the toes, the number of inches (centimeters) between the extended fingers and the tips of the toes (+ or −)
Back scratch	To assess upper-body (shoulder) flexibility, which is important in tasks such as combing hair, putting on overhead garments, and reaching for a seat belt	With one hand reaching over the shoulder and one up the middle of the back, the number of inches (centimeters) between the extended middle fingers (+ or −)
8-foot (2.4 m) up-and-go test	To assess agility and dynamic balance, important in tasks that require quick maneuvering such as getting off a bus in time or getting up to attend to something in the kitchen, go to the bathroom, or answer the phone	Number of seconds required to get up from a seated position, walk 8 ft (2.4 m), turn, and return to a seated position

Adapted, by permission, from R. Rikli and J. Jones, 2001, *Senior fitness test manual* (Champaign, IL: Human Kinetics), 61-73.

test intervals. On the two trials of the sit-and-reach test, he reached a distance of −8 inches (−20 cm) and −7.5 inches (−19 cm). On the back scratch he scored −6.5 inches (−17 cm) on both test trials. He performed all tests with the right arm or leg. Finally, during the 2-minute step test he completed 57 steps at the required height. Several steps were not counted because of his inability to repeatedly raise the right leg to the required step height. To determine how Larry's scores compare with the national norms on each of these test items, consult the *Senior Fitness Test Manual* (Rikli & Jones, 2001). Once you have compared his scores with those of similarly aged men, you will have a better idea of which components of his functional fitness are in need of improvement.

Phoebe's test results show that she has several impairments that need to be addressed immediately if she is to make any significant gains in balance and mobility. She will clearly benefit from activities designed to improve her strength and flexibility, aerobic endurance, and functional mobility. The fact that she scored low on all items of the Senior Fitness Test suggests that she needs to start with activities that are not too challenging for her and that specifically target each of the physical deficits identified by the Senior Fitness Test. Now review Larry's performance on the two strength items of the Senior Fitness Test to identify whether his strength is impaired.

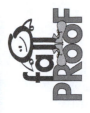

FallProof Program Report Card

Name of participant: Phoebe   Name of facility: Dingley Senior Center   Date: 5/1/2009

Test	Score	Rating	Comments
8-foot (2.4 m) up-and-go test (Best of two test trials)	11.9 Trial 1 11.0 Trial 2	<5th percentile compared with norms, high fall risk based on 8.5 sec cutoff	Mobility is very poor. Need to focus on improving dynamic balance, lower-body strength, and gait pattern. Important program components include COG training, GPEV, and strength (particularly lower body).
Fullerton Advanced Balance (FAB) scale	16/40	High risk for falls based on cutoff of 25 or lower	Phoebe scored poorly (2 or lower) on all test items requiring sensory reception and organization, dynamic COG control, or strength and flexibility. Important program components include COG training, MST, GPEV, strength, and flexibility.
Berg Balance Scale (BBS) (Alternate balance scale for clients with CPF score <12 or other exclusionary criteria)	48/56	Scored above high fall risk cutoff of 45 or lower but has clear balance impairments	Phoebe would perform only one of these balance tests. Note that she is not considered to be at high risk for falls based on her BBS score. However, she scored 13 on the CPF scale, so the FAB scale is the more appropriate test for Phoebe.
30-foot (9 m) walk Preferred speed: Maximum speed:	23 # steps 13.0 Time 21 # steps 10.0 Time	Performance on both conditions of test is below average	Gait speed needs to be improved. Important program components include GPEV, strength, and flexibility.
Walkie-talkie test Positive—stops to respond Negative—does not stop	☐ Positive ☑ Negative	Good	Phoebe is able to divide attention between walking and talking.
30-second chair stand (Record single trial score)	4	<5th percentile, at risk for loss of functional mobility	Phoebe has very poor lower-body strength and possible problems with dynamic COG control. Important program components include dynamic COG training and strength.
Arm curl ☐ Left ☑ Right (check one) (Record single trial score)	6	<5th percentile, at risk for loss of functional mobility	Phoebe has very poor upper-body strength. Important program component is strength (particularly upper body).
Sit and reach (optional) ☐ Left ☑ Right (check one) (Record best of two trial scores)	Trial 1: −6.5 in. (−16.5 cm) Trial 2: −6.9 in. (−17.5 cm)	<5th percentile, at risk for loss of functional mobility	Phoebe has very poor lower-body flexibility. Important program component is flexibility.
Back scratch (optional) ☐ Left ☑ Right (check one) (Record best of two trial scores)	Trial 1: −7.6 in. (−19.3 cm) Trial 2: −7.0 in. (−18 cm)	<10th percentile	Phoebe has poor upper-body flexibility. Important program component is flexibility (particularly upper body).
2-minute step in place (Record single trial score)	Steps 53	<5th percentile	Phoebe has poor aerobic endurance and will need frequent rests during class. Encourage short walks around house between classes.
Balance Efficacy Scale (BES) (Total possible 100%)	40 %	Below average	Phoebe has low self-confidence about her balance, particularly when support is not available. Requires high dose of success early in class to boost confidence.

GPEV = Gait Pattern Enhancement and Variation; MST = Multisensory Training; COG = Center-of-Gravity; CPF = Composite Physical Function.

Figure 3.2 Report card for Phoebe.

Although generally only the two strength test items from the Senior Fitness Test are administered before the start of the FallProof program, you should consider administering the remaining tests of flexibility and aerobic endurance if you have sufficient time before starting the program. While flexibility is not as important a risk factor for falls as strength is (particularly in the lower body), low flexibility in the upper or lower body negatively affects an older adult's functional mobility and ability to perform many ADLs (e.g., climb stairs, negotiate curbs). Poor aerobic endurance adversely affects how long an activity can be performed as well as the ability to be out and about in the community, especially if the older adult no longer drives a car or has limited access to transportation.

Assessment of Balance-Related Self-Confidence

The Balance Efficacy Scale (BES) evaluates how confident the older adult feels when performing various ADLs that require balance. Participants are asked to rate, on a scale of 0 to 100, how confident they are that they can successfully perform a given task (e.g., rise from a chair) without losing their balance. The BES consists of 18 questions that assess an individual's perceived confidence when performing a variety of daily activities with or without assistance. The total score obtained on the test is divided by 18 to yield a mean BES score. Program participants should complete the BES *before* they attempt any of the physical performance tests so that their self-evaluation of their abilities is not influenced by a recent performance on a physical test. The BES form generally is included with other program materials that participants bring to the first class session. Alternatively, participants can complete the form while they are waiting to perform the physical tests associated with the program assessment (preferably participants should sit away from the testing area and have an assistant present to answer questions). Participants who score below 50 on the scale should be considered to have low self-confidence, and every effort should be made to present activities early in the program that foster confidence through success. Decisions on how much to challenge participants should be guided by how confident they feel in their balance abilities. A copy of the BES is presented in form 3.8 on pages 104-106.

> **Key Point**
>
> Program participants should complete the BES before they perform any of the physical tests associated with the initial assessment for a balance and mobility program.

Consistent with her response to question 13 of the health and activity questionnaire, which asks how concerned she is about falling, Phoebe scored very low on the BES. She is extremely concerned about falling in general, as indicated by her score of 7 (extremely concerned) on question 13 of the health and activity questionnaire, as well as has very low balance-related self-confidence, as indicated by her score of 40 out of 100 on the BES. She exhibits the greatest lack of self-confidence when asked about performing ADLs requiring balance *without* assistance. On each item of the BES that asked Phoebe to rate how confident she feels about performing a certain activity (e.g., climbing or descending stairs, getting into and out of a shower or bathtub, putting on a pair of trousers) without assistance, she indicated that she is not at all confident, a response that equates to a score of 0 on a scale of 0 to 100.

Larry stated he was very concerned about falling (that is, 5 out of 7) on question 13 of the health and activity questionnaire, and he scored a 53 on the BES. Although his score is not as low as Phoebe's, Larry also demonstrates low self-confidence (0-20 percent) when asked to rate how confident he feels about performing any of the daily activities described *without* assistance. On the items of the scale that described activities in which assistance was available, however, he generally indicated that he was absolutely confident. This response equates to scores ranging between 90 and 100 percent on the BES.

SUMMARY

The goal of this chapter was to introduce you to the screening and assessment tools administered as part of the FallProof balance and mobility program. By administering each of the tests described, you will obtain a better understanding of each client's level of disability, nature of pathology, physical activity patterns, and functional limitations contributing to the disability observed. The possible underlying impairments that contribute to the observable functional limitations can also be identified in some cases. Collectively, the test results serve as the basis for developing a balance and mobility program that addresses the individual needs of each participant.

Retesting participants at regular intervals (every 2-3 months) is a means of determining the overall effectiveness of the program and whether the program adequately addresses each participant's balance and mobility impairments. Regular testing also provides participants with valuable feedback as to their progress and motivates participants to set new goals as they accomplish previous ones. Each of the tests described in this chapter is intended to help you, the instructor, learn more about the various dimensions of the balance system and provide more targeted instruction as a result.

A review of the health and activity questionnaire and the various test results for Phoebe provided you with a wealth of information that you can now use to design a program that will meet her specific needs. As the health and activity questionnaire revealed, Phoebe has several medical conditions that adversely affect her balance and mobility. The physical impairments associated with Phoebe's various medical conditions (e.g., heart attack, diabetes, chronic asthma, arthritis) have resulted in a number of functional limitations that require Phoebe to seek assistance in order to accomplish ADLs. These functional limitations have so limited her participation in regular physical activity and other social and recreational activities that her level of disability has increased significantly as well. As a result of her declining abilities and fall history, Phoebe has a very high fear of falling and very low balance-related self-confidence. These issues must be addressed immediately if any significant improvement is to occur with respect to her physical impairments.

Larry will benefit from participation in the FallProof program. Although his functional abilities are higher than Phoebe's, he could improve in several areas and thereby lower his overall fall risk. You should select higher-level exercises for Larry earlier in the program so that the balance challenge is better matched to his capabilities.

Can Phoebe benefit from participation in a balance and mobility program? Absolutely! Although she must contend with a number of permanent impairments that cannot be ameliorated (e.g., peripheral neuropathy, asthma, arthritic joints), the more temporary impairments she is experiencing (e.g., lack of strength, flexibility, dynamic balance) can be improved significantly. A targeted program of exercises that address each of the temporary impairments and compensate for the permanent impairments will lead to significant improvements in her ability to engage in daily activities that require balance and mobility. A better overall quality of life will result.

Test Your Understanding

1. Which of the following is *not* true regarding the Fullerton Advanced Balance scale?
   a. It is composed of 10 items that measure multiple dimensions of balance.
   b. It is a standardized test with good reliability and validity.
   c. It is designed to measure impairments in balance and gait.
   d. It addresses functional limitations contributing to balance impairments.
   e. It does not require specialized equipment.

2. If a client performs poorly on item 10 of the Fullerton Advanced Balance scale, an appropriate interpretation is that the client
   a. has reduced limits of stability
   b. has poor anticipatory postural control
   c. has poor reactive postural control
   d. does not use surface information adequately to maintain balance
   e. has poor lower-body flexibility

3. The primary purpose of the Berg Balance Scale is to determine if your client
   a. has a gait problem
   b. has lower-body muscle weakness
   c. needs further medical testing
   d. has the ability to perform functional tasks associated with daily living that require balance
   e. is appropriate for your community-based balance program

4. Your client has difficulty performing the sit-to-stand item on the Berg Balance Scale. All of the following could be potential impairments except
   a. lower-body muscle weakness
   b. poor sensory integration
   c. poor dynamic COG control
   d. abnormal weight distribution during the transfer to standing
   e. upper-body muscle weakness

5. The Senior Fitness Test measures the following physical impairments associated with functional mobility:
   a. lower- and upper-body strength and flexibility, aerobic endurance, dynamic balance and agility
   b. lower-body strength and flexibility, upper-body strength and flexibility, aerobic endurance
   c. aerobic endurance, dynamic balance and agility, lower-body strength, upper-body flexibility
   d. lower- and upper-body strength, dynamic balance and agility, lower- and upper-body flexibility
   e. lower- and upper-body strength, lower- and upper-body flexibility, gait speed, aerobic endurance

6. The walkie-talkie test measures a client's ability to
   a. divide attention between two tasks
   b. ask and answer a question while walking

   c. walk while carrying on a conversation
   d. hear another person ask a question while walking
   e. respond quickly to a question that is asked during walking

7. Which of the following is *not* true of the Senior Fitness Test?
   a. It is quick and easy to administer.
   b. It requires very little equipment to administer.
   c. It has norm-referenced standards that can be used for comparison.
   d. It is a highly valid and reliable test.
   e. It can be used only for measuring older adults who are relatively healthy.

8. An individual who takes 15 seconds and 18 steps to complete the 30-foot walk (9 m) walk at preferred speed would score the following values for Gait Velocity (GV), Stride Length (SL), Cadence (C), and Gait Stability Ratio (GSR):
   a. GV = 2 ft/sec; SL = 3.33 ft/stride; C = 1.2 step/sec; GSR = 1.67
   b. GV = 2 ft/sec; SL = 1.67 ft/stride; C = 0.83 step/sec; GSR = 1.67
   c. GV = 2 ft/sec; SL = 3.33 ft/stride; C = 1.2 step/sec; GSR = 0.6
   d. GV = 0.5 ft/sec; SL = 1.67 ft/stride; C = 1.2 step/sec; GSR = 1.67
   e. GV = 0.5 ft/sec; SL = 3.33 ft/stride; C = 0.83 step/sec; GSR = 0.6

9. The Balance Efficacy Scale measures
   a. how worried a person is about falling
   b. how confident a person feels about performing basic ADLs
   c. how confident a person feels about performing instrumental ADLs
   d. how confident a person feels about performing various ADLs that require balance

10. The Composite Physical Function (CPF) scale is used to assess a person's
   a. self-perceived ability to perform basic, instrumental, and advanced ADLs
   b. ability to perform a wide variety of daily activities
   c. ability to perform basic ADLs only
   d. ability to perform instrumental ADLs only

Practical Problems

1. Familiarize yourself with the instructions associated with each of the physical performance tests described in this chapter and administer at least three of the tests to an older adult for practice.

2. Complete a report card for Larry (see form 3.3 on pp. 93-94). Use the completed report card for Phoebe as a guide and the data about Larry provided in this chapter. Develop a prioritized list of problems for both Phoebe and Larry that you plan to address during your program. Be sure to indicate which problems you think are changeable or temporary (e.g., strength) and which you think are more permanent or less amenable to change (e.g., peripheral neuropathy). Doing this may help you better prioritize your efforts during the early stages of a balance and mobility program.

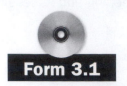

Form 3.1

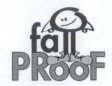

FallProof Health and Activity Questionnaire

Name _____ Date _____

Address _____

City _____ State _____ Zip _____

Home phone # (_____) _____ Gender: Male ❑ Female ❑

Date of birth _____ Height_____ Weight _____

Person to contact in a case of emergency _____ Phone # (____) _____

Name of your physician _____ Phone # (____) _____

1. Have you ever been diagnosed as having any of the following conditions?

			If yes, year of diagnoses
Heart attack	❑ Yes	❑ No	_____
Transient ischemic attack	❑ Yes	❑ No	_____
Angina (chest pain)	❑ Yes	❑ No	_____
High blood pressure	❑ Yes	❑ No	_____
Stroke	❑ Yes	❑ No	_____
Peripheral vascular disease	❑ Yes	❑ No	_____
Diabetes	❑ Yes	❑ No	_____
Neuropathies (problems with sensations)	❑ Yes	❑ No	_____
Respiratory disease	❑ Yes	❑ No	_____
Parkinson's disease	❑ Yes	❑ No	_____
Multiple sclerosis	❑ Yes	❑ No	_____
Polio/post-polio syndrome	❑ Yes	❑ No	_____
Epilepsy/seizures	❑ Yes	❑ No	_____
Other neurological conditions	❑ Yes	❑ No	_____
Osteoporosis	❑ Yes	❑ No	_____
Rheumatoid arthritis	❑ Yes	❑ No	_____
Other arthritic conditions	❑ Yes	❑ No	_____
Visual/depth perception problems	❑ Yes	❑ No	_____
Inner ear problems/recurrent ear infections	❑ Yes	❑ No	_____
Cerebellar problems (ataxia)	❑ Yes	❑ No	_____
Other movement disorders	❑ Yes	❑ No	_____
Chemical dependency (alcohol or drugs)	❑ Yes	❑ No	_____
Depression	❑ Yes	❑ No	_____

2. Have you ever been diagnosed as having any of the following conditions?

Cancer   ❑ Yes   ❑ No

If yes, describe what kind: _____

_____

_____

Joint replacement   ❑ Yes   ❑ No

If yes, how many times?_____   ❑ Right hip
                                            ❑ Left hip
                                            ❑ Right knee
                                            ❑ Left knee

Cognitive disorder   ❑ Yes   ❑ No

If yes, describe condition: _____

_____

_____

Uncorrected visual problems   ❑ Yes   ❑ No

If yes, describe type:_____

_____

_____

Any other type of health problem?   ❑ Yes   ❑ No

If yes, describe conditions:_____

_____

_____

3. Do you currently experience any of the following symptoms in your legs or feet?

Numbness   ❑ Yes   ❑ No

Tingling   ❑ Yes   ❑ No

Arthritis   ❑ Yes   ❑ No

Swelling   ❑ Yes   ❑ No

4. Do you currently have any medical conditions for which you see a physician regularly?

                                           ❑ Yes   ❑ No

If yes, describe conditions:_____

_____

_____

(continued)

5. Do you require eyeglasses?   ❏ Yes   ❏ No

     If yes, what type of glasses do you wear?   ❏ Bifocals

                                                  ❏ Graded lenses

                                                  ❏ Magnification only

                                                  ❏ Trifocals

6. Do you have your eyesight checked at least once a year?

                                                  ❏ Yes   ❏ No

7. Do you require hearing aids?   ❏ Yes   ❏ No

     If yes, which ear?   ❏ Left   ❏ Right   ❏ Both

8. Do you use an assistive device for walking?   ❏ Yes   ❏ No   ❏ Sometimes

     If yes or sometimes, what type of assistive device do you use?

     ❏ Single-point cane   ❏ Rolling stand walker

     ❏ Three-point cane   ❏ Three-wheel walker with seat

     ❏ Quad cane

9. List all medications that you currently take (including all over-the-counter and alternative medicines)

Type of Medication	For what condition?
_____	_____
_____	_____
_____	_____
_____	_____
_____	_____
_____	_____
_____	_____
_____	_____
_____	_____
_____	_____

10. Have you required emergency medical care or hospitalization in the last year?

                                             ❏ Yes   ❏ No

     If yes, please list when this occurred and briefly explain why. _____

     _____

     _____

     _____

11. Have you ever had any condition or experienced any injury that has affected your balance or ability to walk without assistance? ❑ Yes ❑ No

If yes, please list when this occurred and briefly explain condition or injury.

_____

_____

_____

12. How many times have you fallen *within the past 6 months?* _____

If you have fallen in the past 6 months, please give a detailed description of the incident.

   a. Date:_____

   b. Location (i.e., indoors, outdoors): _____

   c. Reason for fall (i.e., uneven surface, going down stairs): _____

      _____

      _____

   d. Did you require medical treatment? ❑ Yes ❑ No

   e. Please provide some details for any additional fall you had in the past 6 months:

      _____

      _____

      _____

13. How concerned are you about falling?

❑ 1	❑ 2	❑ 3	❑ 4	❑ 5	❑ 6	❑ 7
Not at all	A little		Moderately	Very	Extremely	

14. As a result of this concern, have you stopped doing some of the things you used to do or liked to do?

                                        ❑ Yes ❑ No

15. How would you describe your overall health?

   ❑ Excellent ❑ Very good ❑ Good ❑ Fair ❑ Poor

16. In general, how would you rate the quality of your life?

❑ 1	❑ 2	❑ 3	❑ 4	❑ 5	❑ 6	❑ 7
Very low	Low		Moderate	High	Very high	

(continued)

17. Please indicate your ability to do each of the following. (Place a ✔ in the most appropriate box.)

	Can do	Can do with difficulty or with help	Cannot do
a. Take care of own personal needs (e.g., dressing yourself	❏ 2	❏ 1	❏ 0
b. Bathe yourself, using tub or shower	❏ 2	❏ 1	❏ 0
c. Climb up and down a flight of stairs (e.g, second story)	❏ 2	❏ 1	❏ 0
d. Do light household activities (e.g., cooking, dusting, washing dishes, sweeping a walkway)	❏ 2	❏ 1	❏ 0
e. Do heavy household activities (e.g., scrubbing floors, vacuuming, raking leaves)	❏ 2	❏ 1	❏ 0
f. Do own shopping for groceries or clothes	❏ 2	❏ 1	❏ 0
g. Walk outside (one or two blocks)	❏ 2	❏ 1	❏ 0
h. Walk 1/2 mile (0.8 km, 6-7 blocks)	❏ 2	❏ 1	❏ 0
i. Walk 1 mile (1.6 km, 12-14 blocks)	❏ 2	❏ 1	❏ 0
j. Lift and carry 10 pounds (4.5 kg, e.g., a full bag of groceries)	❏ 2	❏ 1	❏ 0
k. Lift and carry 25 pounds (11 kg, e.g, medium to large suitcase)	❏ 2	❏ 1	❏ 0
l. Do strenuous activities (e.g., hiking, calisthenics, moving heavy objects, bicycling, aerobic dance activities, strenuous digging in garden)	❏ 2	❏ 1	❏ 0

18. In general, do you currently require household or nursing assistance to carry out daily activities?

❏ Yes   ❏ No

If yes, please check the reasons.

❏ Health problems
❏ Chronic pain
❏ Lack of strength or endurance
❏ Lack of flexibility or balance
❏ Other reasons: _____

_____

_____

19. In a typical week, how often do you leave your house (to run errands, go to work, go to meetings, classes, church, social functions, etc.)?

❏ less than once   ❏ 3-4 times

❏ 1-2 times   ❏ almost every day

20. Do you *currently* participate in regular physical exercise (such as walking, sports, exercise classes, housework, or yard work) that is strenuous enough to cause a noticeable increase in breathing, heart rate, or perspiration?

❏ Yes   ❏ No

If yes, how many days per week?

❏ One   ❏ Two   ❏ Three   ❏ Four   ❏ Five   ❏ Six   ❏ Seven

21. When you go for walks (if you do), which of the following best describes your walking pace?

❏ Strolling (easy pace, takes 30 minutes or more to walk a mile)

❏ Average or normal (can walk a mile in 20-30 minutes)

❏ Fairly brisk (fast pace, can walk a mile in 15-20 minutes)

❏ Do not go for walks on a regular basis

22. Did you require assistance in completing this form?

❏ None (or very little)   ❏ Needed quite a bit of help

Reason: _____

_____

_____

_____

From D. Rose, 2010, *FallProof!* 2nd ed. (Champaign, IL: Human Kinetics). Reprinted by permission, from the Center for Successful Aging at California State University, Fullerton. Question 17 of this form is reprinted, by permission, from R. Rikli and J. Jones, 1998, "The reliability and validity of a 6-minute walk test as a measure of physical endurance in older adults," *Journal of Aging and Physical Activity*, 6: 363-375.

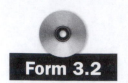

Form 3.2

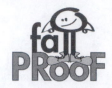

FallProof Health and
Activity Questionnaire Short Form

Name_____

Address _____

City_____ State_____ Zip _____

Home phone # (_____) _____ Gender: Male ❑ Female ❑

Date of birth _____ Height_____ Weight _____

Person to contact in a case of emergency _____ Phone # (_____) _____

Name of your physician _____ Phone # (_____) _____

1. Have you been diagnosed with any new medical conditions since the start of the program?

   ❑ Yes   ❑ No

   If yes, please indicate name of condition below: _____

   _____

   _____

   _____

2. Have you had a joint replaced since the start of the program?

   ❑ Yes   ❑ No

   If yes, please indicate which joint was replaced. _____

   _____

   _____

   _____

3. Have there been any changes in your medication since the start of the program (dosage or type)?

   Type of medication   **Dosage**

   _____   _____

   _____   _____

   _____   _____

   _____   _____

   _____   _____

   _____   _____

4. In general, how would you currently rate the quality of your life?

❏ 1   ❏ 2   ❏ 3   ❏ 4   ❏ 5   ❏ 6   ❏ 7
Very low   Low   Moderate   High   Very high

5. How much bodily pain have you generally had during the past 4 weeks while doing normal activities of daily living?

❏ 1   ❏ 2   ❏ 3   ❏ 4   ❏ 5   ❏ 6   ❏ 7
None   Very little   Moderate   Quite a bit   Severe

6. How concerned are you about falling?

❏ 1   ❏ 2   ❏ 3   ❏ 4   ❏ 5   ❏ 6   ❏ 7
Not at all   A little   Moderately   Very   Extremely

7. In a typical week, how often do you leave your house (to run errands, go to work, go to meetings, classes, church, social functions, etc.)?

❏ less than once   ❏ 1-2 times   ❏ 3-4 times   ❏ almost every day

8. Do you currently participate in regular physical exercise (such as walking, sports, exercise classes, housework, or yard work) that is strenuous enough to cause a noticeable increase in breathing, heart rate, or perspiration?

❏ Yes   ❏ No

If yes, how many days per week?

❏ One   ❏ Two   ❏ Three   ❏ Four   ❏ Five   ❏ Six   ❏ Seven

(continued)

9. Please indicate your ability to do each of the following.
   (Place a ✔ in the most appropriate box.)

	Can do	Can do with difficulty or with help	Cannot do
a. Take care of own personal needs (e.g., dressing yourself	❑ 2	❑ 1	❑ 0
b. Bathe yourself, using tub or shower	❑ 2	❑ 1	❑ 0
c. Climb up and down a flight of stairs (e.g, second story)	❑ 2	❑ 1	❑ 0
d. Do light household activities (e.g., cooking, dusting, washing dishes, sweeping a walkway)	❑ 2	❑ 1	❑ 0
e. Do heavy household activities (e.g., scrubbing floors, vacuuming, raking leaves)	❑ 2	❑ 1	❑ 0
f. Do own shopping for groceries or clothes	❑ 2	❑ 1	❑ 0
g. Walk outside (one or two blocks)	❑ 2	❑ 1	❑ 0
h. Walk 1/2 mile (0.8 km, 6-7 blocks)	❑ 2	❑ 1	❑ 0
i. Walk 1 mile (1.6 km, 12-14 blocks)	❑ 2	❑ 1	❑ 0
j. Lift and carry 10 pounds (4.5 kg, e.g., a full bag of groceries)	❑ 2	❑ 1	❑ 0
k. Lift and carry 25 pounds (11 kg, e.g, medium to large suitcase)	❑ 2	❑ 1	❑ 0
l. Do strenuous activities (e.g., hiking, calisthenics, moving heavy objects, bicycling, aerobic dance activities, strenuous digging in garden)	❑ 2	❑ 1	❑ 0

10. When you go for walks (if you do), which of the following best describes your walking pace?
    ❑ Strolling (easy pace, takes 30 minutes or more to walk a mile)
    ❑ Average or normal (can walk a mile in 20-30 minutes)
    ❑ Fairly brisk (fast pace, can walk a mile in 15-20 minutes)
    ❑ Do not go for walks on a regular basis

Form 3.3

FallProof Program Report Card

Name of participant: _____ Name of facility: _____ Date: _____

Test	Score	Rating	Comments
8-foot (2.4 m) up-and-go test (Best of two test trials)	____ Trial 1 ____ Trial 2		
Fullerton Advanced Balance (FAB) scale	____/40		
Berg Balance Scale (BBS) (Alternate balance scale for clients with CPF score <12 or other exclusionary criteria)	____/56		
30-foot (9 m) walk Preferred speed: Maximum speed:	____ # steps ____ Time ____ # steps ____ Time		
Walkie-talkie test Positive—stops to respond Negative—does not stop	☐ Positive ☐ Negative		
30-second chair stand (Record single trial score)			

(continued)

93

FallProof Program Report Card *(continued)*

Test	Score	Rating	Comments
Arm curl ❑ Left ❑ Right *(check one)* (Record single trial score)			
Sit and reach *(optional)* ❑ Left ❑ Right *(check one)* (Record best of two trial scores)	___ Trial 1 ___ Trial 2		
Back scratch *(optional)* ❑ Left ❑ Right *(check one)* (Record best of two trial scores)	___ Trial 1 ___ Trial 2		
2-minute step in place (Record single trial score)	___ Steps		
Balance Efficacy Scale (BES) (Total score possible 100%)	___ %		

From D. Rose, 2010, *FallProof!* 2nd ed. (Champaign, IL: Human Kinetics). Reprinted by permission, from the Center for Successful Aging at California State University, Fullerton.

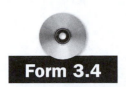

Score Sheet for
Fullerton Advanced Balance Scale

Name: _____ Date of test: _____

1. Stand with feet together and eyes closed
   - ❏ 0 Unable to obtain the correct standing position independently
   - ❏ 1 Able to obtain the correct standing position independently but unable to maintain the position or keep the eyes closed for more than 10 seconds
   - ❏ 2 Able to maintain the correct standing position with eyes closed for more than 10 seconds but less than 30 seconds
   - ❏ 3 Able to maintain the correct standing position with eyes closed for 30 seconds but requires close supervision
   - ❏ 4 Able to maintain the correct standing position safely with eyes closed for 30 seconds

2. Reach forward with outstretched arm to retrieve an object (pencil) held at shoulder height
   - ❏ 0 Unable to reach the pencil without taking more than two steps
   - ❏ 1 Able to reach the pencil but needs to take two steps
   - ❏ 2 Able to reach the pencil but needs to take one step
   - ❏ 3 Can reach the pencil without moving the feet but requires supervision
   - ❏ 4 Can reach the pencil safely and independently without moving the feet

3. Turn 360 degrees in right and left directions
   - ❏ 0 Needs manual assistance while turning
   - ❏ 1 Needs close supervision or verbal cuing while turning
   - ❏ 2 Able to turn 360 degrees but takes more than four steps in both directions
   - ❏ 3 Able to turn 360 degrees but unable to complete in four steps or fewer in one direction
   - ❏ 4 Able to turn 360 degrees safely taking four steps or fewer in both directions

4. Step up onto and over a 6-inch (15 cm) bench
   - ❏ 0 Unable to step up onto the bench without loss of balance or manual assistance
   - ❏ 1 Able to step up onto the bench with leading leg but trailing leg contacts the bench or swings around the bench during the swing-through phase in both directions
   - ❏ 2 Able to step up onto the bench with leading leg but trailing leg contacts the bench or swings around the bench during the swing-through phase in one direction
   - ❏ 3 Able to correctly complete the step up and over in both directions but requires close supervision in one or both directions
   - ❏ 4 Able to correctly complete the step up and over in both directions safely and independently

(continued)

5. Tandem walk

   ❑ 0 Unable to complete 10 steps independently

   ❑ 1 Able to complete the 10 steps with more than five interruptions

   ❑ 2 Able to complete the 10 steps with three to five interruptions

   ❑ 3 Able to complete the 10 steps with one or two interruptions

   ❑ 4 Able to complete the 10 steps independently and with no interruptions

6. Stand on one leg

   ❑ 0 Unable to try or needs assistance to prevent falling

   ❑ 1 Able to lift leg independently but unable to maintain position for more than 5 seconds

   ❑ 2 Able to lift leg independently and maintain position for more than 5 but less than 12 seconds

   ❑ 3 Able to lift leg independently and maintain position for more than 12 but less than 20 seconds

   ❑ 4 Able to lift leg independently and maintain position for the full 20 seconds

7. Stand on foam with eyes closed

   ❑ 0 Unable to step onto foam or maintain standing position independently with eyes open

   ❑ 1 Able to step onto foam independently and maintain standing position but unable or unwilling to close the eyes

   ❑ 2 Able to step onto foam independently and maintain standing position with eyes closed for 10 seconds or less

   ❑ 3 Able to step onto foam independently and maintain standing position with eyes closed for more than 10 seconds but less than 20 seconds

   ❑ 4 Able to step onto foam independently and maintain standing position with eyes closed for 20 seconds

Do not perform test item 8 if score is 2 or lower on test item 4. Also do not introduce test item 8 if test item 4 was not performed safely and/or it is contraindicated to perform this test-item (review test administration instructions for contraindications). Give test item 8 a score of 0 and proceed to test item 9.

8. Jump with both feet

   ❑ 0 Unable to attempt jump or attempts to initiate jump but one or both feet do not leave the floor

   ❑ 1 Able to initiate jump with both feet but one foot either leaves the floor or lands before the other

   ❑ 2 Able to perform jump with both feet but unable to jump farther than the length of feet

   ❑ 3 Able to perform jump with both feet and achieve a distance greater than the length of feet

   ❑ 4 Able to perform jump with both feet and achieve a distance greater than twice the length of feet

9. Walk with head turns

- ❑ 0 Unable to walk 10 steps independently while maintaining 30-degree head turns at an established pace
- ❑ 1 Able to walk 10 steps independently but unable to complete required number of 30-degree head turns at an established pace
- ❑ 2 Able to walk 10 steps but veers from a straight line while performing 30-degree head turns at an established pace
- ❑ 3 Able to walk 10 steps in a straight line while performing 30-degree head turns at an established pace but head turns less than 30 degrees in one or both directions
- ❑ 4 Able to walk 10 steps in a straight line while performing required number of 30-degree head turns at established pace

10. Demonstrate reactive postural control

- ❑ 0 Unable to maintain upright balance; makes no observable attempt to step; requires manual assistance to restore balance
- ❑ 1 Unable to maintain upright balance; takes two or more steps and requires manual assistance to restore balance
- ❑ 2 Unable to maintain upright balance; takes more than two steps but is able to restore balance independently
- ❑ 3 Unable to maintain upright balance; takes two steps but is able to restore balance independently
- ❑ 4 Unable to maintain upright balance but able to restore balance independently with only one step

From D. Rose, 2010, *FallProof!* 2nd ed. (Champaign, IL: Human Kinetics).

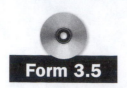

Score Sheet for Berg Balance Scale

Name: _____ Date of test: _____

1. Sit to stand

Instructions: Please stand up. Try not to use your hands for support.

Grading: Mark the lowest category that applies.

❑ 0 Needs moderate or maximal assistance to stand

❑ 1 Needs minimal assistance to stand or to stabilize

❑ 2 Able to stand using hands after several tries

❑ 3 Able to stand independently using hands

❑ 4 Able to stand with no hands and stabilize independently

2. Stand unsupported

Instructions: Please stand for 2 minutes without holding onto anything.

Grading: Mark the lowest category that applies.

❑ 0 Unable to stand 30 seconds unassisted

❑ 1 Needs several tries to stand 30 seconds unsupported

❑ 2 Able to stand 30 seconds unsupported

❑ 3 Able to stand 2 minutes with supervision

❑ 4 Able to stand safely for 2 minutes

If person is able to stand 2 minutes safely, score full points for sitting unsupported (item 3) and proceed to item 4.

3. Sit with back unsupported with feet on floor or on stool

Instructions: Sit with arms folded for 2 minutes.

Grading: Mark the lowest category that applies.

❑ 0 Unable to sit without support for 10 seconds

❑ 1 Able to sit for 10 seconds

❑ 2 Able to sit for 30 seconds

❑ 3 Able to sit for 2 minutes under supervision

❑ 4 Able to sit safely and securely for 2 minutes

4. Stand to sit

Instructions: Please sit down.

Grading: Mark the lowest category that applies.

- ❏ 0 Needs assistance to sit
- ❏ 1 Sits independently but has uncontrolled descent
- ❏ 2 Uses backs of legs against chair to control descent
- ❏ 3 Controls descent by using hands
- ❏ 4 Sits safely with minimal use of hands

5. Transfer

Instructions: Please move from chair to chair and back again. (Person moves one way toward a seat with armrests and one way toward a seat without armrests. Arrange chairs for pivot transfer.)

Grading: Mark the lowest category that applies.

- ❏ 0 Needs two people to assist or supervise to be safe
- ❏ 1 Needs one person to assist
- ❏ 2 Able to transfer with verbal cuing or supervision
- ❏ 3 Able to transfer safely with definite use of hands
- ❏ 4 Able to transfer safely with minor use of hands

6. Stand unsupported with eyes closed

Instructions: Close your eyes and stand still for 10 seconds.

Grading: Mark the lowest category that applies.

- ❏ 0 Needs help to keep from falling
- ❏ 1 Unable to keep eyes closed for 3 seconds but remains steady
- ❏ 2 Able to stand for 3 seconds
- ❏ 3 Able to stand for 10 seconds with supervision
- ❏ 4 Able to stand for 10 seconds safely

7. Stand unsupported with feet together

Instructions: Place your feet together and stand without holding onto anything.

Grading: Mark the lowest category that applies.

- ❏ 0 Needs help to attain position and unable to hold for 15 seconds
- ❏ 1 Needs help to attain position but able to stand for 15 seconds with feet together
- ❏ 2 Able to place feet together independently but unable to hold for 30 seconds
- ❏ 3 Able to place feet together independently and stand for 1 minute with supervision
- ❏ 4 Able to place feet together independently and stand for 1 minute safely

(continued)

The following items are to be performed while standing unsupported.

8. Reach forward with outstretched arm

   Instructions: Lift your arm to 90 degrees. Stretch out your fingers and reach forward as far as you can. (Place a ruler at the end of the fingertips when the arm is at 90 degrees. Fingers should not touch the ruler while reaching forward. The recorded measure is the distance forward that the fingers reach while the participant is leaning forward as much as possible.)

   Grading: Mark the lowest category that applies.

   ❑ 0 Needs help to keep from falling

   ❑ 1 Reaches forward but needs supervision

   ❑ 2 Can reach forward more than 2 inches (5 cm) safely

   ❑ 3 Can reach forward more than 5 inches (13 cm) safely

   ❑ 4 Can reach forward confidently more than 10 inches (25 cm)

9. Pick up object from the floor from a standing position

   Instructions: Please pick up the slipper that is placed in front of your feet.

   Grading: Mark the lowest category that applies.

   ❑ 0 Unable to try or needs assistance to keep from losing balance or falling

   ❑ 1 Unable to pick up shoe and needs supervision while trying

   ❑ 2 Unable to pick up shoe but comes within 1 to 2 inches (2.5-5 cm) and maintains balance independently

   ❑ 3 Able to pick up shoe but needs supervision

   ❑ 4 Able to pick up shoe safely and easily

10. Turn to look over left and right shoulders while standing

    Instructions: Turn your upper body to look directly over your left shoulder. Now try turning to look over your right shoulder.

    Grading: Mark the lowest category that applies.

    ❑ 0 Needs assistance to keep from falling

    ❑ 1 Needs supervision when turning

    ❑ 2 Turns sideways only but maintains balance

    ❑ 3 Looks behind one side only; other side shows less weight shift

    ❑ 4 Looks behind from both sides and weight shifts well

11. Turn 360 degrees

    Instructions: Turn completely in a full circle. Pause, then turn in a full circle in the other direction.

    Grading: Mark the lowest category that applies.

    ❑ 0 Needs assistance while turning

    ❑ 1 Needs close supervision or verbal cuing

    ❑ 2 Able to turn 360 degrees safely but slowly

    ❑ 3 Able to turn 360 degrees safely to one side in less than 4 seconds

    ❑ 4 Able to turn 360 degrees safely to each side in less than 4 seconds

12. Alternate placing left or right foot on bench or stool while standing unsupported

Instructions: Place feet on the bench (or stool) one at a time, alternating feet. Continue until each foot touches the bench (or stool) four times. (Recommend use of 6-inch, or 15 cm, bench.)

Grading: Mark the lowest category that applies.

❑ 0 Needs assistance to keep from falling or is unable to try

❑ 1 Able to complete fewer than two steps, needs minimal assistance

❑ 2 Able to complete four steps without assistance but with supervision

❑ 3 Able to stand independently and complete eight steps in more than 20 seconds

❑ 4 Able to stand independently and complete eight steps in less than 20 seconds

13. Stand unsupported with one foot in front

Instructions: Place one foot directly in front of the other. If you feel that you can't place your foot directly in front, try to step far enough ahead that the heel of your forward foot is ahead of the toes of the other foot. (Demonstrate this test item.)

Grading: Mark the lowest category that applies.

❑ 0 Loses balance while stepping or standing

❑ 1 Needs help to step but can hold for 15 seconds

❑ 2 Able to take small step independently and hold for 30 seconds

❑ 3 Able to place one foot ahead of the other independently and hold for 30 seconds

❑ 4 Able to place feet in tandem position independently and hold for 30 seconds

14. Stand on one leg

Instructions: Please stand on one leg as long as you can without holding onto anything.

Grading: Mark the lowest category that applies.

❑ 0 Unable to try or needs assistance to prevent fall

❑ 1 Tries to lift leg and is unable to hold 3 seconds but remains standing independently

❑ 2 Able to lift leg independently and hold for up to 3 seconds

❑ 3 Able to lift leg independently and hold for 5 to 10 seconds

❑ 4 Able to lift leg independently and hold for more than 10 seconds

Total score   /56

From D. Rose, 2010, *FallProof!* 2nd ed. (Champaign, IL: Human Kinetics). Reprinted, by permission from K. Berg, 1992, *Measuring balance in the elderly: Development and validation of an instrument*, Dissertation. (Montreal, Canada: McGill University).

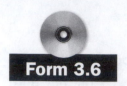

Score Sheet for 30-Foot (9 m) Walk

Name: _____ Date of test: _____

1. Walk at preferred speed

   Time: _____ (in seconds)

   Number steps: _____

   Gait velocity: _____ (in feet or meters per second)

   (Formula: 30 ft or 9 m/time in seconds)

   Cadence: _____ (steps per second)

   (Formula: number of steps/time in seconds)

   GSR: _____ (steps per foot or meter)

   (Formula: ratio of cadence to velocity)

   Stride length: _____ (in feet or meters per stride)

   (Formula: divide number of steps by 2 for the number of strides, then 30 ft or 9 m/number of strides)

2. Walk at maximum speed

   Time: _____ (in seconds)

   Number steps: _____

   Gait velocity: _____ (in feet or meters per second)

   (Formula: 30 ft or 9 m/time in seconds)

   Cadence: _____ (steps per second)

   (Formula: number of steps/time in seconds)

   GSR: _____ (steps per foot or meter)

   (Formula: ratio of cadence to velocity)

   Stride length: _____ (in feet or meters per stride)

   (Formula: divide number of steps by 2 for the number of strides, then 30 ft or 9 m/number of strides)

   Gait adaptation: _____ (in feet or meters per second)

   (Formula: subtract preferred velocity from maximum velocity)

From D. Rose, 2010, *FallProof!* 2nd ed. (Champaign, IL: Human Kinetics).

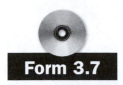

Score Sheet for Walkie-Talkie Test

Name: _____ Date of test: _____

☐ Positive score (stops to respond)

☐ Negative score (does not stop to respond)

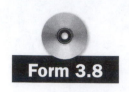

Form 3.8

Balance Efficacy Scale

Name: _____ Date of test: _____

The following are a series of tasks that you may encounter in daily life. Please indicate how confident you are, *today*, that you can complete each of these tasks without losing your balance. Your answers are confidential. *Please answer the way you feel and not how you think you should feel.*

Circle one number from 0-100 percent.

1. How confident are you that you can get up out of a chair (using your hands) without losing your balance?

   0 percent   10   20   30   40   50   60   70   80   90   100 percent

   Not at all confident   Somewhat confident   Absolutely confident

2. How confident are you that you can get up out of a chair (*not* using your hands) without losing your balance?

   0 percent   10   20   30   40   50   60   70   80   90   100 percent

   Not at all confident   Somewhat confident   Absolutely confident

3. How confident are you that you can walk up a flight of 10 stairs (using the handrail) without losing your balance?

   0 percent   10   20   30   40   50   60   70   80   90   100 percent

   Not at all confident   Somewhat confident   Absolutely confident

4. How confident are you that you can walk up a flight of 10 stairs (*not* using the handrail) without losing your balance?

   0 percent   10   20   30   40   50   60   70   80   90   100 percent

   Not at all confident   Somewhat confident   Absolutely confident

5. How confident are you that you can get out of bed without losing your balance?

   0 percent   10   20   30   40   50   60   70   80   90   100 percent

   Not at all confident   Somewhat confident   Absolutely confident

6. How confident are you that you can get into or out of a shower or bathtub (*with* the assistance of a handrail or wall) without losing your balance?

   0 percent   10   20   30   40   50   60   70   80   90   100 percent

   Not at all confident   Somewhat confident   Absolutely confident

7. How confident are you that you can get into or out of a shower or bathtub (with *no* assistance from a handrail or wall) without losing your balance?

   0 percent   10   20   30   40   50   60   70   80   90   100 percent

   Not at all confident   Somewhat confident   Absolutely confident

8. How confident are you that you can walk down a flight of 10 stairs (using the handrail) without losing your balance?

| 0 percent | 10 | 20 | 30 | 40 | 50 | 60 | 70 | 80 | 90 | 100 percent |

Not at all confident   Somewhat confident   Absolutely confident

9. How confident are you that you can walk down a flight of 10 stairs (*not* using the handrail) without losing your balance?

| 0 percent | 10 | 20 | 30 | 40 | 50 | 60 | 70 | 80 | 90 | 100 percent |

Not at all confident   Somewhat confident   Absolutely confident

10. How confident are you that you can remove an object from a cupboard *located at a height that is level with your shoulder* without losing your balance?

| 0 percent | 10 | 20 | 30 | 40 | 50 | 60 | 70 | 80 | 90 | 100 percent |

Not at all confident   Somewhat confident   Absolutely confident

11. How confident are you that you can remove an object from a cupboard *located above your head* without losing your balance?

| 0 percent | 10 | 20 | 30 | 40 | 50 | 60 | 70 | 80 | 90 | 100 percent |

Not at all confident   Somewhat confident   Absolutely confident

12. How confident are you that you can walk across uneven ground (with assistance) when good lighting is available without losing your balance?

| 0 percent | 10 | 20 | 30 | 40 | 50 | 60 | 70 | 80 | 90 | 100 percent |

Not at all confident   Somewhat confident   Absolutely confident

13. How confident are you that you can walk across uneven ground (with *no* assistance) when good lighting is available without losing your balance?

| 0 percent | 10 | 20 | 30 | 40 | 50 | 60 | 70 | 80 | 90 | 100 percent |

Not at all confident   Somewhat confident   Absolutely confident

14. How confident are you that you can walk across uneven ground (with assistance) at night without losing your balance?

| 0 percent | 10 | 20 | 30 | 40 | 50 | 60 | 70 | 80 | 90 | 100 percent |

Not at all confident   Somewhat confident   Absolutely confident

15. How confident are you that you can walk across uneven ground (with *no* assistance) at night without losing your balance?

| 0 percent | 10 | 20 | 30 | 40 | 50 | 60 | 70 | 80 | 90 | 100 percent |

Not at all confident   Somewhat confident   Absolutely confident

16. How confident are you that you can stand on one leg (with support) while putting on a pair of trousers without losing your balance?

| 0 percent | 10 | 20 | 30 | 40 | 50 | 60 | 70 | 80 | 90 | 100 percent |

Not at all confident   Somewhat confident   Absolutely confident

(continued)

17. How confident are you that you can stand on one leg (with *no* support) while putting on a pair of trousers without losing your balance?

0 percent	10	20	30	40	50	60	70	80	90	100 percent
Not at all confident					Somewhat confident					Absolutely confident

18. How confident are you that you can complete a daily task *quickly* without losing your balance?

0 percent	10	20	30	40	50	60	70	80	90	100 percent
Not at all confident					Somewhat confident					Absolutely confident

Lastly, we are interested in understanding what factors affect your confidence levels. On the following lines, please provide reasons for answering the way you did on questions 1 through 18. For example, if you answered that you were not at all confident, why do you feel that way? If you were not at all confident about an activity because you no longer do it very often (e.g., climb stairs, walk on uneven ground), we would like to know that also.

_____

_____

_____

_____

_____

From D. Rose, 2010, *FallProof!* 2nd ed. (Champaign, IL: Human Kinetics). Reprinted, by permission, from the Center for Successful Aging at California State University, Fullerton.

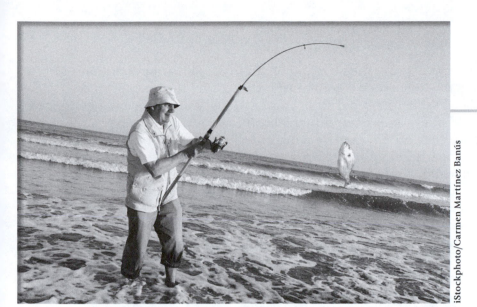

iStockphoto/Carmen Martínez Banús

Chapter 4

Center-of-Gravity Control Training

Objectives

After completing this chapter, you will be able to

- understand how center-of-gravity (COG) control influences balance,
- develop a set of exercise progressions that improve COG control in seated, standing, and moving task situations,
- manipulate the difficulty of a balance activity by altering the task demands, the environmental constraints, or both, and
- manipulate the task demands, the environment, or both in order to ensure safety.

The balance and mobility activities presented in this chapter will improve your participants' ability to (a) maintain a better upright position, whether seated or standing; (b) lean away from and return to a centered position (i.e., posturally aligned with weight evenly distributed across the base of support) with improved postural control; and (c) move the body through space more quickly and confidently. In addition, the exercises improve selected physical and motor skill fitness parameters (e.g., aerobic endurance, strength, power, coordination, flexibility) that are essential to good balance and mobility. To accomplish each of these movement goals, participants must first understand where their COG is located relative to their base of support (i.e., feet and buttocks when sitting or feet when standing) and how to move the COG relative to that base (e.g., rise from a chair, walk up a flight of stairs). These exercises are often labeled the *belly button*

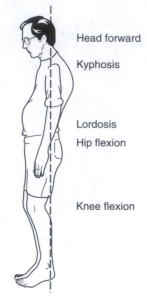

Head forward

Kyphosis

Lordosis

Hip flexion

Knee flexion

Figure 4.1 Maladaptive posture.

control exercises because they conjure up an image of the approximate location of the COG when standing and what part of the body must be manipulated to maintain postural control while performing a variety of daily tasks in various environmental contexts.

Older adults who are experiencing a decline in postural stability often develop inaccurate perceptions of true vertical and begin to adopt abnormal standing postures as a result (see figure 4.1). A commonly observed maladaptive standing posture is one with a forward head position, rounded upper back, and backward tilt of the pelvis. Older adults may also exhibit asymmetrical standing postures in which they place more weight on one side of the body. This posture is common among older adults who have experienced a stroke, have arthritis-related pain in certain joints, or have an uncorrected leg-length discrepancy.

The exercises described in this chapter progress from seated to standing to moving tasks. In a seated position, for example, participants learn to sit upright, shift their weight to various positions in space, and restore an upright seated position following small expected or unexpected perturbations (e.g., pushing or pulling of the body). After describing the core exercise progressions for each level of balance challenge, the chapter will teach you how to further manipulate the level of balance challenge associated with the exercise progressions by varying either the demands of the task being performed or the environment in which it is performed.

Ideas for increasing the overall challenge of the exercise progressions are described in two features, one at the end of the seated balance section and one at the end of the standing balance section. For example, a simple way to increase the balance challenge associated with a set of seated or standing exercises is to instruct participants to either wear dark glasses that reduce their vision or close their eyes and repeat each exercise they were able to perform successfully with their eyes open. This simple environmental manipulation encourages participants to rely more on feeling the contact between their feet and the surface below as well as sensing where their various body parts are in space. By doing so, they develop a more correct internal representation of true vertical that does not rely on vision for maintenance or correction.

Finally, after the seated, standing, and moving balance exercise sections, the chapter presents a set of culminating activities that combine several different core exercises previously practiced in isolation. For example, an activity such as shift around the clock combines multiple directions of seated dynamic weight shifts as individuals shift their weight to different numbers on an imaginary clock.

> ## Key Point
>
> Older adults who are experiencing a decline in postural stability often develop inaccurate perceptions of true vertical and begin to adopt abnormal standing postures as a result.

SEATED BALANCE ACTIVITIES

The type of support surface selected for the seated COG control exercises will depend on the *individual capabilities* of the participants. Although more frail participants may need to begin the exercise progressions while seated on a chair with a firm support surface and back support, most participants in a community-based program will be ready to begin exercising while seated on a chair with no back support and a compliant sitting surface (i.e., easiest level of difficulty). The next levels of difficulty involve sitting on a balance ball with a ball holder beneath it (more difficult) and

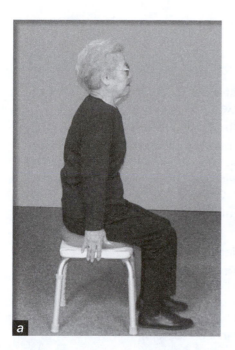 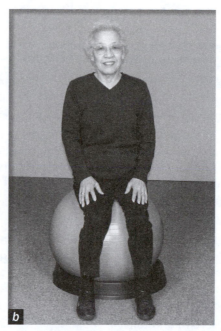 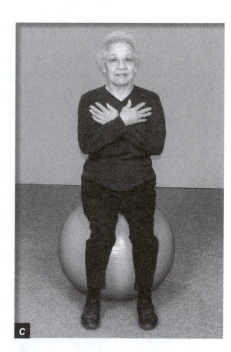

Figure 4.2   Different levels of balance challenge can be introduced by manipulating the seated support surface and the position of the hands during an exercise: *(a)* easiest, *(b)* more difficult, *(c)* most difficult.

then sitting on a ball without a ball holder (most difficult). Hand placement during each exercise also modifies the level of challenge. The easiest position involves placing the hands on the chair or ball surface. Resting the hands on the thighs is more challenging, and folding the arms across the chest is the most difficult hand position. Figure 4.2, *a* through *c,* shows three examples of seated support surfaces and hand positions illustrating the three levels of relative difficulty.

General Safety Guidelines

◆ Following a review of the initial test results for your participants, identify those who are likely to experience difficulty with certain exercises and recommend modifications where appropriate. If you have assistants, tell them as well.

◆ Instruct assistants to closely supervise participants who are likely to have difficulty with an exercise, particularly when the participant is sitting on the balance ball without a ball holder. Two methods of supervising participants are illustrated in figure 4.3.

◆ When not enough assistants are available to guard unstable participants, position chairs on either side of the clients to help stabilize them. If you are working with a large group, consider moving participants who are less stable to easier seated support surfaces.

◆ Increase the angle of knee flexion for participants who have artificial joints, severe lower-body weakness, or medical conditions that cause pain in the hip or knee joints by having them sit on a slightly larger ball or higher chair with a Dyna-Disc beneath their buttocks.

◆ Do not ask participants to perform the next level of a task until they can *safely* perform the preceding level.

◆ Do not ask participants to perform an exercise with their eyes closed if they are not able to perform the task safely with their eyes open. Increasing a participant's postural stability by altering the hand position (i.e., placing hands on support surface versus thighs) or moving

(continued)

the participant to an easier seated support surface may be sufficient to facilitate better performance.

◆ Instruct participants to open their eyes immediately if they feel they are about to lose their balance.

◆ When introducing arm, trunk, or leg movements, select a seated support surface that is challenging but safe so participants can perform the exercises successfully.

◆ Instruct participants to avoid grabbing other participants if they feel unstable.

◆ When a participant is using a balance ball, select a size that allows the person to sit in the middle of the ball and still place their feet flat on the floor. Ideally, the knees should be flexed at a 90-degree angle to the floor. Unless otherwise instructed, participants should place their feet hip-width apart.

◆ Carefully match the size of the balance ball to the height of your clients. The following ball sizes are recommended:

Participant Height	Balance Ball Size
Below 65 inches (165 cm)	18 inches (45 cm)
65 inches (165 cm) to 68 inches (173 cm)	22 inches (55 cm)
69 inches (175 cm) to 75 inches (191 cm)	26 inches (65 cm)
76 inches (193 cm) to 81 inches (206 cm)	30 inches (75 cm)
82 inches (208 cm) and taller	33 inches (85 cm)

◆ Follow these additional guidelines when using a stability ball:

• Always check that the ball is inflated to the specified dimension (check with measuring tape or use a ball-measuring device).

• Check for any scratches or deep cuts on the balance ball that might render it unsafe. Deflate damaged balls, render them unusable, and discard them appropriately.

• Check to see whether you need to alter the size of the balance ball when the participant is using a ball holder or an Airex Balance Pad as a support surface (elevates the feet by 2 inches, or 5 cm). Using an Airex Balance Pad in this way changes the relative angles of the knee and hip joints.

• Consider having clients with total hip replacements use a balance ball that is one size larger than the size recommended for their height (particularly if they are at the high end of the height range) to increase the angle at the hip joint. This will increase their level of comfort during certain activities.

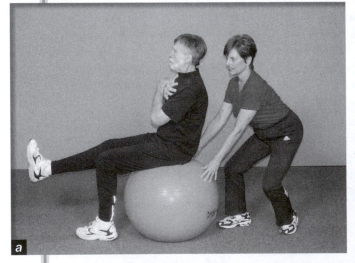 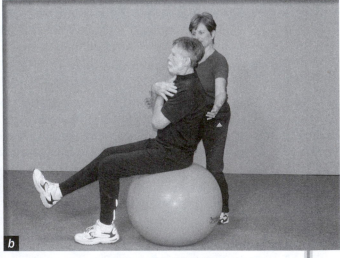

Figure 4.3 Two methods of supervising participants: *(a)* assistant stabilizing the ball while the participant performs an exercise and *(b)* assistant spotting the participant seated on a balance ball.

LEVEL 1: MAINTAINING SEATED BALANCE

The activities described in level 1 teach participants how to (a) develop a more upright seated posture, (b) use vision to improve seated balance, (c) develop a better sensory awareness of the body's position in space, and (d) strengthen the muscles of the trunk. Select the support surface and hand position that are best suited to each individual's capabilities before beginning any of the seated exercises described in this section. The support surface and hand position should require active stabilization by the trunk muscles but should not be so difficult that the participant is unable to maintain balance during the eyes-closed sensory awareness activity in level 1. The introductory activities in level 1 will help you plan for subsequent activities after observing how well participants perform the sequence of exercises while seated on the different support surfaces and with the hands in different starting positions.

Before beginning any of the seated COG balance activities, demonstrate the correct sitting posture for your class participants and then have them practice while they are seated in a straight-back chair. Provide the following verbal cues to your participants as they practice:

- Sit tall with your back resting against the chair and your feet flat on the floor.

- Relax your arms and place your hands on your thighs.

- Hold your head erect with your eyes focused on a vertical target at eye level, and tuck in your chin by gently pulling it straight back (as though it is sliding on a tray held directly beneath it) until your ears are directly above your shoulders.

- Pull your abdominal muscles up and in—try to flatten your stomach.

- Straighten your upper back and raise your chest while moving your shoulders back and down against the chair back.

- Maintain this position for 15 seconds, breathing normally and relaxing the rest of your body at the same time. Relax (but not too much), and repeat the exercise again.

- Move your buttocks toward the front of the chair and repeat the exercise without your back resting against the chair.

Practicing correct sitting posture is an excellent exercise that you can also assign as homework during the early stages of the program. Introducing this exercise before starting any of the seated balance activities will also help you establish the initial level of balance challenge for each individual client. Participants who are unable to achieve a correct sitting posture while seated on a stable surface will not be able to sit on more challenging support surfaces such as a Dyna-Disc or balance ball without further compromising their posture.

Present the following sensory awareness cues to participants during level 1 seated balance activities, particularly during eyes-closed repetitions:

- Imagine there is a string connected to the top of your head that is being pulled toward the ceiling.

- Sense that your ears are directly above your shoulders.

- Sense that your shoulders are directly above your hips.

- Feel equal weight on both sides of your buttocks.

- Sense the angle of your knees relative to your hips and ankles.

- Feel your feet in contact with the floor.

- Feel that the pressure is distributed evenly under both feet.

Note that two types of sensory cues are being used here. Directing clients to *feel* that their feet are in contact with the floor focuses their attention on the type of information (i.e., light touch, pressure, vibration) being provided by the cutaneous receptors. Meanwhile, use of the word *sense* tunes participants into the type of information (i.e., position of body parts relative to other body parts) provided by the proprioceptors within the muscles or joints. Your selective use of these different types of cues is particularly important during the multisensory training activities described in chapter 5.

Exercise Progression

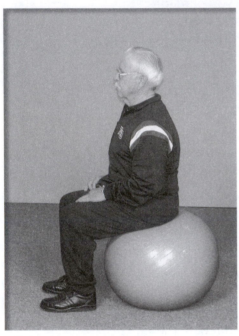

Figure 4.4 An older adult seated on a balance ball that is the correct size for the participant's height.

Seated Balance

The participants' hands should be in one of the three starting positions, as illustrated in figure 4.2.

a. With the feet hip-width apart and flat on the floor, maintain an upright seated position for 30 seconds (figure 4.4).

b. Direct the eyes forward and fix them on a visual target immediately in front and at eye level. (Vertical targets such as doorjambs, window frames, or vertical lines on a wall are particularly helpful for reinforcing an upright postural alignment.)

c. Repeat the exercise with the eyes closed. Move the hands to an easier position (e.g., from thighs to ball or chair) during the first repetition.

d. If the previous repetition was completed with adequate stability, repeat the exercise with the hands in a more difficult position.

LEVEL 2: SEATED BALANCE WITH VOLUNTARY ARM MOVEMENTS

Reminders for Participants

- Sit tall on the chair or ball.
- Keep the eyes directed forward and focused on a vertical target at eye level unless otherwise instructed.
- Move the arms through as complete a range of motion as possible while maintaining upright balance.
- Breathe evenly throughout the exercise.
- Perform each exercise slowly.

Different arm movements are introduced in level 2 to further challenge each participant's seated balance abilities. Subtle movements of the COG are now required as the arms are moved in different directions. At the same time, the trunk and lower body muscles are being used more actively for stabilization, thereby improving strength. The movements in this section also help improve flexibility, particularly at the shoulder joints, as participants are encouraged to move their arms through as complete a range of motion as possible. The development of a good breathing pattern is also emphasized during this set of exercises.

Exercise Progressions

1. Single-Arm Raise

a. Raise and lower the right arm and then the left arm in each of the following directions: forward to shoulder height, forward and up to as vertical a position as possible, laterally to shoulder height, and laterally to as vertical a position as possible (figure 4.5).

b. Hold each arm at the end position for three slow counts and then lower the arm back to the starting position.

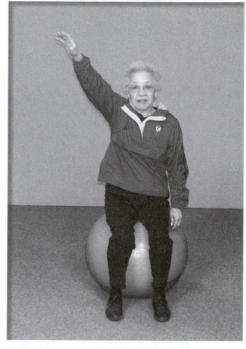

Figure 4.5   Single-arm raise.

2. Double-Arm Raise

a. Raise and lower both arms in each of the following directions: forward to shoulder height, forward and up to as vertical a position as possible, laterally to shoulder height, and laterally to as vertical a position as possible (figure 4.6).

b. Hold both arms at the end position for three slow counts and then lower the arms back to the starting position.

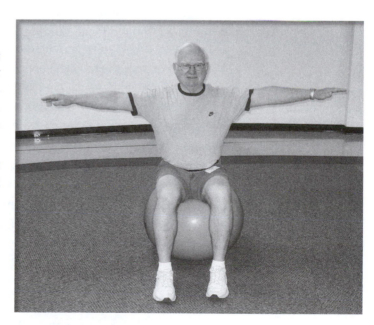

Figure 4.6   Double-arm raise.

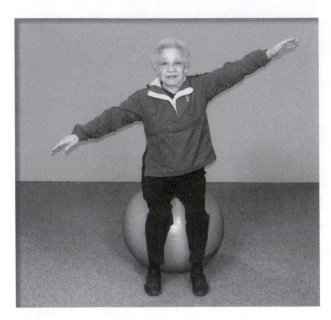

Figure 4.7 Diagonal arm raise.

3. Diagonal Arm Raise

a. Raise one arm diagonally out to the side of the body and toward the ceiling (figure 4.7).

b. Hold for three counts and then lower the arm to the starting position.

c. Repeat with the opposite arm.

d. Repeat the exercise with both arms moving simultaneously, one arm moving diagonally upward and the other moving diagonally downward.

Once your participants become familiar with the movements associated with each of the core exercise progressions in level 2, you can manipulate either the demands associated with the tasks or the environment in which the tasks are performed to further increase the balance challenge. Several ideas are presented in the feature that follows.

Increasing the Seated Balance Challenge by Manipulating the Task and Environmental Demands

Task Demands

◆ Change the difficulty level of the seated support surface (e.g., progress from Dyna-Disc to ball with ball holder to ball with no ball holder).

◆ Require a more difficult starting arm position (e.g., progress from hands on chair or ball to hands on thighs to arms folded across chest).

◆ Reduce or alter the base of support (e.g., progress from feet together to semi- or full tandem to single-leg stance).

◆ Increase the number of repetitions of each exercise.

◆ Increase or decrease the speed at which the exercise is performed.

◆ Follow arm movements with the eyes and head (level 2).

◆ Combine arm and leg movements on certain activities.

◆ Coordinate arm, trunk, or leg movements to music of various tempos.

◆ Perform trunk movements (level 3) while holding a weighted object.

◆ Introduce resistance to selected activities in the form of hand or ankle weights or resistance bands of different tensions (levels 2 and 4).

◆ Alter the shape and weight of the objects being manipulated during an exercise.

◆ Develop a sequence of movements that must be performed in the correct order (also improves memory).

◆ Perturb participants (level 4) simultaneously at hips and shoulders and in opposite directions (e.g., pull left or right hip as left or right shoulder is pushed).

◆ Increase the size of the perturbation (level 4).

◆ Introduce a second task to be performed simultaneously with a balance activity (e.g., progress from counting backward to reading aloud to reaching for objects to catching objects).

Environmental Demands

◆ Perform selected exercises with reduced vision (have participants wear dark glasses) or absent vision (have participants close eyes).

◆ Alter the support surface beneath the feet (e.g., use foam squares, rocker board, Dyna-Disc).

◆ Reduce or remove vision *and* alter the support surface beneath the feet.

◆ Perform certain exercises in a busy visual environment (e.g., have participants perform in front of a striped curtain or while following a checkerboard being moved in front of the face).

LEVEL 3: SEATED BALANCE
WITH VOLUNTARY TRUNK MOVEMENTS

Level 3 exercises further challenge balance by having the participants move their trunk in different directions. Since a larger segment of the body is moving, the movements of the COG increase, requiring greater effort to maintain balance during each movement. These exercises also improve the strength of the trunk, hip, and lower-body muscles by requiring larger and controlled movements away from a centered position and against gravity. Flexibility, particularly in the hip and trunk regions, will also improve during each of these exercise progressions, as participants are encouraged to move through as complete a range of motion as possible. Do not hesitate to reduce the difficulty associated with the starting hand position or move the participants to easier seated support surfaces if you feel they are not ready to perform these exercises on a more difficult support surface.

Reminders for Participants

• Sit tall with the feet flat on the floor before beginning each trunk movement.

• Breathe evenly throughout the exercise.

• Keep the eyes directed forward and focused on a visual target at eye level unless otherwise instructed.

• Perform each trunk movement through as complete a range of motion as possible while maintaining balance.

• Perform each exercise slowly.

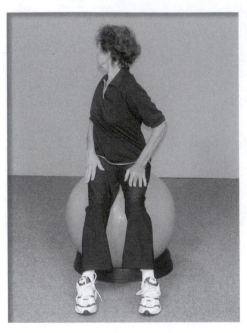

Figure 4.8   Lateral trunk rotation.

Exercise Progressions

1. Lateral Trunk Rotation

   a. Rotate the trunk *slowly* to one side, keeping the hips forward (figure 4.8). The goal is to look over the turning shoulder at the wall behind.

   b. Hold the position for three counts and then return to the starting position at the midline.

   c. Breathe evenly throughout the exercise.

   d. Repeat, rotating to the opposite side.

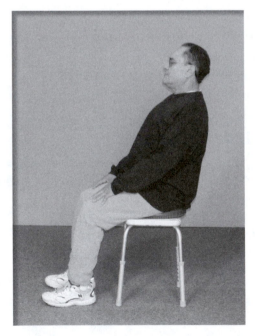

Figure 4.9   Trunk lean in the backward direction.

2. Trunk Lean in Forward and Backward Directions

   a. Lean the trunk forward, beginning at the hips, until the nose is above the knees. The eyes should be directed forward and focused on a target at eye level throughout the lean. Breathe evenly throughout the exercise.

   b. Maintain an extended upper-body position throughout the lean.

   c. Hold for three counts and then return to an upright starting position.

   d. Lean the trunk backward while keeping the upper body extended (figure 4.9).

   e. Hold for three counts and then return to an upright starting position.

3. Trunk Lean in Diagonal Forward and Backward Directions

a. Lean the trunk diagonally forward until the nose is above one knee. The eyes should be directed forward and focused on a target at eye level throughout the lean (figure 4.10). Breathe evenly throughout the exercise.

b. Maintain the upper body in an extended position throughout the lean.

c. Hold for three counts and then return to an upright starting position.

d. Repeat the movement in the opposite forward diagonal direction.

e. Repeat the diagonal trunk movements to both sides of the body, but this time lean the trunk in a backward direction. Keep the eyes directed forward and focused on a target.

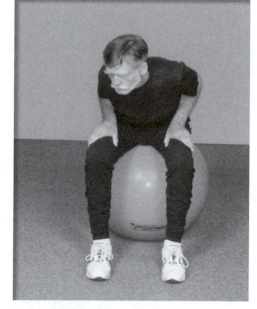

Figure 4.10 Diagonal forward lean on the balance ball.

Once again, refer to the feature on pages 114-115 for additional ideas on how to manipulate the level of balance challenge associated with each set of exercise progressions presented in level 3. Following completion of these core exercises, you might consider incorporating one of the culminating activities that are described on pages 127 through 130 at the end of the seated balance section. Each culminating activity reinforces the many skills that have been acquired at each level. These activities can be performed in small groups and provide a fun way to practice a combination of skills in a gamelike setting. The most appropriate culminating activities to introduce after your class participants have practiced the first three levels of seated balance activities are (a) pass the potato, please; (b) hot potato; and (c) balloon volleyball.

LEVEL 4: SEATED BALANCE WITH VOLUNTARY LEG MOVEMENTS

Level 4 activities increase the challenge of maintaining seated balance by having participants perform various movements with the legs as opposed to the arms and trunk. These lower-body movements are also excellent activities for strengthening the muscles of the trunk, legs, and feet. Performing movements through as complete a range of motion as possible also improves flexibility in the hip, knee, and ankle joints.

Reminders for Participants

- Sit tall on the chair or ball.
- Return the foot to the floor immediately if you start to lose balance.
- Keep the eyes directed forward and focused on a visual target at eye level unless otherwise instructed.
- Perform each exercise through as complete a range of motion as possible while maintaining seated balance and an upright trunk.
- Perform each exercise slowly.

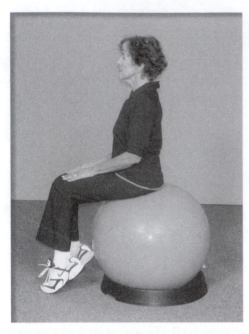

Figure 4.11 Double-heel lift.

Exercise Progressions

1. Heel Lift

    a. Perform continuous heel lifts with both heels lifting simultaneously (weight should shift to the balls of the feet as the heels leave the floor). Perform 10 repetitions (figure 4.11).

    b. Perform alternating heel lifts with each foot 10 times.

    c. Perform double- and single-heel lifts on verbal commands.

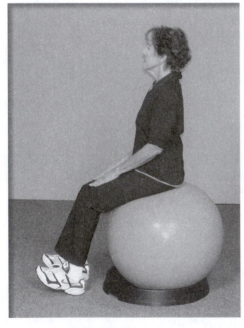

Figure 4.12 Toe lift.

2. Toe Lift

    a. Perform continuous toe lifts with both feet (weight should shift to the heels of the feet as the toes lift from the floor). Perform 10 repetitions (figure 4.12).

    b. Perform alternating toe lifts with each foot 10 times.

    c. Perform double- and single-toe lifts on verbal command.

3. Combination Heel and Toe Lift

a. Combine continuous heel and toe lifts with both feet (weight should shift to the balls of the feet as the heels leave the floor and then shift back to the heels as the toes are lifted off the floor).

b. Perform 10 repetitions.

c. Perform alternating heel and toe lifts with each foot 10 times.

d. Perform double and alternating combination lifts on verbal command.

4. Single-Leg Extension (With Toe or Heel Leading)

a. Extend one leg forward, contacting the floor with the toes of the leading leg (figure 4.13). (Participants who are less stable may need to hold onto the chair or ball during early repetitions.)

b. Perform five repetitions with each leg.

d. Repeat the exercise but alternate legs.

c. Repeat the single-leg extensions with the heel contacting the floor on each extension.

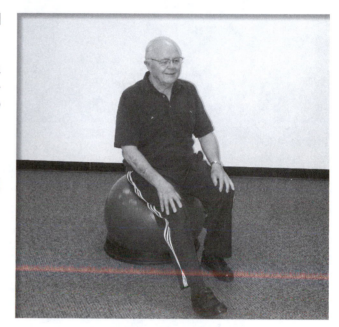

Figure 4.13   Single-leg extension.

5. Seated Knee Lift

a. March in place by alternating knee lifts (the height of the knee lift depends on an individual's capabilities). Shift weight onto the hip of the stance leg before lifting the other leg off the floor. Breathe evenly throughout the exercise.

b. Perform 10 repetitions while maintaining an upright seated position.

c. Repeat the exercise but vary the height of the knee lifts (e.g., low, medium, high).

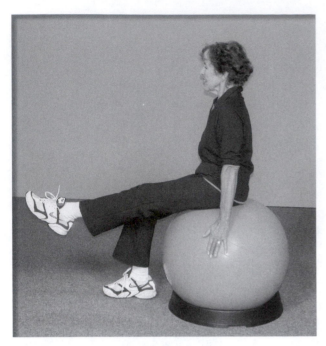

Figure 4.14 Single-leg raise.

6. Single-Leg Raise

a. Extend one leg out until it is as parallel to the floor as possible (figure 4.14). (The height of the raise will be determined by the participant's ability to maintain an erect trunk position.)

b. Hold for three counts and then lower the leg to the starting position. Breathe evenly throughout the exercise.

c. Repeat with the other leg until the exercise has been performed 10 times with each leg.

d. Perform combination knee lifts and leg raises. Begin with multiple repetitions on the same leg and then progress to alternating legs. Hold onto the ball or chair during the early repetitions.

Refer again to the feature on pages 114-115 for ideas on how to increase the balance challenge by manipulating the task and environmental demands associated with the exercise. Two fun culminating activities that can be introduced after the core exercise progressions in this level have been sufficiently practiced are (a) quick feet and (b) seated soccer (see page 129).

LEVEL 5: SEATED BALANCE WHILE RESISTING PERTURBATIONS

Level 5 activities further increase the challenge to maintain seated balance through small and quick perturbations (pushes or pulls) applied in various directions (i.e., forward, backward, lateral, diagonal) to the hips or shoulders. At this level, you are working on the participants' anticipatory *and* reactive postural control abilities. Participants are seated on a support surface (e.g., chair with no back, Dyna-Disc, balance ball with holder) that matches their individual capabilities while adopting one of the three starting arm positions (i.e., hands resting on the chair or ball, hands resting on the thighs, or arms folded across the chest).

When the participant is perturbed, muscles of the trunk and lower body are strengthened as the participant tries to maintain a seated balance position. Level 5 activities challenge the participant to react quickly and efficiently to the perturbation. Look for the participant to respond with the appropriate countermovement (i.e., body movement in a direction that is opposite to the perturbation). Note how quickly the participant begins moving in the opposite direction after the perturbation and the amount of countermovement used. Ideally, the amount of countermovement should be proportional to the size of the perturbation.

Follow these safety guidelines when performing seated perturbation activities:

- Inform assistants of any participant who should not be perturbed due to an existing medical condition.
- Begin with small perturbations (pushes or pulls) applied to the hip region. Administer the push or pull movement quickly and gradually increase the force on each subsequent repetition. Also consider the type of surface on which the participant is seated when deciding how much force to apply. For example, an older adult who is seated on a chair with no backrest and a Dyna-Disc below the buttocks will be able to tolerate more force being applied than an individual who is seated on a balance ball with no ball holder beneath it.
- Do not increase the size of the perturbation if the participant is slow to initiate the countermovement or responds with too small or too large a countermovement for the size of the perturbation applied.
- Wait until the participant recovers from one perturbation before initiating the next.
- Be prepared to provide manual support at this advanced stage of the exercise progression.

Exercise Progressions

1. Predictable Perturbations

a. Inform participants in advance that you (or your assistants) are going to try to disrupt their seated balance by saying, "Don't let me pull or push you off balance." By verbally warning participants in advance of applying the perturbation, you are testing how well they are able to stabilize the body in anticipation of being pushed or pulled off balance. Predictable perturbations test a participant's level of anticipatory postural control.

b. Begin by quickly pushing or pulling each participant's hips in a forward or backward direction. Progress to lateral and diagonal pushes and pulls once the participant is able to respond appropriately to the forward and backward perturbations. You can also push the ball under the client to vary the nature of the perturbation.

c. Apply perturbations to different parts of the body simultaneously (e.g., push the left hip forward as you pull the right shoulder toward you and vice versa).

2. Unpredictable Perturbations

a. With no advance warning, apply perturbations of different sizes. Observe how well the participant is able to respond automatically to the disruption of balance. Unpredictable perturbations test a participant's reactive postural control.

b. Stand behind the participants so it is more difficult for them to predict the direction of the perturbation. Note the ability of participants to scale their response to the size of the perturbation (e.g., a small push should result in a small response in the opposite direction). Also check whether the participants adapt to repeated perturbations of similar force by applying more muscular force in advance of the perturbation. If this is the case, they will not move as far from a centered position following the perturbation. This reduced movement indicates that they are able to establish a good postural set for this activity.

c. Repeat the perturbations, but this time simultaneously push and pull one hip and shoulder in different directions using different levels of intensity (small and medium pushes or pulls). Do not provide advance warning of the perturbations. Vary the interval between perturbations in an effort to increase the unpredictability.

LEVEL 6: SEATED BALANCE WITH DYNAMIC WEIGHT SHIFTS THROUGH SPACE

Seated balance activities requiring self-initiated weight shifts improve dynamic COG control because participants must shift their weight away from a centered position by moving the hips in various directions while maintaining balance. At the same time, the trunk, hip, and lower-body muscles are being strengthened during these isotonic exercises. In addition, these exercises increase flexibility, particularly at the hip joint. As with the exercises described previously, the seated support surface (e.g., balance ball with or without holder) and arm position (e.g., holding seated surface, hands resting on thighs, arms folded across chest) should match each participant's individual capabilities. Performing weight shifts while seated on a Dyna-Disc is very difficult, so it will be necessary to move clients to a ball with a ball holder to perform these next progressions. If clients are not ready to make this transition, have them continue to perform the easier trunk movements until they are stable enough to sit on the more challenging seated support surface.

During all level 6 progressions that your clients perform with their eyes closed, you should present the following sensory awareness cues:

- Can you feel the weight shift under the buttocks as you move in a forward (backward, lateral, diagonal) direction? Imagine you are sliding your hips on a tray beneath you.

- Can you sense that your shoulders are directly above the hips as you shift your weight in a forward (backward, diagonal) direction? (This cue is for forward, backward, or diagonal weight shifts.)

- Can you sense that your shoulder is directly above your hip as you shift your weight to the right or left? (This cue is for lateral weight shifts.)

- Can you feel the pressure increase under (a) the feet and move toward the toes as you shift your weight in a forward direction, (b) the heels as you shift

---

General Reminders for Participants

- Sit tall on the chair or ball.
- Position the feet hip-width apart and flat on the floor.
- Keep the shoulders relaxed and level throughout the exercises.
- Keep the eyes directed forward and focused on a vertical target at eye level unless otherwise instructed.
- Breathe evenly throughout each exercise.
- Perform all exercises slowly and through as complete a range of motion as possible.

your weight in a backward direction, (c) the outside of your right foot as you shift your weight laterally and to the right, (d) the outside of your left foot as you shift your weight laterally and to your left, (e) the toes of the right (left) foot as you shift your weight in a forward and right (left) diagonal direction, (f) the heel of the left (right) foot as you shift your weight in a backward and left (right) diagonal direction?

Exercise Progressions

1. Forward and Backward Weight Shifts

a. Shift weight by moving the hips in a forward direction, hold for three counts, and return to a centered position (figure 4.15a).

b. Shift weight by moving the hips backward, hold for three counts, and return to a centered position (figure 4.15b).

c. Repeat the exercise with the eyes closed (use sensory awareness cues to reinforce correct movement pattern).

d. Repeat the forward and backward weight shifts, but move through a centered position without stopping.

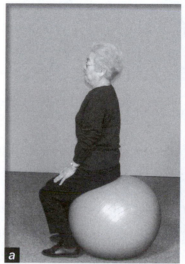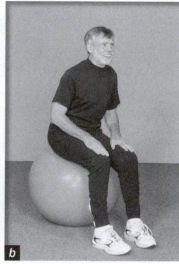

Figure 4.15 Weight shifts on a balance ball. *(a)* Forward weight shifts. *(b)* Backward weight shifts.

2. Lateral Weight Shifts

a. Shift weight in a lateral direction through the hip and away from a centered position (figure 4.16). Be sure to keep the hip leading the action aligned with the shoulder during the weight shift.

b. Return to a centered position and then shift weight laterally in the other direction.

c. Repeat the exercise with the eyes closed (use sensory awareness cues to reinforce correct movement pattern).

d. Repeat the lateral weight shift, but this time move from right to left without stopping in the centered position.

e. Repeat the lateral weight shifts described in the previous step with the eyes closed (use sensory awareness cues to reinforce correct movement pattern).

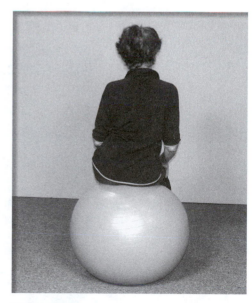

Figure 4.16 Lateral weight shifts on balance ball.

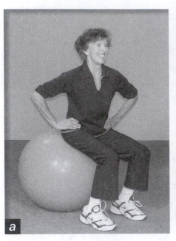
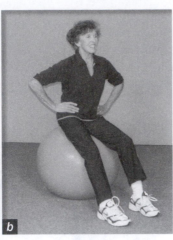

Figure 4.17 Diagonal weight shifts on balance ball. *(a)* Forward weight shifts. *(b)* Backward weight shifts.

3. Diagonal Weight Shifts

   a. Shift weight in a diagonal and forward direction (figure 4.17a).

   b. Return to a centered position and then shift weight diagonally and backward (figure 4.17b).

   c. Repeat the exercise with the eyes closed (use sensory awareness cues to reinforce correct movement pattern).

   d. Repeat the diagonal weight shifts, but this time move diagonally forward and backward without stopping in the center.

   e. Repeat the previous diagonal weight shifts with the eyes closed (use sensory awareness cues to reinforce correct movement pattern).

   f. Repeat diagonal weight shifts in each of the four directions without stopping in the center between movements.

   g. Repeat the diagonal weight shifts in all four directions with the eyes closed (use sensory awareness cues to reinforce correct movement pattern).

Do not have your clients perform the exercise progressions in level 3 during the same class in which you introduce the exercise progressions in level 6. There is a tendency for class participants (and sometimes the instructor) to confuse trunk leans and weight shifts and move the body incorrectly as a result.

Following adequate practice of each of the core progressions in level 6, it is appropriate to increase the task demand by adding resistance (figure 4.18). Wrap a length of resistance band of a given tension low around each participant's hips and then gently pull on the band in a direction opposite to the intended weight

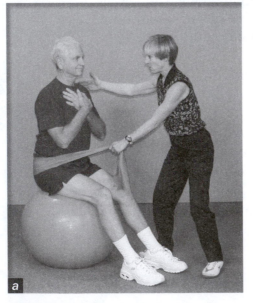
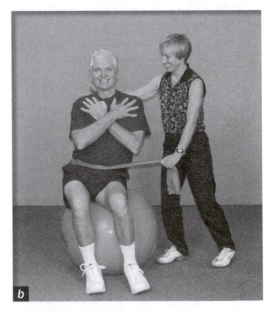

Figure 4.18 Moving against a resistance band in *(a)* backward and *(b)* lateral directions.

shift. In addition to adding more challenge to the activity, the resistance band serves as an excellent tactile feedback device. Participants will be able to feel the band's resistance increase against their hips as they shift weight in each direction. If they do not feel the increased tension, they will know they are not initiating the weight shift through the hips. Adding resistance to level 6 exercise progressions can be time consuming in a group setting so it is recommended that you enlist the help of one or more trained assistants and divide the class into smaller groups. You can also limit these progressions to individual clients who are clearly having difficulties shifting their weight through the hips. The use of resistance in these progressions is best suited to one-to-one training settings.

General guidelines for using resistance bands include the following:

- Use a resistance band that is at least 8 feet (2.4 m) in length.
- Determine the resistance most appropriate for the participant (the color of the band and the amount of pull in the opposite direction are associated with a given tension).
- For all dynamic weight shifts, place the resistance band low around the hips of the participant.
- Apply resistance by gently pulling the band in a direction exactly opposite to the direction in which the participant is shifting weight. Be sure to distribute the tension evenly across the band by keeping it flat against the hips.
- Instruct participants to position the hands on the thighs or fold them across the chest.
- Be sure to select a seated support surface (e.g., chair with no backrest, chair with Dyna-Disc, balance ball with or without holder) that allows participants to perform the exercises safely.
- Resistance bands also serve as excellent tactile cuing devices, reinforcing the importance of initiating the weight shift through the hips.

Refer to the feature on pages 114-115 for other ideas on how to increase the balance challenge for level 6 exercise progressions. An excellent culminating activity to introduce after the core progressions in this level are practiced is shift around the clock. This activity is described in the section on culminating activities on page 130.

LEVEL 7: SEATED BALANCE WITH DYNAMIC WEIGHT SHIFTS AGAINST GRAVITY

The exercise progressions described in level 7 move from practicing weight shifts through space to performing weight shifts against gravity. These exercise progressions are intended to further challenge the balance system and teach class participants how to dynamically control the COG when they are required to bounce in a vertical, horizontal, or diagonal direction. The exercises also strengthen and increase the power of the lower-body muscles, especially the hip flexors and extensors, the quadriceps, and the plantar and dorsiflexor muscle groups.

General instructions and safety guidelines for performing dynamic weight shifts against gravity include the following:

- Instruct participants to position the hands on the thighs or fold them across the chest.

- Provide participants who are less stable with a holder for the balance ball and position them close to a wall or a chair. (Dyna-Disc support surfaces are not appropriate for these activities.)
- Have participants position their feet hip-width apart and flat on the floor.
- Instruct participants to sit tall and focus their eyes on a visual target in front of them and at eye level while bouncing.
- Have participants gradually increase the size of the vertical bounce until their buttocks leave the ball on each bounce.
- Instruct participants to stop bouncing if they feel any discomfort in the hip or knee joints or begin to experience any dizziness.
- Check the level of dizziness in all participants following each exercise progression. Use the 10-point scale described on page 46 in chapter 2 and remember that the level of dizziness reported should not exceed a rating of 4 to 5.
- Encourage participants to reduce the height of the bounce or stop bouncing if they begin to feel unstable on the ball.
- Make sure participants have enough dynamic postural control to perform the level 7 activities, as these activities are advanced.
- Gradually increase the number of repetitions you ask your participants to perform over several classes. Level 7 exercise progressions are more demanding activities, and your more deconditioned class participants will fatigue quickly. Instruct participants with arthritis or total joint replacements to bounce at lower heights during all exercise progressions.

Exercise Progressions

1. Vertical Ball Bounce

a. Push against the floor with the feet to initiate the vertical bounce. The top of the head moves upward toward the ceiling. Repeat the bounce 10 times.

b. Increase the size of the vertical bounce by gradually increasing the speed and force applied against the floor with the feet. The buttocks will begin to lose contact with the ball on the upward bounce. Complete 5 to 10 repetitions, increasing the height of the bounce on each repetition.

c. Repeat low bounces with the eyes closed.

2. Bounces in Forward and Backward Directions

a. Push against the floor with the feet to initiate the bounce while shifting the weight (through the hips) forward and backward during the bounce. Repeat the exercise 10 times.

b. Increase the size of the forward and backward movement by increasing the force applied against the floor with the feet and the range of motion at the hips. Complete 5 to 10 repetitions.

c. Repeat the forward and backward bounces at a low level with the eyes closed.

3. Bounces in Lateral Directions

a. Push against the floor with the feet to initiate the bounce while shifting the weight through the hips in the right and left lateral directions during the bounce. Repeat the exercise 10 times at a low bounce height.

b. Repeat the exercise, gradually increasing the size of each lateral movement by increasing the force applied against the floor with the feet and increasing the range of motion at the hips on each repetition. Complete 5 to 10 repetitions.

4. Bounces in Forward and Backward Diagonal Directions

a. Push against the floor with the feet to initiate the bounce while shifting the weight through the hips in the forward and backward diagonal directions during the bounce. Repeat the exercise 10 times.

b. Increase the size of the forward and backward diagonal movement on each subsequent repetition by using more force against the floor with the leading foot and increasing the range of motion at the hips. Complete 5 to 10 repetitions.

Once participants have mastered each of the exercise progressions in level 7, you can begin to manipulate the task and environmental demands as described in the feature on pages 114-115. Because these exercise progressions are relatively difficult in and of themselves, use caution when selecting a particular task or environmental demand.

Culminating Activities for Seated Balance

The culminating group activities described in this section provide participants with the opportunity to practice the many different exercise progressions they have been introduced to in each of the seven levels of seated balance activities. By introducing an object to be passed and retrieved, whether with the hands or the feet, you are further increasing the task demands by requiring participants to divide their attention between the task of balancing and the task of passing the object. Balance must be more subconsciously controlled as attention is diverted toward reaching, passing, catching, or throwing. The balance level to which these particular culminating activities best apply is indicated at the start of each activity description. The most appropriate culminating activities for each of the seven levels are also named immediately following the discussion of the core exercise progressions for each level. Before introducing any of the culminating activities, be sure to review the following safety tips:

- Do not introduce group activities until participants can safely perform all of the seated balance exercises on one of the seated support surfaces *and* with the arms in the most difficult position (folded across the chest).

- Move some participants onto an easier seated support surface (e.g., chair with backrest, chair with Dyna-Disc, balance ball with holder) so you can introduce this group activity earlier in the program but still maintain a safe exercise environment.

- Restrict the size of your groups to 4 to 6 participants and provide external support (e.g., nearby chairs) for participants.
- Bear in mind that older adults are just as competitive as younger adults in game situations. Continually remind your participants that balance comes first and that they should not attempt to perform a movement during any game if they begin to feel unstable.

Pass the Potato, Please

This is a good culminating activity to introduce after the core exercise progressions associated with levels 2 and 3 have been adequately practiced. This first variation of a passing activity is self-paced so it does not introduce too great a balance challenge too early. Participants are seated on various support surfaces in a circle (no more than four participants in each circle). A ball is passed in different directions (e.g., straight ahead, on the diagonal, clockwise, counterclockwise) as determined by the instructor (figure 4.19). As participants become more comfortable passing the ball in the different directions, the height of the pass and the weight of the ball can be varied. Pass the potato, please allows participants to practice the various trunk movements introduced in level 3. The instructor can also move around the outside of the circle and have the participants retrieve and then pass the ball back from different heights and angles to incorporate more arm and trunk movements.

Hot Potato

A slightly more challenging version of the previous passing activity is called hot potato. This culminating activity can also be introduced to reinforce the exercise progressions practiced in levels 2 and 3. The objective of this activity is to pass the ball around the circle as quickly as possible. Requiring participants to perform the

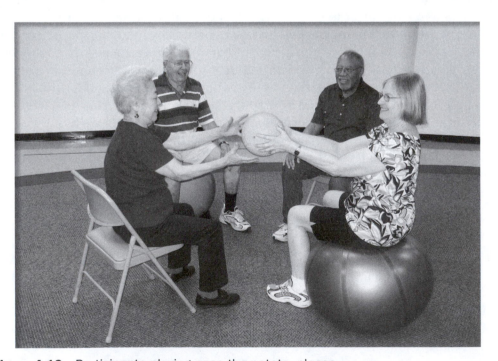

Figure 4.19 Participants playing pass the potato, please.

task more quickly places an added challenge on the postural control system. You can also increase the cognitive demands associated with the activity by periodically calling out a verbal command to change the direction in which the participants are passing. Adding this cognitive demand will give you the opportunity to watch how quickly a participant processes and responds to each verbal command. In addition, a second ball can be introduced to further increase the physical and cognitive demands associated with the task. Balls of different weights can also be used to add a resistance component to the activity.

Balloon Volleyball

This is the most challenging culminating activity to introduce after practicing level 2 and 3 exercise progressions. What makes balloon volleyball more difficult is that it further increases the task demands by adding a more challenging external timing component. As with the previous two culminating activities, small groups of class participants (4 to 6) form a circle. They then attempt to tap a balloon to one another as many times as possible before the balloon contacts the floor. Unlike the ball-passing activities, balloon volleyball requires participants to react more quickly because they do not know when the balloon will reach them. Attention is being further diverted from the task of balancing, requiring that it be controlled at a more subconscious level.

Quick Feet

This activity requires three differently colored spots to be arranged around each participant: one spot directly in front of the right foot, one spot in front of the left foot, and one spot midway between the other two spots. For this activity, the participant must move the foot to the designated spot and back to the starting position as quickly as possible. For example, when the right spot is called, the participant moves the right foot forward to contact the right spot and then immediately returns the foot to its original starting position. When the left spot is called, the participant moves the left foot forward to contact the left spot, and when the middle spot is called, the participant contacts the middle spot with either foot. As the activity progresses, the various spots can be called in combination (e.g., right, middle, right, left) so that the participant must perform a sequence of movements as quickly as possible. This activity improves the participant's central processing speed as well as movement speed. Having participants perform longer movement sequences also stimulates memory. Be sure to encourage your participants to hold onto the seated surface or a nearby chair until they feel stable enough to place their hands on their thighs. It might also be wise to move some of your participants onto an easier seated support surface when they are first learning this culminating activity. Quick feet is good to introduce after level 4 voluntary leg movement progressions have been practiced.

Seated Soccer

This is another excellent but more challenging culminating activity to introduce following completion of the core exercise progressions in level 4. Seated soccer is a fun way to (a) improve seated balance control when the base of support is reduced and (b) divide the participant's attention so that the act of balancing becomes controlled less consciously. Be sure to select a seated support surface that matches each participant's capabilities in order to maximize safety during this activity. Have participants form a circle (3 to 4 in each circle). The objective of the activity is for participants to kick the ball from person to person in the circle. The participants should trap the ball before kicking it; encourage them to stop the ball with one foot and then kick it with the other foot. When introducing this activity to the class, be sure to place chairs next to each person in the circle and encourage participants who are less stable to hold onto a chair while trapping and kicking the ball.

Safety Tips for Seated Soccer

- Do not introduce this culminating activity until your participants can safely perform the most difficult seated balance exercise progression in level 4 (i.e., single-leg raises) with the arms in the most difficult position (folded across the chest). You can also move some participants onto an easier seated support surface (e.g., chair with backrest, chair with Dyna-Disc, balance ball with holder) so you can introduce this group activity earlier in the program but still maintain a safe exercise environment.
- Remind participants that balance comes first and that they should not attempt to perform a movement in the game if they begin to feel unstable.
- Demonstrate the most appropriate way to kick the ball (i.e., instep kick) before starting the activity.
- Instruct participants to stop the ball with one foot before attempting to kick it to another person.
- As their skill improves, encourage participants to stop the ball with one foot and kick it with the other foot.

Shift Around the Clock

Shift around the clock is an excellent culminating activity to introduce after participants have practiced the core progressions described in level 6. Participants are to imagine that they are sitting in the center of a clock face that is directly below them on the floor. Instruct participants to shift their weight forward to 12 o'clock, forward and diagonally right to 1 o'clock, laterally to the right to 3 o'clock and so on until they have shifted all the way around the imaginary clock face. Begin each lean or weight shift from a centered position, and return to the center after each movement. As soon as participants become familiar with moving to each of the positions on the imaginary clock from a centered position, eliminate the return to the center and have participants move from one clock position to another without pausing in the middle. Increase the speed with which the clock positions are announced to further challenge participants. Both memory and motor coordination will improve as an outcome of this activity. As the program progresses, you can add even more challenge to this activity by manipulating certain task demands (e.g., alter the base of support, add a secondary task such as counting or reading) or environmental demands (e.g., alter the support surface beneath the feet, reduce or remove vision) as described in the feature on pages 114-115.

Seated Balance Activities Summary

When introducing any of the exercise progressions described for the seven levels of seated balance activities, remember to match each individual's capabilities to the challenge of the task and the environment in which the task is performed. As participants become more comfortable performing an activity on the selected equipment, consider moving them onto a more challenging surface when they are performing the lower-level exercise progressions. For example, if a participant is able to perform exercises in level 2 while seated on a chair and Dyna-Disc with the arms folded across the chest and the eyes closed, consider changing the chair to a balance ball with a ball holder beneath it when these exercise progressions are repeated in a subsequent class. Participants moving to a new, more challenging seated surface can adopt an easier hand position (on the ball itself) and keep the eyes open until they are ready to accept more challenge. Note that participants may need to return to the chair and Dyna-Disc to perform the more challenging and higher-level exercise progressions.

Several ways to progressively increase the challenge associated with each seated balance activity have been described in the feature on pages 114-115. Remember that you are manipulating the demands imposed by the task or the environment in order to increase the challenge associated with each balance exercise. Given that manipulating these two variables directly affects a participant's ability to perform a task, do so in a way that does not compromise safety or negatively affect a participant's self-confidence. You can further reinforce what participants have learned in each level by incorporating culminating activities that allow participants to practice the many balance skills they have acquired in a fun, gamelike atmosphere. Consider what type of support surface you would have Phoebe and Larry sitting on while performing any of the culminating activities just described. Would you change the type of seated support surface for certain games, and if so, why?

STANDING BALANCE ACTIVITIES

The standing balance exercise progressions you select for your individual class participants will depend on their *individual capabilities*. Some participants may need to begin with the easier exercise progressions described in each of the seven levels of standing balance activities, whereas other participants may be ready to perform the more difficult progressions in a given level.

Once participants are able to perform the core exercise progressions associated with the seven levels of standing balance activities, you can again increase the balance challenge by manipulating either the task demands or the environmental demands in ways similar to those described for the seated balance activities. By manipulating just one or two aspects of the task, you will add variety to the practice session and challenge the sensory, motor, and cognitive systems at the same time. After the descriptions of the seven levels of exercise progressions, this section also includes a set of culminating activities that will enable your clients to practice several different exercise progressions simultaneously in a fun, gamelike atmosphere.

Safety Guidelines for Standing Balance Activities

◆ Alert all assistants to participants who may have difficulty performing standing activities so that these participants can be closely supervised. Also inform assistants of participants with medical conditions (e.g., peripheral neuropathy, joint replacements, osteoporosis) that make it difficult to perform standing exercises on compliant surfaces.

◆ If needed, have certain participants perform the standing exercises with their backs to the wall (participants should stand about 2 feet, or .6 m, away from the wall), with a chair in front of them, or with very close supervision (or with all three).

◆ Do not ask participants to perform the next exercise progression until they can safely perform the task at hand. For example, do not ask participants to perform an exercise with the eyes closed if they are not able to do it safely with the eyes open.

◆ Instruct participants to open their eyes immediately if they feel they are about to lose their balance.

◆ Instruct participants how to safely mount and dismount compliant (foam, half-foam roller, or Dyna-Disc) and moving (rocker board) surfaces.

◆ Have participants practice getting safely on and off foam, roller, or Dyna-Disc surfaces in the forward direction only before beginning the exercise progressions.

LEVEL 1: CHECKING STANDING POSTURE

Before introducing any of the standing balance activities described in this section, teach your class participants how to check their standing posture. Demonstrate the correct standing posture to your class and then have participants practice while standing with their backs against a wall. If you are fortunate enough to have a wall of mirrors in your facility, have participants practice while facing the mirror and then standing sideways to it. Provide the following verbal cues as you observe whether your class participants are standing correctly:

- Stand with your back against the wall and your feet flat on the floor with the heels approximately 6 inches (15 cm) from the wall.
- Relax your arms and let them hang by your sides. (Observe whether the space between the arm and the body is equal on both sides for each client.)
- Hold your head erect and direct your eyes forward to focus on a target. (Check whether the participant's chin is parallel to the floor.)
- Gently move your head straight back until your ears are directly above your shoulders.
- Your upper back should be erect and your chest slightly elevated.
- Pull your abdominal muscles in and up so that your stomach flattens. (Check to see that each client's lower back has a slight forward curve and that the hips are level, the kneecaps are facing forward, and the ankles and feet are straight.)
- Notice that your weight is distributed evenly on your feet.
- Breathe normally and hold this position for 15 seconds with your eyes open. Now close your eyes and try to concentrate on the feeling of standing correctly.

Reminders for Participants

- Stand tall and imagine that the top of the head is being pulled toward the ceiling by a string.
- Keep the eyes directed forward and focused on a vertical target at eye level.
- Try to maintain each standing position for as long as possible (30 seconds maximum).

Your clients can also check their alignment by placing one hand behind their neck with the back of the hand against the wall and the other hand behind their lower back with the palm facing the wall. If they are able to move their hands forward and backward more than an inch, the curves of the spine are not in proper alignment. A good homework assignment to give your clients is to have them practice their standing posture either against a wall or in front of a full-length mirror.

LEVEL 2: STANDING BALANCE WITH ALTERED BASE OF SUPPORT

The exercise progressions described in this level help participants learn how to control the COG when in a standing position. As the base of support changes during this set of exercise progressions, subtle shifts of the COG are necessary for maintaining upright balance. For example, as participants move from a Romberg position (feet together) to a sharpened Romberg position (tandem stance), they must recognize that their base of support has become narrower and longer and adjust the position of the COG accordingly. To maintain stable, upright control in a sharpened Romberg position, the participants must shift the COG forward to a position directly above the heel of the front foot and the toe of the rear foot. The participants must then move the COG once more as they adopt a single-leg stance; this time the COG is directly above the stance leg as the other leg is lifted off the floor. The ultimate goal of the exercise progressions at this level is to teach the participants the strategy for manipulating the COG as the base of support is altered. Once acquired, this strategy should serve the older adult well in daily activities that involve a changing base of support (e.g., walking, stepping into and out of the bathtub, standing in confined spaces).

You can help participants move safely on and off altered support surfaces by providing the following instructions:

- Always test the altered support surface by putting one foot onto the middle of the surface and feeling its level of compliance (in the case of a foam or Dyna-Disc surface) or its direction and amount of tilt (in the case of a rocker board).

- When one foot has been positioned in the center of the altered surface, slowly transfer weight onto that foot and bring the other foot onto the surface (figure 4.20).

- Stand tall with slightly flexed knees (i.e., soft knees) and focus the eyes on a vertical target directly in front and at eye level.

- Step off any altered surface in a forward direction, taking a moment to firmly plant the lead foot on the firm surface before lifting the other foot off the altered surface.

Exercise Progressions

1. Standing Floor Activities

a. Stand with the feet together (Romberg position; see figure 4.21a). Hold the position for 10 to 15 seconds or as long as possible. Repeat with the eyes closed.

b. Move the feet into a split stance (heel of the front foot in front of and to the side of the toes of the rear foot; see figure 4.21b). Hold the position for 10 to 15 seconds or as long as possible. Repeat with the eyes closed.

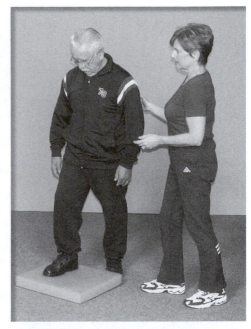

Figure 4.20 Getting safely on and off altered support surfaces.

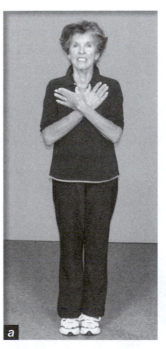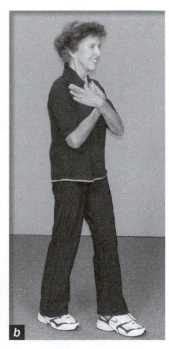

Figure 4.21 Four examples of activity progressions with altered base of support: *(a)* feet together (Romberg), *(b)* feet in split stance, *(continued)*

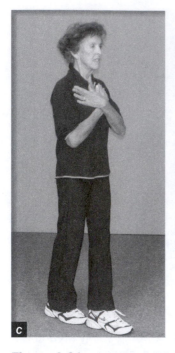
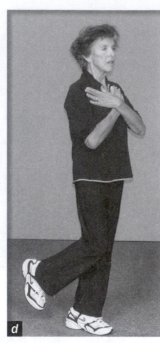

c. Move the feet into a semi-tandem position (front foot directly in front of the rear foot with a small space between the feet). Hold the position for 10 to 15 seconds or as long as possible. Repeat with the eyes closed.

d. Stand in a sharpened Romberg position (heel-to-toe standing position; see figure 4.21c). Hold the position for 10 to 15 seconds or as long as possible. Repeat with the eyes closed.

e. Adopt a single-leg stance, resting the raised leg on the stance foot or against the stance leg (see figure 4.21d). Hold the position for 10 to 15 seconds or as long as possible. Repeat with the eyes closed.

Figure 4.21 *(continued) (c)* feet in sharpened Romberg, and *(d)* single-leg stance.

An easy way to manipulate the balance challenge associated with these exercise progressions is to modify (a) the task demands (e.g., alter the position of the arms during the exercise) or (b) the environmental demands (e.g., alter the support surface beneath the feet). It may be necessary to reduce the balance challenge for some participants by asking them to adopt an easier arm position (e.g., arms at sides), particularly during the eyes-closed exercises. On the other hand, some participants may be able to perform the exercise progressions with the arms folded across the chest or may be able to progress more quickly to a more challenging standing surface (or may be able to do both). See the feature on page 135 for additional ideas.

2. Standing While Performing a Cognitive Task

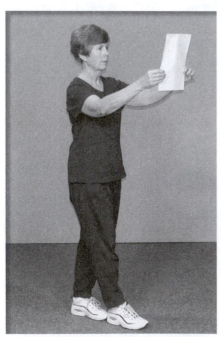

a. Repeat each exercise performed successfully in the first set of progressions in level 2 while performing a secondary cognitive task (e.g., reading aloud, counting backward by 3s; see figure 4.22).

b. Repeat each exercise performed successfully in the first set of progressions in level 2 while standing on a compliant surface and performing a secondary cognitive task.

c. Repeat each exercise performed successfully in the first set of progressions in level 2 while standing on a rocker board and performing a secondary cognitive task.

Figure 4.22 Participant standing in a sharpened Romberg position while reading aloud.

Increasing the Standing Balance Challenge by Manipulating the Task and Environmental Demands

Task Demands

◆ Alter the pacing of the exercise (i.e., increase or decrease the speed of the weight shifts, transfers, stepping sequences) using a hand clap, metronome, or music.

◆ When practicing exercise progressions in level 3, instruct participants to repeat each of the multidirectional weight shifts while gradually increasing the distance over which they shift their weight. You will notice participants beginning to flex at the hips as the distance between the forward lean and the backward lean increases. Do not increase the lean distance beyond the point where participants begin to flex the hips.

◆ Add a secondary task (e.g., count backward, read aloud, reach for objects, catch and throw objects) to be performed simultaneously with the balance activity.

◆ Move participants to the next bench or step height once they are able to perform all exercise progressions in level 7 safely. For example, progress from a 4-inch (10 cm) to a 6-inch (15 cm) bench height.

Environmental Demands

◆ Have participants perform selected exercise progressions with reduced or absent vision.

◆ Alter the standing support surface (e.g., switch to foam, rocker board, Dyna-Disc) during exercise progressions performed in levels 3, 4, and 5.

◆ Have participants perform activities while facing a wall decorated with a busy visual pattern (e.g., hang a vinyl checkerboard tablecloth or a large square of material with a complex pattern). Alternatively, move a checkerboard through the visual field and instruct participants to follow it with the eyes only.

3. Standing While Performing an Upper-Body Task

a. Repeat each exercise performed satisfactorily in the first set of progressions in level 2 while reaching for objects placed at different heights. Manipulate the weight and shape of the objects to increase the challenge.

b. Repeat each exercise performed successfully in the first set of progressions in level 2 while catching and throwing objects of different weights and shapes (see figure 4.23).

c. Repeat each exercise performed successfully in the first set of progressions in level 2 while reaching for objects of different weights placed at different heights, but this time do so on a compliant surface.

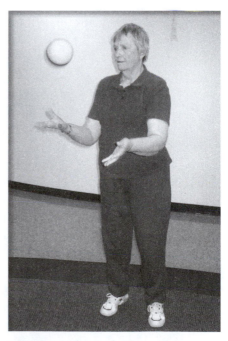

Figure 4.23 Standing while tossing a ball from hand to hand.

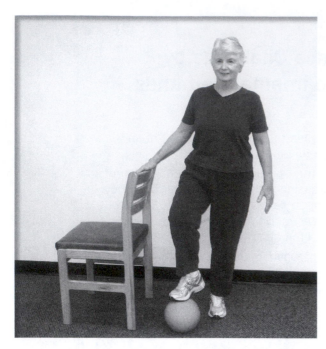

Figure 4.24   Standing with the foot on top of a ball.

4. Standing While Performing a Lower-Body Task

a. Use a foot to draw or write on the floor. For example, draw shapes such as a circle, square, or diamond. Next, ask participants to perform longer movements by having them write their first names with the right foot and their last names with the left foot.

b. Move a small towel in different directions with the foot. Use one foot to push the towel away from and back toward the body in a variety of directions and to scrunch and then spread out the towel. Transfer the towel (using the foot) to the opposite foot and repeat. (This activity is best performed with the shoes removed.)

c. Stand with one foot on a medium-sized ball (figure 4.24). Move the ball in different directions (forward, backward, diagonally, in a circle) while maintaining standing balance. Place the ball under the opposite foot and repeat the activity. Hold onto a sturdy chair for support while lifting the foot onto the ball and during any portion of the exercise.

d. Once the lower-body task exercise progression can be performed without assistance, replace the ball with a more compliant one that does not allow as much weight to be placed on it for support (the most compliant object to place under the foot is a balloon). Repeat the lower-body task exercise progression.

LEVEL 3: MULTIDIRECTIONAL WEIGHT SHIFTS

The exercises described in level 3 expand each participant's limits of stability so that participants can accomplish ADLs that require greater ranges of body motion or extreme leaning (e.g., pulling weeds in the garden, leaning into cupboards or the washing machine). Expanded stability limits also place an individual at a lower risk for losing balance during an unexpected perturbation. These exercises teach participants how to move the body more efficiently through space and in a way that is most appropriate for the task demands. Improved joint flexibility and lower-body strengthening are also promoted, as the distance through which participants are required to shift and transfer weight increases.

To enhance learning, use the following tactile and verbal feedback with participants:

- Place chairs a suitable distance in front of and behind participants or position participants between a wall and a chair.
- Have participants touch the chair in front of them with the hips as they lean forward and touch the wall behind them with the buttocks as they shift their weight backwards. Move the chairs closer to the participants if you observe that they are bending at the hips before reaching the chairs in front of them or they are losing their balance before reaching the wall on the backward weight shifts.
- Watch to see that participants are not rising onto their toes as they lean forward. Instruct them to reduce the lean distance so that their heels remain in contact with the floor.
- Instruct participants to stand tall and keep their eyes focused on a vertical target at eye level in front of them.
- Emphasize weight shifting through the hips (not the head) on backward weight shifts. Instruct participants to keep the shoulders aligned directly above the hips throughout the weight shift. Having a partner stand off to the side and watch for correct alignment of shoulders and hips is helpful.
- To practice lateral weight shifts, have participants turn to one side so they can continue to use the chairs or wall for tactile feedback. The hips should make contact with each chair (or the chair and wall) as they move in a lateral direction. The shoulder should remain directly above the hip and move in the same direction during the weight shift. Some older adults tend to lower the opposite shoulder during the weight shift as though performing a countermovement. Performing this activity in front of a mirror or a partner who is instructed to watch for correct shoulder and hip alignment can be very helpful.
- Instruct participants to relax the shoulders and imagine that they are sliding their hips and shoulders along a horizontal rail as they perform the lateral weight shifts.
- When practicing diagonal weight shifts, encourage participants to feel the changing pressures under their feet as they shift weight in the forward diagonal (pressure moves forward under the toes) and backward diagonal (pressure moves back toward the heel) directions. Again, the shoulders should remain directly above the hips throughout the weight shift.
- Have participants perform a quick visual check to see that the knee is directly above the foot at the end of the forward diagonal weight shift.
- Check to see that participants are maintaining slightly flexed knees on the lateral and diagonal weight shifts. Remind them to use soft knees.

When participants perform any of the progressions in this section with their eyes closed, remember to emphasize the sensory awareness cues that were first introduced during the level 6 seated weight shift progressions on pages 122-123.

Exercise Progressions

1. Forward and Backward Weight Shifts

a. Stand comfortably with feet hip-width apart.

b. Shift weight forward until pressure can be felt under the balls of the feet and the heels begin to lift off the floor. Return to a centered position. Repeat five times, and then repeat with the eyes closed for the same number of repetitions. The upper and lower body should move in the same direction.

c. Shift weight backward through the hips until the toes begin to rise from the floor. Return to a centered position. Repeat five times. Repeat with the eyes closed for the same number of repetitions.

d. Shift weight in the forward and backward directions without pausing in the center. Repeat the movement sequence 10 times. Repeat with the eyes closed for the same number of repetitions.

2. Lateral Weight Shifts

a. Shift weight through the right hip until the inside edge of the right foot begins to lift from the floor. Return to a centered position. Repeat five times before changing sides.

b. Repeat the weight shift to the left side. Return to a centered position.

c. Shift weight from left to right without pausing in the center. The shoulders should be aligned directly above the hips and should remain relaxed and level throughout the exercise.

3. Forward Diagonal Weight Shifts

a. Position the right foot so that the heel of that foot is ahead of and to the side of the toes of the left foot.

b. Slowly shift weight forward through the right hip until the knee is directly above the toes of the right foot. The right knee should bend as the weight transitions forward. The upper body should remain erect and facing forward throughout the weight shift. The shoulders should remain relaxed and level.

c. Hold for a count of three and return to a centered position. Repeat five times.

d. Reverse the position of the feet so that the heel of the left foot is now ahead and to the side of the right foot.

e. Repeat the diagonal weight shift forward and to the left.

f. Hold for a count of three and return to a centered position. Repeat five times.

g. Repeat each forward and diagonal weight shift with the eyes closed.

4. Backward Diagonal Weight Shifts

a. Position the left foot so that the heel is ahead of the toes of the right foot.

b. Shift weight backward and diagonally through the hip until foot pressure is centered over the right heel. Bend the right knee during the backward transition. The upper body should remain erect and facing forward. The shoulders should be directly aligned above the hips and remain relaxed and level.

c. Hold for three counts and return to a centered position.

d. Repeat five times before changing the position of the feet.

e. Repeat the backward and diagonal weight shifts to the left.

f. Repeat the exercise with the eyes closed.

5. Forward and Backward Diagonal Weight Shifts

a. Begin by moving diagonally forward to the right and then diagonally backward to the left without pausing at a centered position.

b. Repeat five times before repositioning the feet and performing the exercise on the opposite diagonal.

c. Repeat the exercise with the eyes closed.

6. Combination Backward Weight Shifts

a. Position the feet hip-width apart and focus the eyes on a forward visual target at eye level. The upper body should remain erect with the shoulders relaxed and level.

b. Shift weight backward through the right hip until the pressure increases under the right heel. Return to a centered position.

c. Shift weight directly backward through both hips until the pressure increases under both heels. Return to a centered position.

d. Shift weight backward through the left hip until the pressure increases under the left heel. Return to a centered position.

e. Repeat the exercise with the eyes closed.

Position participants close to a wall for this last exercise progression so they can use the wall as a tactile cue at the end of each backward movement (figure 4.25). Touching the wall reinforces the need to shift the weight through the hips. A fun set of verbal cues to use during this exercise is, "Right cheek touches, both cheeks touch, left cheek touches."

Refer to the feature on page 135 for other ideas on increasing the balance challenge associated with each of these exercise progressions once the participants have become comfortable performing the progressions on a firm surface with their eyes closed. In addition, a good culminating activity to perform at the end of level 3 exercise progressions is shift around the clock, which is described on page 145.

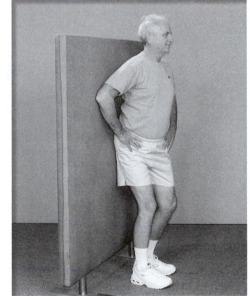

Figure 4.25 Backward weight shifts against a wall.

LEVEL 4: WEIGHT TRANSFERS WITH HEAD AND BODY MOVEMENTS

The marching progressions described in this section challenge motor coordination (e.g., four-corner marching—head turns first) as well as adaptive postural control, particularly when the client is marching in place with the head turned to one side during the marching activity. Level 4 activities improve the client's ability to perform daily activities that require turning the head while walking, such as when checking oncoming traffic before crossing the road or responding to a friend's greeting. Because many older adults become unstable when they perform these types of activities, the marching progressions in this section will be very helpful.

Exercise Progressions

1. Marching in Place on a Firm Surface

    a. Emphasize lifting the knees directly to the ceiling.

    b. Perform this exercise for 30 seconds. Keep the upper body and head erect and the eyes directed forward.

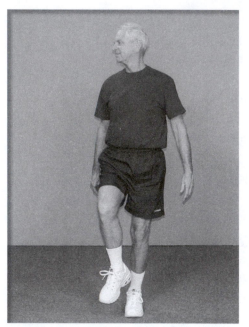

2. Marching in Place With Head Turns

    a. March in place for eight counts with the head erect and the eyes directed forward.

    b. Continue marching for an additional eight counts while turning the head a quarter turn to the right (figure 4.26).

    c. Turn the head back to a forward position while continuing to march for eight counts.

    d. Keep marching, but now turn the head a quarter turn to the left.

3. Four-Corner Marching

    a. March for eight counts with the head and eyes directed forward.

    b. Continue to march for eight counts but turn the head and body a quarter turn to the right.

    c. Continue marching and turning the head and body a quarter turn for eight counts until four turns have been completed.

Figure 4.26 Marching in place with the head turned to the right.

4. Four-Corner Marching—Head Turns First

    a. Repeat the four-corner marching exercise, but now turn the head before turning the body on each quarter turn (i.e., turn the head to the right for eight counts and then turn the body to the right for 8 counts).

    b. Continue gaze fixation on each quarter turn.

Safety Tips
for Marching With Head Turns

- Increase the number of marching counts between turns if the participant experiences any dizziness.
- Encourage gaze fixation with each quarter turn.

LEVEL 5: DYNAMIC WEIGHT TRANSFERS

The progressions described in this section focus on improving anticipatory control skills (weight must be shifted onto the stance leg prior to weight transfer onto the stepping limb) and serve as excellent lead-up activities to the gait pattern enhancement and variation progressions described in chapter 7. These activities also continue to reinforce leading with the trunk as opposed to the head and shoulders. These progressions are similar to the types of lower-body movements characteristic of many basic tai chi exercises.

Exercise Progressions

1. Forward Right and Left Step

   a. Begin with a weight shift through the left hip to unload weight from the right leg. Step forward with the right foot (use colored spots to indicate the desired stepping distance; see figure 4.27). Make sure the right knee is bent as the right foot contacts the floor and that the knee is directly above the right foot at the completion of the forward step. Hold the position for three counts. Then shift weight backward through the left hip until the weight is centered over the left foot. Step backward with the right foot. Perform each forward step activity multiple times before changing the leading leg.

   b. Repeat the exercise with the eyes closed.

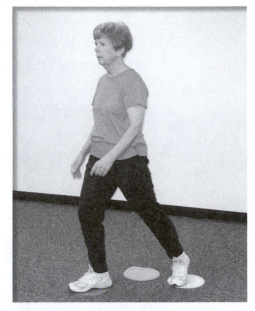

Figure 4.27 Colored spots on the floor are used to guide the desired stepping distance during the forward step.

2. Four-Corner Stepping

   a. Step in a forward direction with the right foot followed by the left foot. Shift weight onto the left foot, and then step back with the right foot followed by the left foot (use colored spots to indicate the desired stepping distance; see figure 4.28).

   b. Repeat the exercise with the eyes closed.

There are many fun ways to increase the balance challenge associated with each exercise progression. Refer to the feature on page 135 for ways to manipulate the task or environmental demands to increase the balance challenge. To help participants practice manipulating the COG during standing activities, you can introduce culminating activities such as line passing, creek crossing, and rock hopping. Each of these activities requires the class participants to dynamically control the COG while leaning in or shifting weight different directions or transferring weight through space.

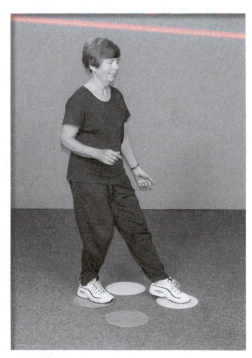

Figure 4.28 Backward weight shift with eyes closed during the four-corner stepping activity.

LEVEL 6: KICKING STATIONARY OBJECTS

The focus in this set of challenging progressions is on further developing the clients' anticipatory postural control skills as well as their ability to perform dynamic weight shifts in a reduced base of support. What makes these progressions even more challenging is the addition of external pacing demands. You will need to be particularly mindful of providing a safe environment when presenting this activity in a group class environment. Please follow the safety tips provided.

Exercise Progression

Ball Kicking

a. Practice kicking a ball against a wall or to a partner who rolls the ball back. When first practicing kicking the ball, hold onto a nearby sturdy chair.

b. As skill level improves, alternate the leg used to kick or trap the ball on each repetition.

> **Safety Tips When Kicking Stationary Objects**
>
> - Position participants who are less accomplished so they are kicking against the wall as opposed to another individual.
> - Instruct participants to stop the ball completely with the foot before attempting to kick it back to the wall or a partner.
> - Position participants who are less stable close to a wall or chair so they can hold on during the trapping and kicking phase of the action.
> - Demonstrate and then encourage participants to kick the ball with the instep for better control.
> - Increase the amount of supervision and support available to participants during this exercise because it requires greater postural control, particularly during the kicking phase.

LEVEL 7: WEIGHT SHIFTS AND TRANSFERS AGAINST GRAVITY

When performing each of the exercise progressions described in level 7, be sure to select the bench height that is best suited to the capabilities of each participant. A good way to determine the best height is to start all the participants at the 2-inch (5 cm) height and observe their overall postural stability while they perform at least four forward and backward toe touches. Progress participants to using the 4-inch (10 cm) bench if they perform the toe touches on the lower-height bench satisfactorily. If a participant begins to lose balance on the forward toe touches or rotates the trunk on the backward toe touches at either of these two bench heights, then do not progress to the 6-inch (15 cm) bench height. Pay close attention to good form during these progressions, particularly when the participants are performing sustained heel raises or step-up, step-down, and swing-through step activities that require the participants to be in a single-leg stance as the leading leg travels up onto and over the bench.

Exercise Progressions

1. Alternating Toe Touches Onto Bench

a. Alternate touching the feet onto a 2-, 4-, or 6-inch (5, 10, or 15 cm) bench. Place only the forefoot on the bench with each toe touch.

b. The knee should be directly above the lead foot on contact.

2. Alternating and Sustained Foot or Forefoot Touches

a. Take weight onto the entire foot touching the bench until the stance leg leaves the floor (see figure 4.29). Hold for 2 to 5 seconds. Imagine that a string tied around the waist is being pulled forward as the foot contacts the bench and assumes the weight of the body.

b. If stability allows, limit foot contact on the bench to the forefoot as was the case for the previous exercise progression. This more challenging form of the toe touch reduces the base of support and requires greater strength in the calf muscles, in particular.

3. Forward Step-Up and Step-Down

Step forward onto and then off of the bench, ending on same side of the bench as the starting position.

4. Forward Step-Up and Step-Down, Opposite Side

a. Step forward onto and then off of the bench, ending on the opposite side of the bench from the starting position.

b. Return to the original position in front of the bench or turn 180 degrees in place and repeat the exercise. Alternate the lead foot on each repetition.

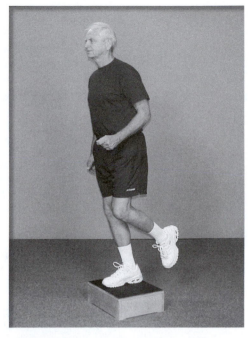

Figure 4.29 Sustained foot or forefoot touches in a forward direction.

5. Forward Swing-Through Step

a. Step forward onto the bench with the lead leg and swing the other leg through, making contact with the bench with only one foot (i.e., step up with the right, swing through with the left, step down with the right; see figure 4.30).

b. Turn in place and repeat the exercise with the opposite leg acting as the lead leg (i.e., step up with the left, swing through with the right, step down with the left).

6. Side Toe Touch

a. Lift the foot closest to the bench up onto the bench and toward the center. Return the foot to its starting position on the ground.

b. Repeat the activity 4 to 5 times with the right foot leading before performing the same progression with the left foot leading the action.

c. Maintain a tall posture with the eyes focused on a vertical target at eye level as the foot is lifted onto the bench.

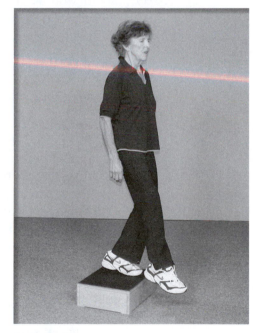

Figure 4.30 Forward swing-through steps on the bench.

7. Sustained Side Raise

a. Lift the foot closest to the bench up onto the bench and shift weight until the other foot is no longer in contact with the floor. Hold for 3 seconds and lower the foot to the floor. Emphasize an erect posture with the eyes directed forward at a visual target during the rising portion of each exercise progression. Watch for excessive hip rotation on the rising phase. The leg in contact with the bench should remain slightly flexed at the knee.

b. Repeat the exercise using the other leg.

8. Side Step-Up and Step-Down

Step sideways onto and then off of the bench, ending on the same side of the bench as the starting position.

9. Side Step-Up and Step-Down, Opposite Side

Step sideways onto and off of the bench, ending on the opposite side of the bench from the starting position.

Once your class participants have practiced each of the progressions in level 7, you can begin to combine the various stepping activities they have been performing into progressively longer step aerobic routines. This culminating activity improves not only dynamic COG control but also memory and attention skills as you lead participants through progressively longer step sequences.

Remember that in order to be a successful instructor of a group-based balance and mobility program, you must be able to modify the exercise progressions in order to appropriately but safely challenge each class participant. The more you practice manipulating the challenge of different balance activities for individual clients, the better you will become at manipulating the task or environmental demands in order to optimize the challenge for the entire group. Since it is much easier to modify exercise progressions when you are working with only a single client, begin practicing with individuals before instructing a group of older adults.

Culminating Activities for Standing Balance

Pass the Potato, Please in Standing Position

Participants stand on a firm surface or various support surfaces and face each other in a circle. There should be a little less than an arm's length between each participant (no more than four participants in each circle). A ball is passed in multiple directions (e.g., directly ahead, on a diagonal, clockwise, counterclockwise) according to the instructor's commands or an individual you designate as the announcer in each group. You can also have participants call another participant's name in advance of passing the ball. By doing this you will encourage class members to learn each other's names. As participants become more comfortable performing the activity, the height of the pass can be varied (e.g., above the shoulders, below the knees). The weight of the ball may also be varied.

Hot Potato in Standing Position

A variation of the passing activity just described is hot potato. The objective of this activity is to pass the ball around the circle as quickly as possible. Alternatively, you can also organize participants into two staggered lines facing each other. Requiring participants to perform the passing task more quickly places an added challenge on the postural control system. Add a second ball to further increase the attentional demands associated with the task. Adding balls of different weights will also improve upper-body strength. Instruct participants to reverse the direction of their passing on the verbal command of "Change." Because you have now added an external timing component to the task, you must remind participants that balance comes first. They should not try to receive or pass the object if they feel they are about to lose their balance. For more competitive class participants who are not that stable, lower the level of challenge (e.g., move them from a compliant to a firm standing surface) so their safety is maximized.

Balloon Volleyball in Standing Position

Participants stand in the same circle formation used in the previous activities (see figure 4.31). Their goal is to tap a balloon to one another as many times as possible before the balloon contacts the floor. Like the seated version of this activity, the standing version further diverts attention from the task of balancing, requiring that balance be controlled at a more subconscious level. Start this activity with everyone standing on a firm surface and note the level of postural control and eye–hand coordination being exhibited by each participant before introducing altered support surfaces in subsequent repetitions. Again, pay close attention to the more competitive class participants. Station an assistant close by to provide a verbal reminder that balance comes first or to provide manual assistance.

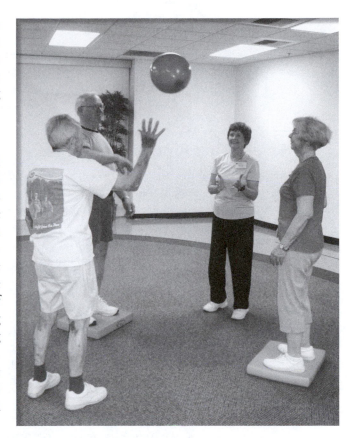

Figure 4.31 Balloon volleyball. This culminating activity can be made more challenging for some participants by altering the support surface.

Shift Around the Clock

While standing with feet flat on the floor and hip-width apart, participants lean to various positions on an imaginary clock face (e.g., 5 o'clock, center, 11 o'clock, center). Participants are to imagine that they are standing in the center of a clock face that is directly below them on the floor. Unlike the sitting version of this activity described on page 130, participants will lean the body toward some positions on the clock (i.e., 12 o'clock, 1 o'clock, and 11 o'clock) and shift their weight through the hips to other clock face positions (i.e., 3 o'clock, 5 o'clock, 6 o'clock, 7 o'clock, and 9 o'clock). Begin each lean or weight shift to a position on the clock from a centered position. Return to a centered position after each movement. Progress the activity by requiring participants to lean or shift from one position on the clock to another without returning back to the center (e.g., 1 o'clock, 7 o'clock). Increase the speed at which the clock positions are announced to further challenge participants. Both memory and motor coordination will improve as an outcome of this activity.

Fast Feet

This group activity encourages class participants to move a little faster when performing weight transfers. Participants stand with their feet flat on the floor and hip-width apart. Begin by asking participants to move the right or left foot away from and back to the starting position in a forward, backward, or lateral direction following your command. For example, you might call out the following sequence: "Right forward, left back, right side, left side." Begin at a slow pace and gradually increase the speed of your verbal commands. You can then progress this activity by instructing your participants to transfer their weight more fully by lunging in each direction as it is called.

Line Passing

This group activity provides participants with an opportunity to practice weight shifts while performing a secondary task of passing an object (figure 4.32). Once participants progress to the point of standing on altered surfaces, this activity will also improve lower-body strength. Upper-body flexibility is enhanced by the different passing activities, as is upper-body strength when the object being passed is weighted.

Participants (4 to 6 per group) form a line, standing one behind the other and approximately an arm's length apart. Organize the line so the shortest person is at the front and the tallest is at the rear. The objective of the activity is to pass an object down the line, beginning with the person at the front. When the object reaches the last person in the line, it is then passed back toward the front. Line passing is performed while participants are standing on different surface types (e.g., compliant, moving). When instructing this activity, have only the odd-numbered people in the line stand on a compliant or moving surface, with the even-numbered participants standing on a firm surface. After several passing rotations, have participants move forward one place (if they are ready to be on a compliant surface) so that the even-numbered participants are standing on the altered surface. The person standing at the front of the line moves to the end.

When leading this group exercise, try the following types of passing activities:

- Pass the ball laterally. The first person in line passes the ball by rotating the trunk to the right and passing the ball at waist height to the person immediately behind. The second person then rotates the trunk to the left and passes

> ### Safety Tips for Line Passing
>
> - Organize participants in the group according to height so that passing is made easier.
> - Make sure that participants remain approximately an arm's length apart when standing in the line.
> - Match the difficulty of the standing surface to the participant's capabilities as the activity is progressed in later classes. For added safety in group environments, alternate the use of firm and altered surfaces between participants standing in the line.
> - Organize the line so that participants are standing near a wall and the last person in line is being well supervised or has a wall behind. Either you or an assistant should walk down the line, providing manual assistance where appropriate.

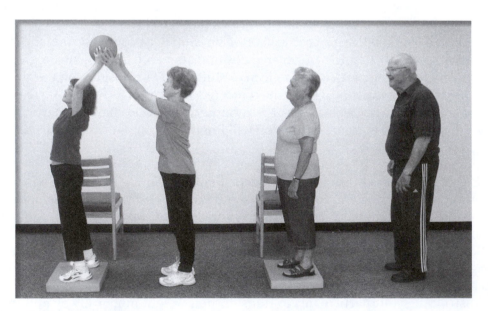

Figure 4.32 Line passing.

the ball to the person behind. Alternate passing sides for the return trip to the front. The weight shift should occur to the side opposite the passing side.

- Pass the ball above and behind the head. This activity requires a forward weight shift as the ball is lifted above and behind the head.
- Pass the ball between the legs. Remind participants to keep the head level and eyes directed forward as the ball is passed between the legs. Their weight should be centered over the feet as much as possible during the passing motion.
- Combine over-the-head and between-the-legs passing.

Increase the challenge of the group activity in any of the following ways:

- Increase the weight of the ball being passed.
- Alter the support surface on which the participant is standing. When teaching a group of participants, do not have all participants stand on an altered surface simultaneously. Rather, have every other person in the line stand on an altered surface and then have participants switch to the firm surface after a certain number of repetitions.
- Add a timing constraint (i.e., aim for a maximum number of successful passes in 30 seconds).
- Add a secondary cognitive task such as counting by 3s (3, 6, 9, 12) along the line or calling out the name of an animal beginning with a letter announced by the instructor.

Creek Crossing

Lay out two lines of masking tape that are approximately 5 to 6 feet (1.5-1.8 m) in length and grow from approximately 6 inches (15 cm) to 18 inches (46 cm) apart. The area between the two lines is the creek, and the areas beyond each line are the creek banks. The goal for the participants is to see how many times they can cross the creek, beginning at its narrowest end, before getting their feet wet (i.e., before touching the floor in the space between the two lines). Following is a suitable exercise progression:

a. Instruct participants to step forward across the creek, turn, and step back to the starting side until they are unable to take a long enough step to avoid getting their feet wet.

b. Instruct participants to place only one foot on the opposite bank (i.e., beyond the second tape line) and then return it to the same side of the creek without getting it wet (equates to a forward lunge of increasing distance). Have them alternate the lead leg on each repetition.

c. Place objects in the creek (i.e., on the floor between the two lines) for participants to pick up as they cross it. On the return trip, they place the objects back in the creek.

d. Instruct participants to step forward across the creek and then step backward when returning to the starting side. (This is an advanced activity suitable only for your more accomplished clients.)

Rock Hopping

Place colored spots at different intervals between the two tape lines representing the creek. The spots represent rocks, and the participants' goal is to reach the other

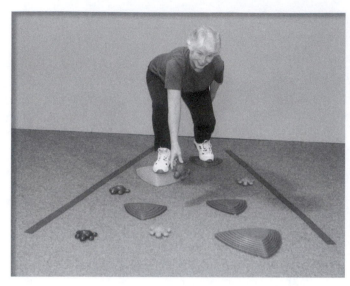

Figure 4.33 Rock hopping. The activity can be made more challenging by requiring participants to pick up objects from the creek bed.

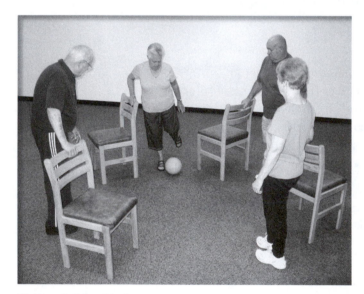

Figure 4.34 Circle soccer.

end of the creek by stepping on the rocks and the creek banks without getting the feet wet. Increase the balance challenge in the following ways:

a. Substitute Dyna-Discs for some of the colored spots so that the surfaces of certain rocks are more unstable as participants move down the creek.

b. Place objects in the creek that participants must bend down to retrieve on their way down the creek (figure 4.33).

Circle Soccer

Organize 4 to 5 participants into a circle in which they are at a comfortable distance from one another. Have the participants kick a soccer ball to one another, keeping the ball within the circle as it is passed among the group members (figure 4.34). Have participants call a person's name before kicking the ball to that person. One point is scored for every successful trap and kick within the circle. Instruct participants who are less stable to hold onto a chair as they trap and kick the ball. Alternatively, divide your class into groups based on stability level and have the participants who are less stable enjoy the game from a seated position while the participants with greater stability perform it in a standing position (with a sturdy chair nearby).

FLOOR-TO-STANDING TRANSFERS

All participants must practice floor-to-standing transfers many times throughout the program (figure 4.35). Many older adults are unaware of the procedures for rising safely from the floor. Safe rising is an important skill to teach your participants in case they fall when alone at home. It has been well documented that morbidity and mortality rates associated with falls increase in proportion to the length of time a person lies after falling. In the following section, the floor-to-standing progression is divided into levels of difficulty from easiest to most difficult. You will also notice that two different floor-to-standing transfer strategies are described under the more difficult category. The first strategy emphasizes upper-body strength, whereas the second strategy emphasizes lower-body strength and hip flexibility. The most difficult transfer strategy is described but not illustrated because it is very difficult for most older adults to use successfully unless they are well conditioned and free of injury.

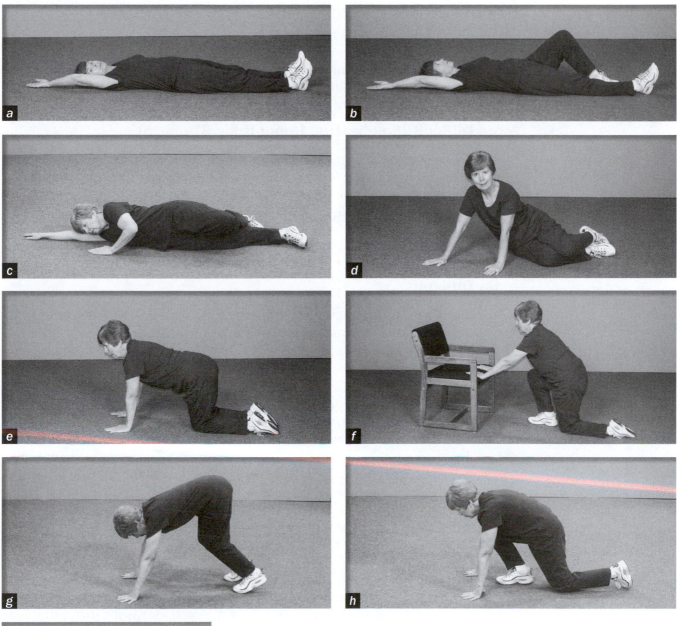

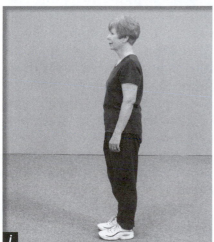

Figure 4.35 Floor-to-standing transfers: *(a)* Begin in supine or prone position, with one arm extended. *(b)* Flex the opposite knee. *(c)* Roll toward the extended arm until a side-lying position is reached. *(d)* Push up into a side-sitting position. *(e)* Rotate the body until kneeling with the hands on the floor. *(f)* Walk, using the hands, to external support (easiest transition to standing) or *(g)* walk, using the hands, to standing (requires good upper-body strength) or *(h)* half-kneel to standing (requires good hip range of motion and lower-body strength). *(i)* Finish in standing position.

Floor-to-Standing Progressions

Easiest

Move from a supine or prone position to a side-lying position to a side-sitting position. From there, move to kneeling with the hands on the floor. Then crawl to an external support to pull up to standing.

More Difficult (Emphasizes Upper-Body Strength)

Move from a supine or prone position to a side-lying position to a side-sitting position. From there, move to kneeling with the hands on the floor. Then walk, using the hands, to standing.

Still More Difficult (Emphasizes Lower-Body Strength)

Move from a supine or prone position to a side-lying position to a side-sitting position. From there, move to kneeling to half-kneeling to standing.

Most Difficult

Move from a supine or prone position to a symmetrical sit-up. Then move from a squat to leg reliance to standing (not pictured).

SUMMARY

This chapter describes progressive balance activities in seated, standing, and moving environments that will help the older adults in your program better understand how to control the COG when they are required to stand steadily in space, lean through their limits of stability, or perform a variety of weight transfers. Participants learn not only how to consciously control the COG in static and dynamic balance environments but also how to control it subconsciously when they are unexpectedly perturbed or performing a second task that forces them to divide their attention between it and balancing. Many of the exercise progressions presented here, particularly the bench activities in level 7, also improve anticipatory postural control.

Once participants have adequately practiced each of the core exercise progressions, you can increase the balance challenge by altering the task or environmental demands associated with the various exercises. Several ideas for increasing balance challenge were presented on pages 114-115 and 135. As important as it is to maximize the balance challenge associated with a set of exercise progressions, it is equally important to minimize the risk of injury. Throughout the chapter are safety tips and exercise precautions that you should carefully review and follow whenever you are presenting a set of exercise progressions. Also remember that the FallProof program is designed to be taught in group settings, so not all class participants will be ready for the same level of balance challenge when performing a set of activities. Here is where your knowledge of the client and your interpretation of their preprogram test results will help you determine what types of COG activities each client requires and the level at which each client should begin practicing those activities.

Test Your Understanding

1. To achieve a stable standing posture, the COG should be positioned such that
   a. it is outside of the base of support
   b. it is contained within the base of support
   c. it is close to the anterior border of the base of support
   d. it is close to the posterior border of the base of support
   e. the base of support is contained within the COG

2. You could lower the challenge for an individual who has difficulty performing the dynamic weight shift exercise progressions while sitting on a balance ball with the hands folded across the chest by having the individual perform the progressions
   a. while sitting on a chair with a Dyna-Disc
   b. while sitting on the balance ball with a ball holder
   c. while sitting on the ball with the hands resting on the thighs
   d. while sitting on the balance ball with the hands resting on the ball
   e. b and c

3. During seated COG control training, task difficulty can be manipulated by altering hand placement. The order of difficulty, from easiest to most difficult, is as follows:
   a. hands on ball, hands held above head, hands folded across chest
   b. hands folded across chest, hands on thighs, hands on ball
   c. hands holding onto assistant, hands on ball, hands folded across chest
   d. hands on ball, hands on thighs, hands folded across chest
   e. hands on thighs, hands on ball, hands folded across chest

4. Which of the following culminating activities is not an effective way to practice various seated activities that require dynamic COG control?
   a. pass the potato, please
   b. hot potato
   c. seated soccer
   d. balloon volleyball
   e. walk the gauntlet

5. Which of the following is an example of changing the environment to increase the level of difficulty?
   a. performing a continuous sequence of movements
   b. altering the type of support surface beneath the feet
   c. performing the selected movement while holding a weighted object
   d. changing the starting arm position from holding the seated surface to hands resting on thighs
   e. changing the seated support surface from a balance ball to a chair with a Dyna-Disc

6. Which of the following is not an appropriate example of an exercise involving dynamic weight transfers through space?
   a. marching in place
   b. rock hopping
   c. forward stepping

    d. four-corner stepping

    e. creek crossing

7. Which of the following is an example of changing the task demands to increase the balance challenge?

    a. reducing the amount of vision available

    b. altering the support surface beneath the feet

    c. performing the activity with a reduced base of support

    d. moving the participant from a ball to Dyna-Disc

    e. performing the activity in front of a busy background (e.g., a checkerboard)

8. Which of the following is an appropriate culminating activity for standing COG control training with weight shifts?

    a. fast feet

    b. line passing

    c. seated soccer

    d. walk the gauntlet

    e. rock hopping

9. Which of the following is a way to increase the task demands of a seated balance activity?

    a. changing the seated support surface

    b. changing the starting arm position from resting on the thighs to holding onto the seated support surface

    c. reducing the amount of vision available

    d. altering the support surface beneath the feet

    e. performing a secondary task at the same time

Practical Problems

1. Experiment with performing the various exercise progressions presented in the chapter so you can better understand how the difficulty of an exercise changes with each variable (i.e., task or environmental demand) that you manipulate. To an outside observer, many of these exercise progressions look very simple; however, once you try them yourself, you can appreciate just how challenging many of them can be, even for a younger adult.

2. Develop a set of seated and standing exercise progressions suitable for Phoebe and Larry, who are members of the same group class. Assume it is the first week of class and you are preparing your 10-minute COG training component to be presented during the skills section of the class. Indicate how you would structure the practice environment in order to optimize the level of balance challenge for each participant. Finally, indicate what types of support surfaces you would have Larry and Phoebe work on during the culminating activities you select for each class. Be sure to review the possible underlying impairments you identified from Larry and Phoebe's test results (presented in chapter 3) so that you can optimize balance challenge while ensuring the safety of both clients.

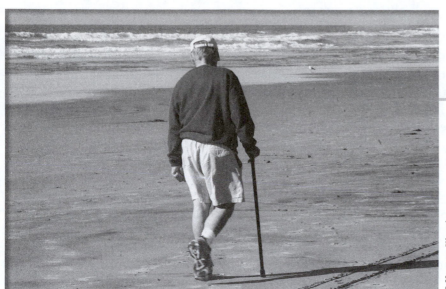
© Human Kinetics

Chapter 5

Multisensory Training

Objectives

After completing this chapter, you will be able to

- describe how each of the three sensory systems (visual, somatosensory, vestibular) contributes to postural control in different sensory environments,
- understand how a given sensory system impairment will affect exercise selection and progression,
- develop a set of exercise progressions to improve the use of the three sensory systems to control balance, and
- structure a safe practice environment.

Our ability to perceive where we are and how we should respond to changing sensory conditions during our daily lives is heavily dependent on (a) the amount and quality of information we receive from our peripheral sensory receptors and (b) how we organize and integrate that information once it has reached the CNS. Each of the three sensory systems (visual, vestibular, and somatosensory) contributing to balance and mobility experiences significant changes as a function of the aging process. Visual acuity, contrast sensitivity, and depth perception decline; the threshold for detecting vibration and joint movement increases; and the number of sensory receptors (hair cells) within the vestibular apparatus drops (Rose, 2005). A reduction in the gain of the vestibulo-ocular reflex (VOR) with advancing age has also been documented (Wolfson, 1997).

Although older adults generally are able to compensate for small age-related changes occurring in each of these systems, impairments associated with particular medical diagnoses (e.g., macular degeneration, peripheral sensory neuropathy,

Ménière's disease) and severe deconditioning will adversely affect their postural control system and limit both the types of activities they can perform successfully and the environments in which they can function safely. The activities presented in this chapter optimize the functioning of the unimpaired sensory systems while compensating for the systems that are known to be permanently impaired. The effectiveness of sensory training programs on selected measures of balance has already been demonstrated for healthy older adults (Hu & Woollacott, 1994a, 1994b), providing a strong rationale for including sensory training in a multidimensional program targeting older adults who are at increased risk for falls.

The use of vision is optimized by teaching gaze-stabilization strategies during seated, standing, and locomotor activities. Performing balance activities on a compliant or moving support surface also promotes the use of vision for controlling balance by compromising the somatosensory system, thereby making it more difficult to obtain accurate sensory information from the surface. Conversely, the use of the somatosensory system as the primary source of sensory information is optimized by compromising vision and maximizing the quality and quantity of somatosensory information obtained by having clients perform balance activities with the feet in contact with a firm, broad surface. Having the participant wear dark glasses or engaging vision by introducing a second task such as reading, tracking objects, reaching for objects, or catching objects is an effective way to reduce the older adult's reliance on vision to control balance. Vision can also be removed by having participants perform activities with the eyes closed once they reach a higher level of performance and feel comfortable performing activities in the absence of vision.

Finally, an increased reliance on vestibular input for balance can be achieved by manipulating both the visual *and* the somatosensory systems. Performing a variety of balance activities on compliant or moving surfaces while vision is distracted (by introducing movement in the field of view), engaged in performing a second task, or absent encourages greater reliance on vestibular information. Of course, knowing which multisensory activities are most appropriate for each participant requires a careful review of the participant's medical history completed at the outset of the program (to ascertain whether certain sensory systems are permanently impaired due to an existing pathology) and the participant's performance on certain test items on the FAB scale (items 1, 3, 7, and 9, in particular) that was conducted as part of the screening and assessment described in chapter 3.

In addition to describing exercises that improve each of the three sensory systems contributing to balance and mobility, this chapter introduces several exercises that improve the older adult's ability to coordinate head and eye movements. These exercises involve the visual system alone or the visual and vestibular systems working together. For example, when the head is stationary and the eyes are moving as they track an object through the visual field (i.e., smooth pursuit), the visual system is being exercised. Once the head begins to move, however, the vestibular system is also activated. As described in chapter 1, the VOR becomes important when turning the head quickly to focus on a target or acknowledge a friend who has called our name. In these situations, the VOR is activated to prevent retinal slip (when the speed of eye movement is not equal to the speed of head movement) by moving the eyes at the same velocity but in the opposite direction as the head (Herdman, 2007). This reflex helps us perceive that the world is stable as we move through space. Older adults with an abnormal VOR often experience vertigo (i.e., an illusion that oneself or the environment is moving). In other situations, when the head and eyes are tracking an object, the VOR must be canceled so that the head and eyes move in the same direction. Individuals who are unable to effectively cancel the VOR do not exhibit smooth eye movements as they track objects. The eyes may periodically jump in order to catch up with the moving object and bring it back into focus.

The exercises in this chapter improve the older adult's ability to use the available sensory information to better control balance and to improve coordination of eye and head movements. More specifically, the goals of multisensory training are as follows:

- Improve the functioning of the somatosensory system by manipulating or removing vision
- Improve the use of visual inputs for balance by manipulating the somatosensory system
- Improve vestibular system function by manipulating both the somatosensory and visual systems
- Enhance the coordination between the visual and vestibular systems

Two guiding principles should be followed when selecting exercises intended to force the use of each of the three sensory systems contributing to balance. You should (1) force the use of systems when the impairments are temporary or changeable and (2) compensate or substitute for system impairments that are permanent or progressive.

Safety Reminders

◆ Review the health history of each participant before introducing *any* multisensory training activities to ensure that you are not asking participants to perform any activities that might compromise their safety. Be sure to review the test results and interpretation sheet associated with the FAB scale before choosing any of the multisensory activities that are intended to force the use of a particular sensory system.

◆ Ask participants to cease performing any activity if they become dizzy or disoriented. If certain clients regularly experience dizziness during a class, recommend that they pay a visit to their primary care physician to discuss the problem.

◆ Remember that for sensory systems with temporary impairments, the goal is to introduce activities that force their use, whereas for permanent sensory system impairments, the goal is to compensate for the loss by introducing activities that improve function in the remaining systems.

◆ Do not introduce the next exercise progression in any level until the previous one can be performed with good balance.

◆ Be aware that some participants may be able to perform the more advanced activities associated with one set of sensory exercises but not those associated with another set of exercises due to an impairment in a different sensory system.

FORCING THE USE OF THE SOMATOSENSORY SYSTEM TO CONTROL BALANCE

Participants who do not have a medical diagnosis indicating that their somatosensory system is permanently or progressively impaired (e.g., peripheral sensory neuropathy or loss of sensation in the feet or lower limbs) should derive considerable benefit from engaging in balance activities that force them to select somatosensory (touch and proprioception) inputs to control balance. To decide whether forcing the use of the somatosensory system is desirable, you must first review the health and activity questionnaire completed by each participant in conjunction with the FAB scale results. Take a moment to review the health and activity questionnaires completed by our two case study participants to determine if they have any impairments that are likely to affect their use of the somatosensory system. You'll find Phoebe's questionnaire on pages 18 through 23 and Larry's questionnaire on pages 25 through 30.

After checking the health and activity questionnaire for any medical diagnosis or self-report of sensation loss in the feet and ankles, review the results obtained for test item 1 (stand with feet together, eyes closed) on the FAB scale or test item 6 (stand unsupported with eyes closed) on the BBS if you conducted that test for some of your lower-functioning clients. Recall that participants who perform poorly (i.e., demonstrate a large amount of sway or prematurely open their eyes) when standing on a firm surface with their eyes closed are not using somatosensory inputs effectively to control their balance—they are visually dependent. In the absence of any information on the health and activity questionnaire that suggests participants are experiencing a loss of sensation, you can be reasonably sure that introducing activities designed to force the use of the somatosensory system will be helpful, albeit challenging, during the early stages of practice. Now take a moment to review the scores obtained by Phoebe and Larry on test item 1 of the FAB scale or test item 6 on the BBS to determine if they are using somatosensory inputs appropriately.

Improving the use of somatosensory inputs is particularly important for older adults when they must perform daily activities in situations of reduced or absent lighting (e.g., walking in the community at night, entering a dark room, or getting up to go to the bathroom at night). The older adult who has significant changes in vision due to age or pathology will also benefit significantly from this type of sensory training. At the Braille Institute, we have found that older adults, even those who have lived with serious visual impairments for many years, do not use somatosensory inputs for balance as well as one might think. Despite their serious visual impairments, they do not automatically switch to using somatosensory inputs as their primary information source.

In order to force the use of the somatosensory system to control balance, you must structure the practice environment to ensure the surface below the feet is firm and to alter the visual environment. The following are four simple ways to alter the visual environment:

- Reduce vision by having the participants wear dark glasses during an activity.
- Remove vision by asking participants to close their eyes during an activity (figure 5.1).

- Engage vision by asking participants to read aloud or reach for or catch objects while performing an activity.

- Distract vision by having participants perform activities while in front of a busy visual pattern (e.g., checkerboard) or while a busy pattern is being moved through their visual field.

Seated Exercise Progressions

Many of the progressive seated balance activities presented in levels 1 through 4 and in level 6 of the COG training chapter are suitable activities for multisensory training. Just be sure that your clients are introduced to the selected progressions during COG training before introducing the progressions for multisensory training. For example, you should present and practice some, if not all, of the level 3 seated trunk lean progressions for COG training before introducing trunk leans into multisensory training. Introducing the selected progressions and observing participants practice them in an earlier class will help you decide whether you need to lower

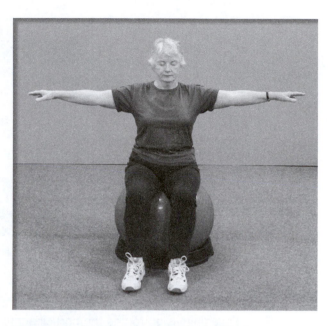

Figure 5.1   Performing activities with the eyes closed forces the participant to rely on somatosensory inputs for balance.

the level of challenge for participants who have a medical condition that affects sensory system function or who performed poorly on the sensory tests conducted during the initial assessment. Because the balance challenge increases as soon as you begin to manipulate the amount or quality of sensory information available to the participants, it will be helpful to know in advance how to structure the task demands so that participant safety is maximized.

Providing the sensory awareness cues listed on page 111 will be particularly important when you are trying to force the use of the somatosensory system. Instead of relying on vision to control balance, your clients will be relying on information from the cutaneous receptors and proprioceptors that make up the somatosensory system. Recall that the cutaneous receptors provide information about touch and pressure, while the proprioceptors tell us where our limbs are relative to one another. When you ask participants to feel the pressure under their feet move toward their toes as they lean forward, you are encouraging them to consciously attend to the information coming from the cutaneous receptors. In contrast, when you cue participants to sense that their shoulders are moving in front of their hips as they lean forward, you are encouraging them to use proprioceptive information to tell them where the shoulders are relative to the hips during the trunk lean.

The following are specific examples of how you can manipulate the visual environment to force the use of the somatosensory system for balance:

- Engage vision by having participants reach for objects of different sizes, weights, and shapes while sitting on a compliant surface with their feet in contact with a firm surface. Hold the objects at various distances and heights (figure 5.2). Encourage trunk movement in a variety of directions. Progress to throwing light objects to participants, varying the throwing heights and the weights of the objects according to the participants' individual capabilities. These activities force the use of the somatosensory system by using a second

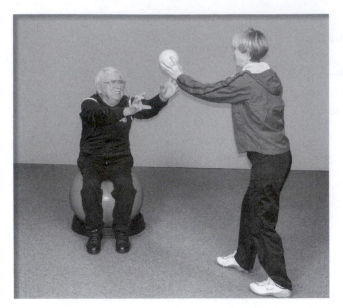

Figure 5.2 Engaging vision forces the participant to rely on somatosensory inputs for balance control.

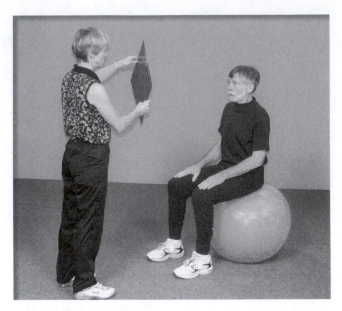

Figure 5.3 The participant must rely on somatosensory inputs to control balance when vision is distracted by an object with a busy surface pattern moving through the visual field.

task to engage the vision. The challenge of the activity can be increased by moving from a self-paced (i.e., reaching) to externally paced (i.e., throwing) practice environment.

- Reduce or remove vision by having participants practice seated weight shifts in a forward, backward, lateral, and diagonal direction while wearing dark glasses or closing their eyes.
- Distract vision by moving an object with a busy surface pattern (e.g., a checkerboard) quickly through the visual field while participants are seated with their feet in contact with a firm surface and hip-width apart (figure 5.3). Participants remain seated in a stable, upright position, keep their head stationary, and try to ignore the object moving through their field of view. This activity distracts vision and makes it impossible for participants to stabilize their gaze by focusing on a stationary target.

You can increase the balance challenge associated with a set of exercise progressions by manipulating several different task demands (see table 5.1). An easy way to increase the balance challenge is to move the client to a more difficult seated support surface. Although performing exercises while seated on a Dyna-Disc or balance ball reduces the amount and quality of the somatosensory information received at the level of the buttocks, the goal of the exercise is not compromised as long as the participant's feet are in contact with a firm ground surface. In addition, you have just learned in this section how to manipulate the environmental demands to force the use of the somatosensory system.

Table 5.1 Multisensory Training at a Glance

Core program components	Additional task demands	Environmental manipulations
Stimulate use of the somatosensory system: Reduce, remove, or engage vision while performing exercise progressions. Have feet in contact with a firm, broad surface.		
Sitting with feet on a firm surface Performing trunk leans in different directions Reaching for objects Catching and throwing objects Resisting perturbations	Altered base of support (e.g., Romberg, semi-tandem, tandem) Altered hand position (e.g., hands on object, thighs, across chest) Compliant surface (e.g., Dyna-Disc, balance ball) under buttocks External timing demand Second task to engage vision	Reduced or absent vision
Standing on a firm surface Performing dynamic weight shifts Marching in place	Altered base of support Altered hand position (folded across chest) Head movements (e.g., lateral, up and down) Second task to engage vision (e.g., ball toss, target search)	Reduced or absent vision
Moving on a firm surface Practicing altered gait patterns	Altered base of support External timing demand	Reduced or absent vision
Stimulate use of the visual system: Perform exercise progressions on compliant or moving surfaces.		
Seated on compliant surface with altered surface beneath feet	Altered base of support (e.g., Romberg, tandem, single leg)	Altered type of support surface beneath feet (e.g., change from foam to Dyna-Disc)
Standing on altered surface	Altered base of support Marching in place	Altered type of support surface (e.g., change thickness of foam beneath feet)
Walking across compliant surface	Altered base of support (e.g., toes, heels) Varied gait pattern (e.g., backward, long steps)	Altered type or thickness of support surface
Stimulate use of the vestibular system: Reduce, remove, engage, or distract vision. Have feet in contact with compliant or moving support surface while performing exercise progressions.		
Seated on compliant surface with reduced vision and altered surface beneath feet	Secondary task to engage vision Reduced base of support	Absent vision Altered type or thickness of support surface
Standing on altered surface with reduced vision	Secondary task to engage vision Marching in place	Absent vision Altered type of support surface (e.g., change from foam to Dyna-Disc)
Walking on altered surface with reduced vision	Secondary task to engage vision Reduced base of support Varied gait pattern	Absent vision Altered type of support surface (e.g., increased thickness of compliant surface)

Standing Exercise Progressions

Just as you did with the seated balance progressions, you can reintroduce selected standing exercise progressions from the COG training component of the program. Most if not all of the standing exercise progressions presented in levels 1 through 5 in the COG training chapter are suitable for multisensory training. In some cases, the standing exercise progressions will have been practiced in altered visual environments, as is the case with progressions 2 (standing while performing a cognitive task) and 3 (standing while performing an upper-body task) in level 2 (standing balance with altered base of support). However, the focus during the COG training was on increasing the challenge of the activity as opposed to forcing the use of the somatosensory system. Providing the same sensory awareness cues you delivered during the earlier seated balance progressions will shift the focus of the activity from increasing the balance challenge to relying on somatosensory inputs to control upright balance.

Moving Exercise Progressions

Once your participants have mastered the standing exercise progressions, you can introduce moving activities that increase the balance challenge and simulate the types of environments older adults might occasionally find themselves in, such as walking in a crowded mall or moving about in the dark. You will find other suitable activities in chapter 7, which describes the gait pattern enhancement and variation component of the program.

Walking Across the Room

a. Walk across the room on a firm surface while reading a poem or story out loud (see figure 5.4).

b. Walk across the room on a firm surface while passing objects back and forth to a partner.

c. Walk across the room on a firm surface while throwing and catching an object with and without a partner. Keep the height of the object's trajectory below the head so it is not necessary to tilt the head to track the object.

d. Walk across the room on a firm surface while wearing dark glasses or closing the eyes.

Do not progress participants to a higher-level exercise progression until they are able to perform the lower-level progression satisfactorily.

As with the seated and standing exercise progressions, you can increase the balance challenge during the moving activities by manipulating the demands of the task (see table 5.1). Good ways to increase the balance challenge during moving activities are to (a) introduce an external timing component (hand clap or metronome to pace the exercise), (b) alter the type of gait pattern used, or (c) alter the arm position (e.g., folded across the chest).

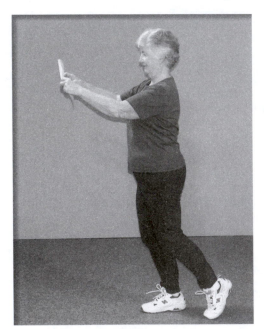

Figure 5.4 Walking while reading aloud.

In summary, the most important things to remember when selecting any exercise intended to make the somatosensory system the primary source of sensory information, whether in a seated, standing, or moving environment, is to ensure that the surface beneath the feet is firm and broad and that vision is manipulated in some way.

> **Safety Tip**
>
> Position participants close to a wall when they are walking with the eyes closed. Allow more fearful participants to open their eyes or lightly touch the wall periodically to enhance somatosensory input. To reduce participants' anxiety levels during early repetitions, you can also walk beside participants and positively reinforce them as they travel across the room.

FORCING THE USE OF THE VISUAL SYSTEM TO CONTROL BALANCE

In the previous set of exercises, you learned that in order to force your clients to rely more on the somatosensory system for controlling balance, you must provide a firm, broad surface for all activities and manipulate vision in some way. The goal in this section is just the reverse. To teach participants how to use their visual system more effectively to maintain balance, you must alter the type of surface on which they are standing to make it more difficult to use somatosensory information. Many of the exercise progressions described in the COG control training chapter and used to force the use of the somatosensory system are appropriate to include here. Three examples of balance activities you can use to encourage clients to use vision to control balance are the following:

- Sit tall on a compliant surface with the feet hip-width apart and in contact with a foam surface. Focus on a forward visual target that is vertical and at eye level for 10 to 15 seconds (figure 5.5).

- Stand on a compliant or moving surface (figure 5.6) with an altered base of support (i.e., Romberg position, split stance, semi-tandem position). Focus the eyes on a vertical target at eye level for 10 to 30 seconds.

- Walk across a foam surface (i.e., thin foam surface, large Airex Balance Pad) on the toes while focusing the eyes on a vertical target at eye level and directly ahead (figure 5.7).

Again, you can increase the balance challenge associated with a set of exercise progressions by manipulating several different task demands. Refer to table 5.1 (on page 159) for ideas.

Review the health and activity questionnaires completed by Phoebe and Larry to determine whether either participant has any diseases of the eye that would make it difficult to use vision to maintain balance. As you may recall from an earlier discussion in this chapter, it is not beneficial to force the use of a sensory system that is permanently impaired or becoming progressively more impaired over time (e.g., macular degeneration). Rather, you would select exercises that would force the use of other, non-impaired sensory systems, so that the older adult can compensate for the loss in one sensory system by maximizing the function of

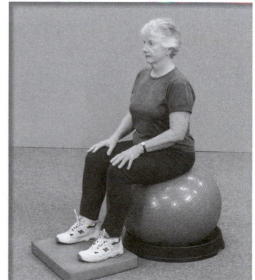

Figure 5.5 Altering the support surface beneath the feet and encouraging participants to focus on a visual target will improve their use of vision to control balance.

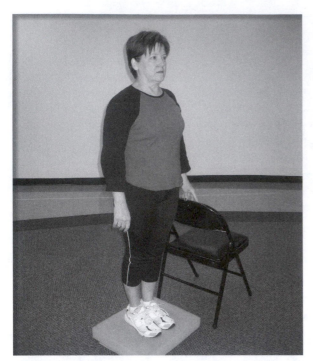

Figure 5.6 Standing on a foam surface while focusing on a visual target.

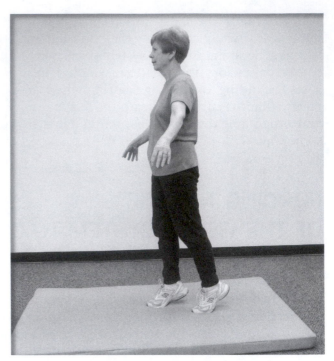

Figure 5.7 Walking across a foam surface on the toes while focusing on a visual target.

the other sensory systems. Maximizing the function of the somatosensory system would be particularly important if permanent or progressive impairments in the visual system were evident.

FORCING THE USE OF THE VESTIBULAR SYSTEM TO CONTROL BALANCE

To encourage participants to use the vestibular system as the primary system for maintaining balance, you must manipulate both the visual *and* somatosensory systems. You can accomplish this by varying the environmental constraints in one of the following ways:

- Perform exercises with reduced or absent vision on an unstable or compliant surface.
- Perform exercises on an unstable or compliant surface while vision is engaged by a second task (e.g., reading, tracking objects with the eyes only). The support surface must be compliant or moving to make it more difficult to distort somatosensory information and make it not as useful to the client for controlling balance.
- Perform exercises on an unstable or compliant surface while vision is being distracted. Visually focus on a busy background or a checkerboard or other busy display moving through the visual field.

Before proceeding, take a moment to review the health and activity questionnaires completed by Phoebe and Larry and determine whether they have any permanent impairments in the vestibular system that would contraindicate performing activities that force the use of the vestibular system. Then review their performances on item 7 (stand on foam with eyes closed) of the FAB scale to see if they experienced any difficulties maintaining balance in a sensory environment that requires using the vestibular system to maintain upright balance. Because there is no item on the BBS that can provide you with any information about vestibular system function, it is recommended that you conduct test item 7 on the FAB scale to obtain this type of information. In the case of very unstable participants, use only one Airex Balance Pad when conducting test item 7. Doing so will reduce the overall challenge of the test while still providing you with valuable information about your client's balance abilities when the surface below the feet is compliant and vision is no longer available.

Seated Exercise Progressions

Many of the exercise progressions presented in the chapter on COG training can be used to force the use of the vestibular system. Just be sure to manipulate vision in one of the three ways identified earlier and have clients perform all exercise progressions with the feet in contact with a compliant or moving surface. Because you must alter the environment so that two of the three sensory systems are not providing accurate information for balance, the degree of difficulty associated with each individual exercise progression is much higher. For that reason, the following individual exercise progressions within each level of the COG training are the most suitable for including in this section of the multisensory training:

a. Maintain an upright, stable posture while seated on a compliant surface (e.g., Dyna-Disc on chair, balance ball) with the feet also placed on a compliant or moving surface. Close the eyes and maintain balance for 10 to 15 seconds. (The exercise can be made less difficult by asking unsteady participants to wear dark glasses rather than close the eyes.)

b. Repeat the exercise with the feet in a reduced base of support (e.g., feet together, split stance, semi-tandem position).

c. Maintain seated balance while performing voluntary arm or leg movements. Remove or compromise vision and place the feet on a compliant or moving surface.

d. While seated on a compliant surface with an altered surface (e.g., foam pad, Dyna-Disc, rocker board) beneath the feet, toss an object from one hand to the other while visually tracking its movement (figure 5.8). Gradually increase the height of the toss between the hands until the head begins to move.

e. While seated on a compliant surface with an altered surface (e.g., foam pad, Dyna-Disc, rocker board) beneath the feet, reach for objects placed at different heights and distances from the body. Use multicolored objects, if available.

f. While seated on a compliant surface with an altered surface (e.g., foam pad, Dyna-Disc, rocker board) beneath the feet, use only the eyes to follow the movement of a checkerboard (held by the instructor or an assistant) through the visual field. The checkerboard should be moved in vertical, horizontal, and diagonal directions.

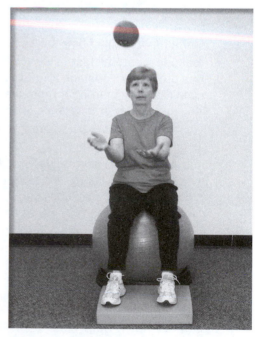

Figure 5.8 The vestibular system becomes an important source of balance information when the eyes are engaged in performing a secondary task and the support surface beneath the feet is altered.

Standing Exercise Progressions

Because it is necessary to disadvantage two of the three sensory systems in order to force the use of the vestibular system, it is important that your individual clients have mastered the seated activities before moving on to the more challenging set of standing activities described here. Check regularly for dizziness as the standing activities become more dynamic in nature.

a. Repeat each of the seated exercise progressions in a standing position.

b. While standing on a compliant surface (e.g., large foam pad), begin marching in place while vision is reduced (e.g., sunglasses are worn) or absent. If clients perform this activity with the eyes closed, begin by having them march no more than four steps with the eyes closed, followed by four steps with the eyes open. Increase the number of marches performed with eyes closed as stability improves (figure 5.9).

Moving Exercise Progressions

Before you introduce these higher-level activities to your clients, you must determine how to organize the practice environment to ensure the safety of the group. When working with a group on moving activities, particularly when vision is being manipulated, one of two strategies will maximize the safety of the group:

• Set up the compliant surfaces along a wall in your facility and have participants perform the activities sequentially as you verbally cue them to lightly touch the wall if they become unstable. You should also follow the more unstable clients in a close supervisory position.

Safety Tips

• Position the foam pad on a surface that will prevent it from sliding (e.g., a nonslip or carpeted surface) during the marching activities.

• Because postural instability increases when the eyes are closed, position clients close to a wall with a chair directly in front of them that they can touch lightly when performing the eyes-closed activities.

• To increase safety, ensure that there is adequate space between clients.

• Instruct participants to lightly hold onto the chair in front of them during the early eyes-closed repetitions. Observe the postural stability individual clients display when support is provided and decide whether clients may perform the marching activity without holding onto the chair or should continue using the chair in subsequent repetitions.

• Check to see that clients are not experiencing high levels of dizziness during this activity. If dizziness is a problem, instruct participants to reduce the height of the marching step, close their eyes for a shorter length of time, or hold onto the chair until they are able to perform the activity without experiencing dizziness. If none of these strategies work, ask the participant to stop performing the activity with the eyes closed.

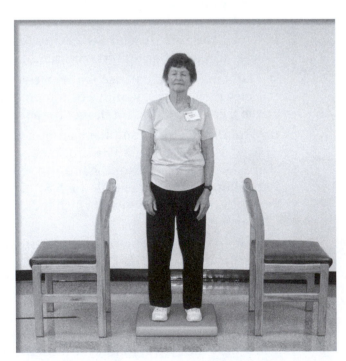

Figure 5.9   The vestibular system provides important information for balance when the surface beneath the feet is altered and vision is absent.

- A second strategy that is often effective is to divide the group and position half of the participants at one end of the room and the other half at the other end, with the groups facing each other. Then have a row of participants (two to three) begin by performing the moving activity until they reach the opposite end of the room and take a position as the last row of the group on that end. The first row of that group then begins the exercise in the opposite direction. You can follow behind each row of performers to monitor their safety. Make sure that you distribute your more unstable participants in different rows to make supervising them easier.

Walking Across Compliant Surface

a. Walk across a compliant surface (i.e., egg crate foam, floor mats) with vision reduced or absent (figure 5.10).

b. Walk forward across a compliant surface with vision reduced or absent using an altered base of support (e.g., toes, heels, tandem).

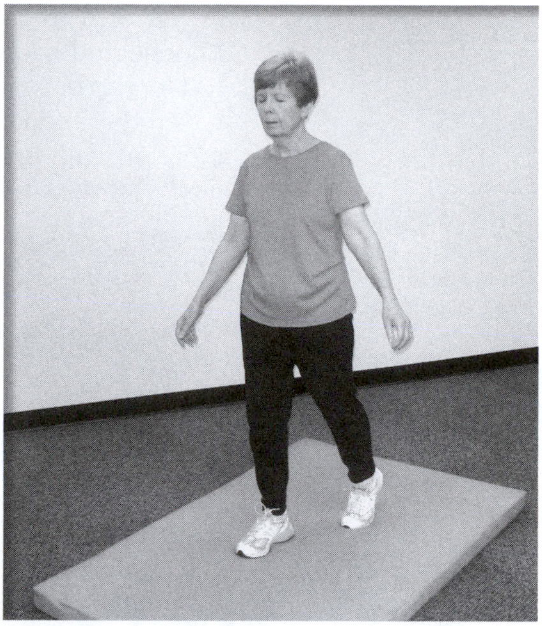

Figure 5.10 Walking across foam with eyes closed is a challenging vestibular activity for some older adults.

Culminating Activities

When you have practiced each of the individual exercise progressions for forcing the use of the somatosensory, visual, or vestibular systems, you can introduce culminating activities so that the participants can practice what they have learned in a fun, gamelike atmosphere. Several of the culminating activities described in the previous chapter can be introduced again in this component of the program. Games such as pass the potato, please; hot potato; and balloon volleyball can be used to force the use of the somatosensory system if played while clients are standing on a firm surface or the use of the vestibular system if played while clients are seated with feet on a compliant surface or standing on a compliant surface. In both variations of these games, vision is the system being manipulated because the client must track a moving object while playing. Shift around the clock is a good culminating activity for reinforcing what clients have learned in the visual training section as long as their feet are in contact with a compliant or moving surface so that the somatosensory system is manipulated. Although you may have involved clients in these games in earlier classes to reinforce various aspects of COG control, reintroducing the games here will reinforce the many skills that have been learned during the multisensory training. The games remain the same; the reason for playing has changed.

EXERCISES COORDINATING EYE AND HEAD MOVEMENTS

The exercises presented in this section improve a participant's ability to (a) move the eyes smoothly while focusing on a moving target, (b) move the head and eyes smoothly while focusing on a moving target, and (c) quickly move the head and eyes from one target to another without losing visual focus. These are excellent exercises to incorporate into the cool-down of the class or as a station activity. As you read through the following exercise progressions, which require participants to perform in seated, standing, and finally moving situations, be thinking of Phoebe and Larry and how they performed on the individual test items on the FAB scale that tested their ability to use the various sensory systems for balance. Given these test results, identify any exercises in this section that are likely to be more difficult for either Phoebe or Larry and note how you might modify the difficulty of the balance activity to ensure their safety and success.

LEVEL 1: EYE MOVEMENTS WITH STATIONARY HEAD WHILE SEATED

The progressions described in this level are designed to improve the older adult's ability to effectively track objects that are moving in space without moving the head or to rapidly move the eyes only between two targets. These exercises are intended to improve the functioning of the visual and vestibular systems that control, either alone or in combination, a wide range of eye and head movements.

Exercise Progressions

1. Smooth Pursuit (Slow) Eye Movements

  a. Move the eyes slowly through space while the head remains stationary. Hold a single target directly in front of the eyes and at arm's length from the face.

  b. Visually follow the target with the eyes as it is slowly moved from side to side, up and down, or diagonally while keeping the head still (figure 5.11). Perform the exercise in a seated position and continue for 30 seconds before resting.

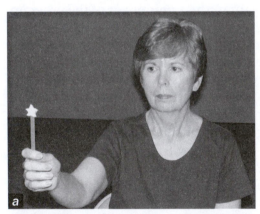
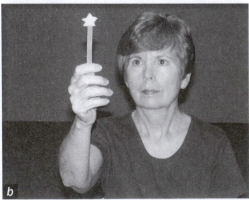
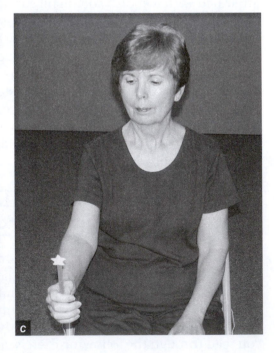

Figure 5.11 An object is slowly followed with the eyes (a) from side to side, (b) up and down, and (c) diagonally.

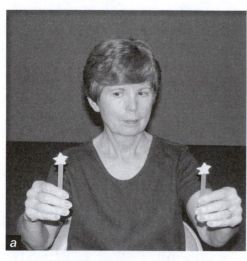 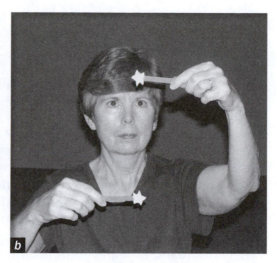

Figure 5.12 Activities requiring quick eye movements in different directions such as *(a)* side to side and *(b)* up and down are an important part of multisensory training.

2. Saccadic (Quick) Eye Movements

a. Hold or focus on two targets in front of the face (at eye level) and approximately 4 to 6 inches (10-15 cm) apart horizontally. Move the eyes *quickly* from target to target while the head remains still (figure 5.12).

b. Repeat the exercise with the targets positioned 4 to 6 inches (10-15 cm) apart vertically. Move the eyes up and down between the targets.

c. Repeat the exercise with the targets positioned 4 to 6 inches (10-15 cm) apart diagonally. The eyes now move diagonally.

d. Quickly move the eyes from one visual target to another visual target (e.g., numbers, letters) placed on a blank wall directly in front of the eyes. Follow verbal cues or move the eyes at your own pace.

e. Sit directly in front of a busy background (e.g., checkerboard pattern, floral pattern) with targets placed at different points on the background. Move the eyes from one target to the next on a given command. Or, move the eyes to targets set at positions of the clock face (e.g., 12 o'clock, 3 o'clock, 8 o'clock) on command or spell out words by finding letters posted against the busy background.

Once participants have adequately practiced each of these exercise progressions in a seated position, you can have them repeat the same set of progressions in a standing position. This will add a balance component to the activities. You can further increase the balance challenge by altering certain task or environmental demands associated with each progression. For example, you can have your class participants repeat the level 1 eye movement exercises while standing on an altered surface or base of support. Because each of the eye exercises in level 1 engages vision, standing balance must be controlled at a more subconscious level and the participant must rely on the other sensory systems (somatosensory and vestibular) to control upright balance.

LEVEL 2: COMBINATION HEAD AND EYE MOVEMENTS IN A SEATED POSITION

The exercises presented in this level improve the ability to visually focus on targets when the head is also moving. Good gaze-stabilization skills are needed when shopping for groceries or walking in busy malls. We are constantly moving our head and eyes in different directions as we scan the shelves for various food items or look at window displays as we move through a shopping mall. The fact that we are usually walking and perhaps dodging people as we perform these different head and eye movements adds to the difficulty of the task. The exercise progressions presented in this section simulate these types of sensory environments.

Although these exercises primarily are designed to teach participants how to coordinate the movements of the head and eyes when performing tasks in a variety of situations, many of the activities requiring head turns also activate the vestibular system. Participants who have a diagnosed vestibular impairment or who performed poorly on FAB test items 7 (stand on foam with eyes closed) or 9 (walk with head turns) during the preprogram assessment will find many of the standing and walking activities to be difficult if not impossible to perform. You will need to identify those participants who are likely to experience difficulty and make the necessary adjustments to the exercise progressions. Remember that the faster the head turns, the more the vestibular system is activated. Reducing the speed or number of head turns will reduce the difficulty of the task. It will also be important to reinforce the need for participants to focus their eyes on a target during the various head turns to minimize instability. Do not allow participants who are experiencing instability during the seated exercises to progress to the standing or moving activities until they are ready.

If any participants report that they feel dizzy during or shortly after an activity, ask them how dizzy they are feeling using the dizziness scale described in chapter 2. Do not ask any client to repeat an exercise until the dizziness has subsided, and if the dizziness increases on the next repetition, have the client stop performing the activity altogether. If participants experience repeated dizziness during any class, encourage them to pay a visit to their primary care physician to discuss the matter. Many older adults experience repeated bouts of dizziness that are dismissed as an inevitable part of the aging process when they are actually the result of an underlying vestibular impairment or, in some cases, cardiovascular problem. Certain medications can also cause dizziness, so be sure to check the participant's medication list.

Exercise Progressions

a. Slowly move the head in a lateral or vertical direction while focusing the eyes on a stationary visual target held directly ahead and at eye level. Gradually increase the speed of the head turns while maintaining a clear visual focus on the target. Stop increasing the head speed once the visual target becomes blurred.

b. While in a seated position, fix the eyes on a visual target (e.g., checkerboard) being moved through the field of vision (see figure 5.3 on p. 158). Use both the head and the eyes to follow the moving target up and down, side to side, and diagonally for 60 seconds before resting.

c. Move the eyes between two horizontal targets that are held an arm's length away and at eye level. The targets should be close enough together that when one target is focused on, the other can be seen in the periphery. Align the head and eyes with one of the targets, move the eyes to focus on the second target, and then move the head to that target (figure 5.13). Repeat in the opposite direction. Vary the speed of the head movement while maintaining a clear focus on the target at all times. Perform at least 10 to 20 head and eye excursions before resting.

d. Repeat the previous exercise but with the two targets positioned vertically. One target should be at the height of the forehead and the other at the height of the chin.

e. Move the eyes quickly between targets set against a busy background (e.g., numbers or letters affixed to a busy background that fills the visual field). For a more challenging task, search for numbers in sequential order or create a word by searching for letters. The word is announced once completed.

After your clients have practiced each of the exercise progressions in this level, you can repeat the progressions with the clients in a standing position. You can also increase the balance challenge by altering the base of support or the support surface beneath the feet once your clients are able to do the exercises well.

> ### Key Point
>
> Combining head and eye movements is difficult for many older adults, so start slowly. You may have to cue the movements verbally early in the repetitions until your clients learn to coordinate the head and eye movements.

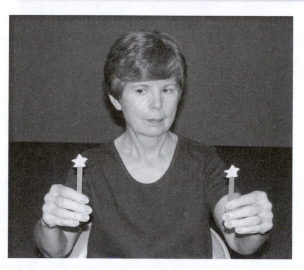

Figure 5.13   The goal of this activity is to move the eyes to a new visual target and then move the head to the target.

LEVEL 3: HEAD AND EYE MOVEMENTS WHILE SHIFTING WEIGHT IN A STANDING POSITION

A more complex level of motor coordination is needed to perform the exercise progressions described in level 3. Not only do participants have to control the movements of the head or eyes but they must also control the movements of the body as they perform weight shifts in different directions or walk across the room. Make sure that individual clients are able to perform the previous progressions in a standing position before introducing the more dynamic activities that are described in this level.

Exercise Progressions

a. Perform lateral weight shifting with head turns. Begin with turning the head in the same direction as the weight shift and progress to turning the head opposite to the weight shift.

b. Repeat the activity with forward and backward weight shifts and diagonal forward and backward weight shifts combined with head movements that are up and down (weight shift forward with head tilted up, weight shift backward with head tilted down, or vice versa).

LEVEL 4: HEAD AND EYE MOVEMENTS WHILE WALKING

Start each of the walking exercises described in this level with a higher number of steps per head turn. For some participants, difficulty may vary depending on the direction of the head movements. If you observe large gait deviations during any of these exercises, increase the number of steps per head turn until little or no deviation is observed. Reduce the number of steps as dynamic balance improves. Encourage rapid eye fixation on a visual target with each head turn.

Exercise Progressions

1. Walking With Head Turns to Right, Center, and Left

a. Begin walking on a firm surface with the head and eyes directed forward. After a set number of steps (1 to 4), turn the head to the right for the same number of steps and then return the head to center with the eyes directed forward (figure 5.14). Repeat the walking activity, but this time direct the head to the left and then back to center. (In some cases you may need to lower the challenge of this activity by verbally indicating when and in what direction participants should turn their head so they are relieved of the task of counting as they walk. For many participants, having to count in addition to moving creates a dual task situation.)

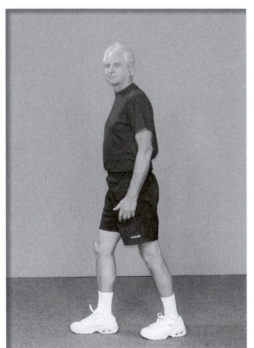

b. Repeat the previous exercise, but this time do not pause the head in the center position at any time. (Again, you might verbally lead this activity for your participants).

c. Repeat the previous exercise, but this time call out the number or word that is posted at regular intervals along the wall on either side of the room. Reading off the numbers or words requires the gaze to be stabilized with each head turn.

d. Walk across the room while turning to catch and then throw a ball on command. Alter the walking pattern (e.g., toes, heels, tandem) to increase the challenge of the activity.

2. Walking With Vertical Head Movements

a. Repeat exercise 1, but this time tilt the head up to the ceiling, back to a vertically centered position with the eyes directed forward, down to the floor, and then back to the centered position for a set number of steps.

b. Repeat the previous step without pausing the head in a centered position.

Figure 5.14 Walking while turning the head requires good adaptive postural control.

3. Walking With Diagonal Head Movements

a. Repeat exercises 1 and 2, but this time move the eyes and head diagonally up and to the right, back to a centered position, and then diagonally down and to the left.

b. Repeat this progression by moving the head and eyes diagonally up and to the left, back to a centered position, and then diagonally down and to the right.

c. Repeat the activity in both directions without pausing the head in a centered position.

Although many of the exercise progressions described in level 4 are sufficiently challenging in and of themselves, you can increase the balance challenge for your more accomplished class participants. These exercises, especially when performed on altered support surfaces, at faster speeds, and with an altered base of support, are challenging even for very healthy older adults who have no apparent balance problems.

Culminating Activity

The culminating activity described in this section is intended to create the type of busy visual environment that older adults often encounter when they attempt to navigate their way through a busy shopping mall or supermarket. Not only is the visual system challenged in these complex environments but so too is the motor system that must respond to the external timing demands created by the often unpredictable movements of other people in the environment. Limit the number of players when first introducing this activity so that the safety of all players can be maximized.

Walk the Gauntlet

This activity is an excellent way to introduce sensory conflict into the practice situation and reinforce several of the exercise progressions introduced during the first section of this chapter, as well as the section on coordinating eye and head movements. The participants are confronted with a complex and moving visual scene as they try to move quickly but safely in a forward direction. Before starting this culminating activity, have your class participants form two lines approximately 6 to 8 feet (1.8-2.4 m) apart. Then have participants turn to face the person directly opposite them in a staggered fashion (see figure 5.15). Position one participant at one end of the two lines.

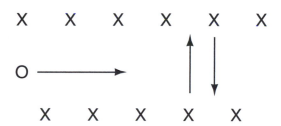

Figure 5.15 Formation for walk the gauntlet.

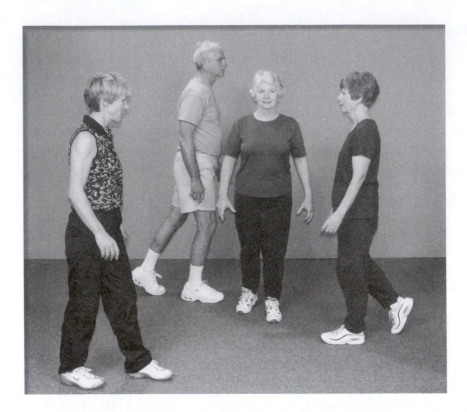

Figure 5.16   Walk the gauntlet simulates the type of sensory conflict encountered in crowded malls and on busy sidewalks.

On your instruction to go, the participant at the end begins walking quickly and safely down the middle of the two lines as each person in a line attempts to cross to the other side just before the participant reaches him/her (figure 5.16). If the participants standing in line time their movements appropriately, they will force the participant walking the gauntlet to change speed or direction repeatedly to avoid body contact. This activity attempts to simulate the sensory conflict that arises when walking through a crowded shopping mall or along a busy sidewalk.

For this game, you need to remind participants not to touch one another. Emphasize the need for body control at all times during this activity. It is also a good idea to follow closely behind the more unstable participants as they walk the gauntlet so you can provide a manual assist if they are inadvertently bumped or simply become disoriented while moving through the complex and changing visual scene. Walk the gauntlet is perhaps the most frequently requested culminating activity and one that promotes good cooperation and socialization among class members.

SUMMARY

The multisensory training exercise progressions improve the older adult's ability to select the appropriate sources of sensory information to control balance and to organize the sensory inputs derived from each sensory system so that the motor response generated is appropriate. Several of these exercise progressions also help the older adult select the most appropriate sensory inputs when the information provided by certain sensory systems is inaccurate. In these situations of sensory conflict, the older adult must be able to ignore the inaccurate sensory inputs (usually provided by vision) in preference to other sensory systems (somatosensory or vestibular) that are providing more accurate sensory information.

Once you have carefully reviewed each client's health and activity questionnaire and certain test items on the FAB scale that emphasize the use or activation of sensory inputs for balance (e.g., walking with head turns, standing on foam with eyes closed, turning 360 degrees in a circle), you can determine whether you should choose exercises that force the use of a sensory system that may be only temporarily impaired or choose exercises that improve function in the intact sensory systems to compensate for a permanent impairment or progressive impairment (e.g., macular degeneration, peripheral neuropathy, bilateral vestibular dysfunction) in another sensory system. A review of these test items will also help you make wise decisions about setting the initial level of difficulty associated with a balance exercise.

Finally, keep in mind that even if your older adult participants perform well on individual FAB scale items that require good sensory reception and integration skills, they will still benefit from practicing the multisensory activities presented in this chapter. This is because the aging process leads to an overall decline in the quality of information provided by each of the three sensory systems. This is particularly true for the vestibular system, which is not activated as much as when the older adult was much younger because older adults tends to stop engaging in the high-velocity head movements they enjoyed as a young person (e.g., twirling in circles, jumping, hopping, skipping, skiing, roller-skating, surfing). Given the plasticity of the sensory systems that has been demonstrated in a number of research studies, all older adults will benefit from regularly engaging in activities that tune up the sensory systems.

Test Your Understanding

1. The primary purpose of multisensory training is to improve
   a. the ability to maintain a better upright position
   b. use of the ankle, hip, and step strategies to maintain balance
   c. gait pattern and stability in gait
   d. the use of visual, somatosensory, and vestibular information for maintenance of upright posture
   e. the use of both motor and sensory systems for the maintenance of balance

2. The major goals of multisensory training include all of the following except
   a. identifying permanent sensory loss and compensating for it
   b. identifying temporary sensory loss and stimulating its use
   c. stimulating sensory systems in an intentional, systematic way
   d. manipulating the environment to encourage the use of the targeted system
   e. altering task demands to facilitate improved motor coordination

3. The assessment tool that provides the most information about sensory organization and integration is the
   a. BBS
   b. Balance Efficacy Scale
   c. FAB Scale
   d. Walkie-Talkie Test
   e. Senior Fitness Test

4. Which of the following is an activity that stimulates the use of somatosensory cues?

    a. walking on grass while focusing on a target

    b. standing on a firm surface while tossing a ball

    c. standing on foam while tossing a ball

    d. standing on a rocker board with the eyes closed

    e. walking on a firm surface while focusing on a target

5. When attempting to alter the information provided by the somatosensory system, you can make an exercise more difficult by manipulating the base of support. Which of the following is an appropriate progression, from easiest to most difficult? Standing with the eyes closed and

    a. feet shoulder-width apart, feet together, feet in split stance, feet in tandem stance

    b. feet together, feet in tandem stance, feet in split stance, feet shoulder-width apart

    c. feet shoulder-width apart, feet in tandem stance, feet in split stance, feet on foam

    d. feet shoulder-width apart, feet together, feet in tandem stance, feet in split stance

    e. feet shoulder-width apart, feet together, feet in single-leg stance, feet on foam

6. Which of the following is an appropriate activity to stimulate the use of vision for upright balance?

    a. walking on a firm surface while turning the head

    b. walking on grass while turning the head

    c. standing on foam and looking at a target on the wall

    d. standing on foam and tossing a ball

    e. playing balloon volleyball while standing on foam

7. Which of the following tasks is the least effective for stimulating use of the vestibular system?

    a. walking on grass while turning the head

    b. standing on a firm surface while tossing a ball

    c. standing on foam while tossing a ball

    d. standing on a rocker board with the eyes closed

    e. walking on a treadmill while reading

8. Which of the following is an appropriate verbal cue to encourage gaze stabilization during a task?

    a. Direct your eyes forward and focus on a visual target.

    b. Can you feel that your head is directly above your shoulders?

    c. Close your eyes and feel where your body is in space.

    d. Try to turn your head and scan the environment with your eyes as you are walking.

    e. Feel your feet in contact with the floor.

9. Which of the following is an inappropriate starting activity for a client who loses balance immediately on test item 7 (stand on foam with eyes closed) on the FAB scale?
   a. walking on a firm surface while turning the head
   b. walking on grass while turning the head
   c. standing on foam and looking at a target on the wall
   d. standing on a firm surface and tossing a ball
   e. standing on a firm surface with the eyes closed

10. Which of the following activities is the most appropriate for a client who is unable to keep the eyes closed during test item 1 (stand with feet together, eyes closed) on the FAB scale or test item 6 (stand unsupported with eyes closed) on the BBS?
   a. walking on egg crate foam while turning the head
   b. standing on a firm surface while reading
   c. standing on a firm surface in tandem stance with the eyes closed
   d. standing on a rocker board while counting backward by 3s
   e. marching in place while standing on foam

Practical Problems

1. Familiarize yourself with the activities presented in each section of this chapter so you can better understand how the use of a sensory system is forced during a particular activity. Practicing each of the activities with additional balance challenges will help you better appreciate how difficult many of these activities will be for your older adult clients.

2. Develop a set of multisensory activities for Larry or Phoebe that reflect the sensory systems you consider most in need of being exercised. Provide a rationale for the exercises you selected based on your review of their completed health and activity questionnaires and their results on selected test items on the FAB scale.

3. Develop a 10-minute presentation that you would deliver to a group of instructors who work with healthy older adults in physical activity settings to justify the need for including multisensory training activities in activity classes for older adults. What precautions would you add during this presentation?

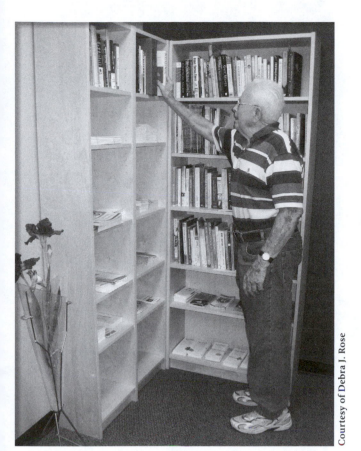

Courtesy of Debra J. Rose

Chapter 6

Postural Strategy Training

Objectives

After completing this chapter, you will be able to

- understand how the task demands and environmental context influence the type of postural strategy used to maintain or restore balance,
- manipulate the challenge of a balance activity by altering the task demands or environmental constraints (or both),
- develop a set of exercise progressions that improve the voluntary and involuntary use of the ankle, hip, and step strategies, and
- manipulate the task or environmental demands (or both) to ensure a safe practice environment.

The progressive balance activities presented in this chapter improve each of the three postural control strategies (ankle, hip, and step) discussed at length in chapter 1. These postural control strategies (figure 6.1) are most commonly used to assist us in maintaining and controlling our balance while performing daily tasks at home or while moving about the community. Not only will the demands associated with the task influence the type of postural strategy used, but so too will the environment in which the task is performed. Helping the older adult become more efficient in selecting and implementing the most appropriate postural strategy for the task demands and environmental situation is the primary reason for incorporating this set of exercise progressions into the program.

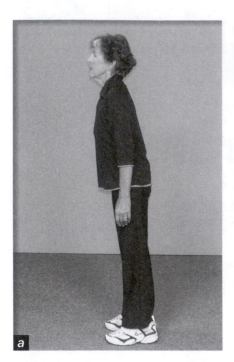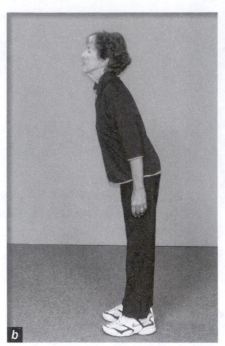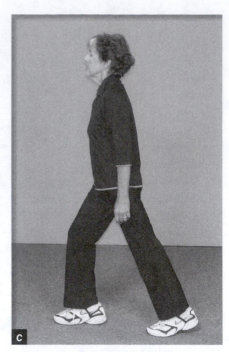

Figure 6.1 Three postural control strategies have been identified: *(a)* ankle, *(b)* hip, and *(c)* step.

PRACTICE REQUIREMENTS

The postural strategies required for maintaining and controlling balance can be practiced by manipulating the task or the environment (table 6.1) in three different ways: (1) maintaining balance while standing on different support surfaces, (2) voluntarily swaying through an increasingly larger distance in multiple directions while standing on different support surfaces, and (3) minimizing or controlling the amount of sway in response to progressively stronger applications of external force.

Just manipulating the type of support surface on which a person is standing can lead to the spontaneous use of a particular postural strategy. For example, when standing quietly on a firm, broad surface, we control our sway by using an ankle strategy. When standing on a narrow (e.g., balance beam) or unstable (e.g., foam, wobble board) surface, however, we often use a hip strategy to maintain balance. This change in strategy is necessary because the surface against which we are pushing is narrower than the length of our feet or gives as we push, making it more difficult for us to maintain balance using the smaller muscle groups of the ankle. When people are experiencing balance and mobility problems, standing on these more difficult surfaces may result in the immediate use of a stepping strategy rather than a hip strategy. The stepping strategy may be prompted by a heightened sense of fear as the amount of sway increases or by the absence of a hip strategy.

Balance activities that require progressively larger movements of the COG through space are another way to practice the ankle, hip, or step strategies. The ankle joints generally are able to control sway only through a small sway envelope in a forward or backward direction. As the sway distance increases, the control moves up to the hip joints, as the larger and stronger hip muscles are required to prevent a loss of balance. Increasing the sway distance still further results in the

Table 6.1 Postural Strategy Training at a Glance

Core program components	Additional task demands	Environmental manipulations
Ankle strategy		
Standing position (voluntary)	Increased distance of anterior–posterior excursion	Reduced or absent vision
Standing position (involuntary)	Small perturbation (push or pull) at hips	
Hip strategy		
Standing position (voluntary)	Increased distance of anterior–posterior excursion Increased speed of sway (i.e., metronome, clap)	Altered support surface (i.e., narrow, compliant) using a half-foam roller, foam pad, or rocker board
Standing position (involuntary)	Moderate perturbation at hips	
Step strategy		
Forward step (voluntary)	Increased forward lean beyond limits of stability Altered direction of step—backward, lateral	Altered support surface (i.e., foam)
Forward step (involuntary)	Large manual perturbation (push or pull) at hips or resistance band release maneuver at different lean angles	Altered support surface (i.e., foam)

need to take one or more steps and establish a new base of support. The speed at which a person sways also determines which postural strategy is selected. Swaying at a slow speed triggers the ankle strategy, whereas swaying at a higher speed in most cases leads to the hip strategy or to the step strategy if the hip strategy is not currently part of an individual's repertoire of postural control strategies.

Externally applied forces, particularly when unexpected, require a more automatic postural adjustment and therefore make up the most advanced set of progressions presented in this chapter. When an external force is applied, a person with good balance selects the postural strategy that best matches the amount of applied force. For example, a person usually responds to a small force (i.e., light push or pull) with rotation about the ankle joints. As the amount of force increases, the larger muscles in the hip region are recruited because the ankle joints can no longer generate enough torque to counter the destabilizing force. Finally, a large external force (i.e., strong push or pull) results in a stepping action to quickly reestablish a good, stable base of support. This chapter will also present activities that require participants to make subtle and not-so-subtle adjustments in body position in anticipation of a destabilizing limb movement.

Daily activities that require the use of postural strategies include stepping onto and off of curbs, climbing and descending stairs, avoiding obstacles, stepping onto and off of escalators or moving walkways, and recovering from an unexpected loss of balance. As you can see from these examples, learning how to select and efficiently execute the most appropriate postural strategy for the task or environmental context is a requirement for successful community ambulation. Knowing what to do in any situation, whether on a conscious or subconscious level, decreases an older adult's risk of falling.

PROGRESSIVE EXERCISE ACTIVITIES

The activities in this section are designed to progressively challenge your client's ability to select and then scale the most appropriate postural strategy for the task or environmental demands presented during practice. Do not progress your clients to the next level of the progression until the previous one has been mastered.

LEVEL 1: VOLUNTARY POSTURAL STRATEGIES

The activities described in level 1 help participants learn when to use a particular postural strategy. Through simple manipulation of certain task variables such as distance and speed, different strategies will spontaneously emerge. For example, if you ask an individual to sway forward and backward through a small distance while you clap your hands slowly (once per second), you will see that the sway is controlled by the ankle joints. As you instruct the participant to sway through a greater distance while you increase the speed of the clap (to twice per second), however, you will see a spontaneous switch from ankle to hip control as the larger hip muscles become active. Involvement of the hip muscles is necessary because the distance and speed of the sway exceed the capabilities of the ankle joints to generate enough force to control the sway. The movement of the body will also change from in phase (upper and lower body move in the same direction) to out of phase (upper and lower body move in opposite directions; compare the different body positions in figure 6.2 *a-b)*. Finally, if you ask the participant to further increase the distance

> ### Safety Tips
>
> - Instruct assistants to supervise participants standing on narrow or compliant support surfaces. When possible, position participants close to a wall or sturdy chair to maximize participant safety.
> - When using resistance bands during activities invoking the step strategy, wrap the band around the hips so that it is flat against the body and hold onto it firmly. Do not release your grip on the band after you release the tension to force the step. Because this activity is time consuming and requires close supervision, it is best suited to a one-to-one training situation.

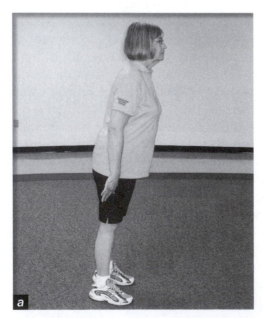 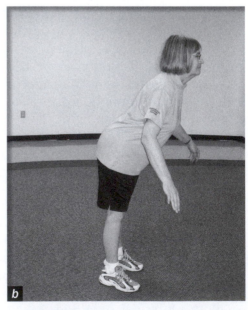

Figure 6.2 As a person moves from *(a)* an ankle strategy to *(b)* a hip strategy, the upper and lower body switch from in-phase to out-of-phase movement.

of the sway while keeping time with the faster clapping speed, you will see the step strategy come into play as the person's stability limits are exceeded. What is interesting about this scenario is that you never have to tell participants which strategy to use at any given time—a given strategy will simply emerge as a function of how you manipulate the demands of the task.

Exercise Progressions

1. Ankle Strategy

a. Have the participants stand on the floor and sway slowly between closely spaced objects (e.g., wall, chairs; see figure 6.3). Look to see that the ankle muscles are controlling the sway and that the upper body and lower body move in the same direction (in phase). Position the objects closer together if you see the heels or toes leave the floor during the forward or backward sway or the movement pattern shift from in phase to out of phase, which indicates that the sway is being controlled by the hip muscles. Recognize that participants with weak ankle muscles or other ankle and foot abnormalities, such as peripheral neuropathy or severe RA in the toes, will find this activity difficult to perform.

b. Instruct participants to practice the previous exercise with the eyes closed so that they can focus on how the pressure under the feet changes as the body sways forward and backward. Use the sensory cues you used when forcing the use of the somatosensory system during multisensory training (see chapter 5).

c. Have participants repeat the exercise with the eyes open but now use a metronome (set at 50-60 beats per minute, depending on client capabilities) or a slow hand clap (once per second) to externally pace the movement.

d. Once participants are able to sway comfortably at the speed of the metronome or hand clap, have them close the eyes while swaying at this speed.

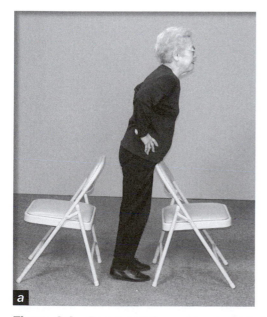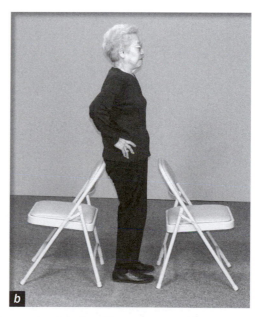

Figure 6.3 Practicing the ankle strategy between two chairs. The upper and lower body move in the same direction, or in phase.

e. Have the participants step out from between the chairs or supports and practice swaying forward and backward without external supports providing tactile cues.

f. Have the participants repeat the previous exercise with the eyes closed. Use the sensory cues introduced during multisensory training (chapter 5) to focus their attention on the somatosensory system and the information it provides relative to touch and proprioception.

2. Hip Strategy

a. Instruct the participants to sway forward and backward while increasing first the distance and then the speed of the sway. As the distance and speed increase, the participants will spontaneously move into the hip strategy to control the sway (if the hip strategy is part of their repertoire). Encourage participants to feel the pressure increase under the toes as they lean forward and then increase under the heels as they lean backward. They will begin to notice the changing angle of the hips as they move into a hip strategy.

b. Have the participants stand on a compliant surface (e.g., foam pad) or on a surface narrower than the length of their feet (e.g., have them stand sideways on a beam or half-foam roller; see figure 6.4). The more unstable participants will immediately begin using the larger hip muscles as opposed to the ankle muscles to control their sway. To trigger the hip strategy in more stable participants, instruct them to begin swaying back and forth. Participants will step off the foam pad or narrow surface if the hip strategy is not part of their repertoire or not being effectively used to control higher levels of sway. This latter problem is caused by an inability to scale the movement pattern to the size of the internal perturbation generated. Having participants grab objects held at a distance that requires reaching with the upper body can also lead to spontaneous use of a hip strategy.

c. Repeat the previous exercise while the participants stand on a rocker board oriented in a forward and backward direction. Instruct the participants to try

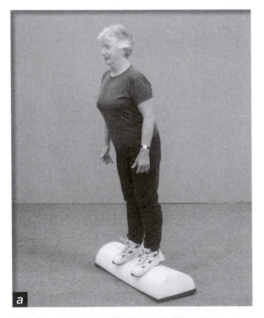 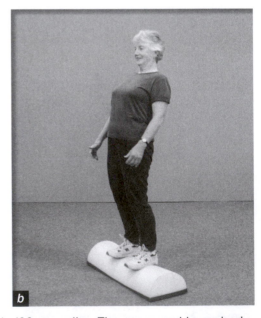

Figure 6.4 Practicing the hip strategy on a half-foam roller. The upper and lower body move in opposite directions, or out of phase.

to keep the platform of the rocker board horizontal to the floor. This exercise often results in a premature stepping strategy if participants cannot control their sway with hip strategy or exceed their maximum limits of stability because they cannot appropriately scale the hip strategy.

3. Step Strategy

a. Begin with a step in the forward direction. Instruct participants to lean forward until they think they have reached their stability limits and then take as many steps as needed to regain their balance. Have them practice initiating the step first with the right leg and then with the left leg. Notice the angle of lean at which an individual chooses to initiate the step and the number of steps and length of each step taken. To increase safety and reduce anxiety, position yourself or an assistant in front and to the side of the participant performing the exercise. Extend the arm closest to the participant's body so that it is level with the chest and can be used to stop the participant's forward momentum if necessary. Instruct participants to look straight ahead and not at the floor as they step. To maximize safety, allow only one participant to perform this exercise at any given time.

b. Repeat the voluntary step activity in a backward direction. Position yourself behind and slightly to the side of participants to increase safety. Make sure participants lean back through the hips before initiating the step. If they begin the backward lean from the head, stop the movement immediately by placing your hand on the upper back and verbally cuing them to begin the backward lean from the hips. In some cases you may need to provide a manual cue by placing your hand in the middle of the lower back and instructing the participant to push against your hand.

c. Repeat the voluntary step activity in a lateral direction. Observe the type of step selected by participants (side step or crossover step). Again, make sure participants shift their weight through the hip before initiating the step. Use a spotting strategy similar to one used while practicing the backward step if a participant initiates the lateral lean from the shoulder (i.e., manually block the shoulder lean and verbally cue the participant to shift weight through the hip). Have participants practice stepping in both lateral directions. For the lateral step exercise progression, stand behind and to the side of the intended lean direction with the arm extended at the height of the participant's shoulder. This position will enable you to stop the movement immediately if the participant initiates the lateral lean from the shoulder.

When teaching these stepping exercises to a group of participants, organize them in a line and then move down the line, asking each participant to step in the desired direction while you are in the correct spotting position. Have the waiting participants move to where they can watch and provide feedback as to whether the step was initiated correctly based on the movement cues you have instructed them to monitor. (The value of having participants engage in observational learning is discussed further in chapter 10.)

> **Reminder**
>
> Do not progress participants to level 2 activities until they are able to initiate a voluntary step in each direction both confidently and efficiently. A sign that participants are ready to progress is that they consistently shift weight through the hip on the backward and lateral step activities. It may take several sessions before participants perform consistently in certain directions (e.g., backward), so participants may need to continue practicing certain level 1 activities in combination with level 2 activities.

LEVEL 2A: INVOLUNTARY POSTURAL STRATEGY TRAINING

In the previous section, clients initiated each of the postural control strategies internally in response to changing task or environmental demands. In this section, the goal will be to externally perturb the client by applying different levels of force at the hips. The type of postural strategy produced should match the level of force applied. Low levels of force should automatically trigger an ankle strategy while higher levels of force should trigger a hip or stepping strategy. Because this set of activities can be anxiety-inducing for clients who are more fearful of falling, it will be important to progress slowly. Note that improvement in the use of subconsciously invoked postural strategies is often not observed until sufficient strength and flexibility have been achieved. Therefore, you should include activities that increase lower-body strength and flexibility during the class and as assigned homework between class sessions. Several upper- and lower-body strength activities are described in chapter 8.

Exercise Progressions

1. Manual Perturbations of Increasing Force

a. Introduce manual perturbations of progressively greater forces. A small perturbation should result in a countermovement with the ankle muscles while a medium perturbation should result in a countermovement with the hip muscles. Applying a large perturbation to the hips should cause the participant to take one or more steps to reestablish balance. An alternative method of facilitating use of the step strategy is to apply manual perturbations to the hips and shoulders. In many cases, you will see the participant take a step even when the amount of force applied is small. This indicates a scaling issue and should be considered less problematic than a failure to make any response at all. With adequate and variable amounts of practice, participants should begin to scale the movement response more appropriately. Reintroducing a movement strategy that has been lost from the repertoire will require much more time and, in some cases, may not be possible for a variety of reasons.

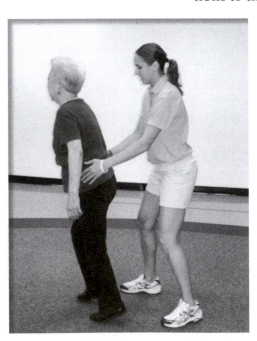

Figure 6.5 Introduce quick perturbations to the hips to elicit a stepping strategy in multiple directions.

b. To elicit the step strategy in multiple directions, stand behind the participant and introduce quick perturbations at the hips (see figure 6.5). Pull the hips back quickly and watch for a countermovement in the forward direction. Alternatively, push the hips forward and see whether the participant counters the pushing action with a backward movement. You can also apply the manual perturbation to the side of the hips to trigger a lateral step. While you should perform this activity with only one client at a time, you can still perform it more efficiently than the resistance band activities described in the next section because it requires less preparation. A good idea is to divide your class into two or more groups and have the groups not involved in this activity engage in other activities that do not require your close supervision. Given that adequate strength and flexibility are required to perform a step strategy, it would be appropriate to have the waiting groups perform lower-body strength and flexibility exercises in a seated position. You need apply only 4 to 6 manual perturbations before moving onto the next client in the group. Again, having the waiting participants watch how the person you are perturbing responds to the loss of balance will better prepare them for their turn at the activity.

LEVEL 2B: INVOLUNTARY POSTURAL STRATEGY TRAINING WITH RESISTANCE BANDS

The resistance band release maneuver described in this section is an alternative method for eliciting an involuntary step strategy but is best suited for use when working with individual clients as opposed to groups. Similar to the manual perturbations used to elicit the stepping strategy in Level 2a, the resistance band release maneuver should not be introduced until your clients are able to initiate a voluntary step in each direction both consistently and effectively. You also must practice the release maneuver with the resistance band many times before working with participants so that they feel well supported as they practice this challenging activity.

Resistance Band Release Maneuver

◆ Wrap a 6- to 8-foot (1.8-2.4 m) length of resistance band (medium to heavy resistance) around the participant's hips. Ensure that the full width of the band is flat against the body and that both ends are of equal length once you grasp the band in your hands.

◆ When performing either the forward or backward release maneuver, position yourself to the side of the client, as shown in figure 6.6. Hold onto both ends of the band with one hand and position the other arm (a) in a guarding position directly in front of the client's chest during the forward release or (b) in a guarding position directly behind the upper back during the backward release.

◆ When performing the lateral step activities, position yourself slightly behind and to the side of the client. Hold both ends of the resistance band firmly in one hand and position the other hand in a guarding position next to the shoulder on the side to which the client will execute the lateral step.

◆ Increase the tension on the band as the client begins to lean into it by slowly pulling it in a direction opposite to the one in which the client is leaning.

◆ When the client reaches the desired angle, quickly release the tension on the band by reversing the direction in which you were originally pulling it so that the hand holding the band is now moving in the same direction as the client. Do not release the band itself.

◆ As the client initiates a step, move with the client so you can provide a manual assist if needed. The arm that is guarding the client should remain in the original position until the client has stopped moving.

◆ For your own safety, do *not* perform this release maneuver with any client whose height or weight would make it difficult for you to provide a manual assist.

Although the resistance band activities described are extremely effective for retraining the step strategy, they should not be performed unless you feel competent in releasing the tension on the resistance band during the step activity. The safety of your clients is your number one concern, so if you do not think you have the ability to perform this technique efficiently and safely, then use the alternative method of applying manual perturbations to elicit a step strategy.

Exercise Progressions

1. Forward Step Strategy From a Leaning Position

The forward step can be practiced with different tensions of resistance band or sport cord attached to a waist belt. The participant stands on a firm surface and leans forward against the resistance band or sport cord. The head and eyes are directed forward (see figure 6.6a). Release the tension on the band unexpectedly (using the release maneuver described earlier) when the participant reaches different lean angles so that you can observe how early in the lean the individual initiates a step. Step forward with the participant to further decrease the tension on the band and control the participant's amount of sway after the step (figure 6.6b). Look to see that participants take one or more steps to regain balance and that they step with each foot on different attempts.

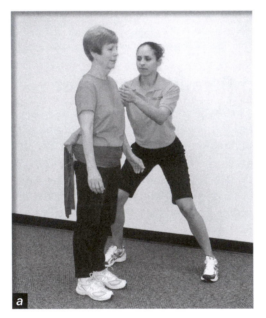 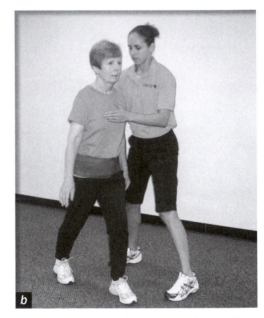

Figure 6.6 The correct release maneuver for using a resistance band on a forward step, from (a) the starting position to (b) the ending position.

If a client fails to lift one or both feet very high during the swing phase when stepping, you might consider using a 2- to 4-inch (5-10 cm) bench in the early repetitions of this progression to make it easier to perform the activity. Raising participants a few inches off the floor minimizes the need for a swing phase because they step down as opposed to forward (figure 6.7 a-b). Before beginning

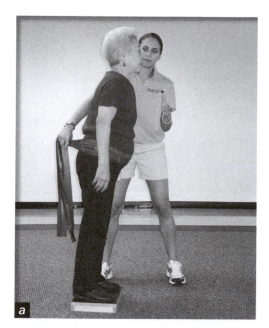 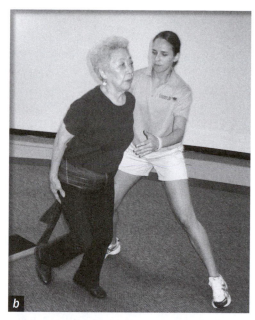

Figure 6.7 The forward step strategy can be made easier by having the participant stand on a small bench to minimize the need to lift the lead leg as high during the stepping phase. *(a)* Starting position. *(b)* Ending position.

this activity, ensure that the bench does not slide on the floor surface. Place a piece of nonslip material (one that extends beyond all sides of the bench) between the floor and the bench to prevent it from moving during the activity.

2. BACKWARD STEP STRATEGY FROM A LEANING POSITION

Repeat the stepping exercise on a firm, level surface, but this time have participants step backward. Stand in front and to the side of the participant while holding onto a resistance band wrapped low around the hips (see figure 6.8). Position the free hand behind the participant's upper back in a guarding position. Use the guarding hand to stop the backward movement of the participants who begin to lean backward from the head. Encourage participants to lean backward through the hips until they feel the tension of the resistance band increase across the buttocks. You can also manually reinforce the need to lean back through the hips by pulling on the band to briefly increase the tension felt across the buttocks and cuing participants to feel the resistance increase as the hips move backward into the band. Do not release the tension on the band until the participant is clearly initiating the backward lean from the hips. Also watch that the shoulders do not fall forward as the hips move back—the goal is to keep the shoulders in line with the hips. You should observe the toes lift off the floor just before the participant initiates the step. Unexpectedly release the tension on the band at different angles of lean to elicit a backward step.

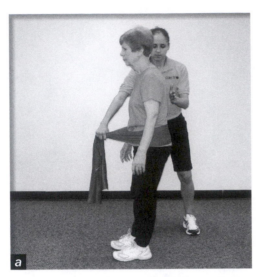
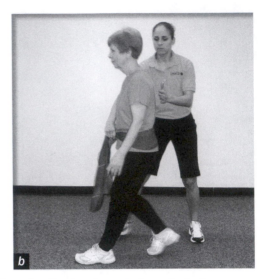

Figure 6.8 *(a)* Starting and *(b)* ending positions for the backward step strategy. Instruct the participant to lean backward through the hips during this exercise.

3. SIDE STEP STRATEGY FROM A LEANING POSITION

Repeat the stepping exercise against resistance on a firm, level surface, but this time have participants lean laterally. Stand to the side of the participant, holding the ends of a resistance band wrapped around the participant's hips. The participant leans to the side, feeling tension from the band at the level of the hips (figure 6.9a). Unexpectedly release the tension on the band at different angles of lean. Two types of side steps may be observed during this exercise. The same-leg step strategy requires a quick weight shift back onto the other leg before the leading leg is lifted (figure 6.9b), whereas the crossover strategy involves crossing the weighted leg over the midline and subsequently stepping with the initially weighted leg to reestablish a wide base of support (figure 6.9c).

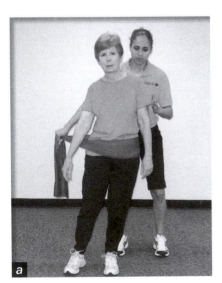
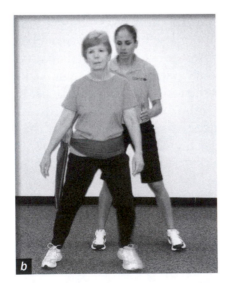
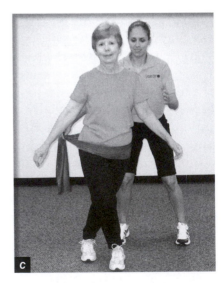

Figure 6.9 From *(a)* an initial leaning position, a loss of balance in a lateral direction may result in *(b)* a same-leg step strategy or *(c)* a crossover strategy.

Verbal Cues

Use specific verbal cues to help your clients better understand what they should be feeling and sensing as they perform the stepping strategy. Here are some examples:

Specific Cues

◆ For the forward step: Feel the pressure increase under the toes as you lean forward; keep your head erect and eyes focused on a vertical target at eye level in front of you. Take as many steps as you feel you need in order to regain your upright balance.

◆ For the backward step: Lean backward through your hips until you begin to feel your toes lifting off the floor. Keep your shoulders in line with your hips as you move backward and your eyes focused on a vertical target at eye level. Take as many steps as you feel you need in order to regain your upright balance.

◆ For the lateral step: Feel the pressure increase under the foot of the lead leg as you lean sideways through the hip. Try and keep your shoulder in line with your hip as you lean to the side. Focus your eyes on a vertical target directly in front of you and at eye level. Take as many steps as you feel you need in order to regain your upright balance.

◆ For the resistance band release maneuver: Feel the tension of the resistance band increase as you lean into it before the step. Take as many steps as you feel you need in order to regain your upright balance after the band is released.

SUMMARY

The exercise progressions presented in this chapter improve your older adult clients' ability to select the appropriate movement strategy when the task or environment demands it. You can manipulate the task or environment in at least three different ways to enable your older adult clients to practice the ankle, hip, and step strategies. Manipulating the task demands by increasing the distance and speed through which you ask an older adult to sway forward and backward will determine whether an ankle or hip strategy is used to control sway. Changing the support surface your clients are standing on from one that is firm and broad to one that is unstable or narrower than the length of the feet will often be sufficient to lead them to spontaneously use the hip strategy to control balance. Finally, the step strategy will be the movement strategy of choice when the task requires older adults to lean beyond their maximum limits of stability. Each of these strategies can also be activated at a subconscious level simply by increasing the amount of force applied during a perturbation, progressing from small (ankle strategy) to medium (hip strategy) to large (step strategy).

Practicing each of the progressions described for the ankle, hip, and step strategies will also help the older adult learn how to perform each strategy efficiently so it can be reproduced consistently when needed. Although it will take much longer for many older adults to learn to reproduce the correct strategy subconsciously when they are unexpectedly perturbed, repeated practice of the three strategies at a conscious level will certainly be helpful. In addition to constructing the appropriate practice environment and manipulating the demands of a task so that a particular strategy is more likely to be selected, you will need to have your clients practice regularly the various lower-body strength activities described in chapter 8. Even though the older adult may have the ability to produce the correct movement strategy, adequate strength is still required to ensure that it is scaled appropriately and executed effectively.

Test Your Understanding

1. When standing quietly on a firm, broad surface, a person controls postural sway by using
   a. an ankle strategy
   b. a hip strategy
   c. a step strategy
   d. a suspensory strategy
   e. a standing steady strategy

2. If you want to encourage participants to use a hip strategy to control postural sway, you would ask them to
   a. sway slowly and over a short distance
   b. step over obstacles of different heights
   c. reach for objects while standing sideways on a narrow beam
   d. attempt to remain standing while you perturb them with a large amount of force
   e. march in place while throwing objects from hand to hand

3. The primary goal of postural strategy training is to improve an individual's ability to
   a. move the COG efficiently and confidently through space
   b. perform each of the four identified movement strategies with efficiency
   c. select and execute each of the three movement strategies required to maintain or restore upright balance
   d. alter the gait pattern to meet the goals of the task being performed
   e. maintain upright balance when the base of support is altered

4. To elicit a stepping strategy,
   a. the COG must be within the base of support
   b. the COG must move beyond the individual's limits of stability
   c. the base of support must be reduced
   d. an external force must be applied to the body
   e. the participant must first be able to demonstrate a hip strategy

5. When practicing the voluntary backward step strategy, it is important that the participants
   a. initiate the backward lean from the head
   b. initiate the backward lean from the shoulders
   c. initiate the backward lean from the hips
   d. initiate the backward lean from the ankles
   e. turn the head to see where they are stepping

6. Practicing the forward step strategy while standing on a 2- to 4-inch (5-10 cm) bench can make it easier to perform because
    a. the participant can see the floor easier
    b. the swing phase of the stepping leg is minimized
    c. the trailing leg does not need to lift as high during the step
    d. standing on a bench makes the participant less fearful of stepping
    e. forward momentum is maximized

7. When asked to sway over a greater distance and at a faster speed, an individual is most likely to use a _____ strategy to prevent a loss of balance.
    a. hip
    b. stepping
    c. ankle
    d. suspensory
    e. mixed

8. In order to get an older adult to initiate an involuntary forward or backward hip strategy, how large a force should you apply by pushing or pulling the client at the level of the hips?
    a. Medium
    b. Large
    c. Small
    d. You should apply the force at the level of the shoulders versus hips.
    e. A combination of (a) and (b).

9. When using a resistance band to elicit a step strategy, the instructor should
    a. tell the participant when tension on the band is about to be released
    b. completely release the band as the participant steps
    c. increase the tension on the band by pulling it away from the participant as the step is initiated
    d. increase the tension on the band by pulling it away from the participant as the lean is initiated and then quickly release the tension at a lean angle likely to lead to a step
    e. not release the tension on the band until the participant reaches a lean angle of at least 45 degrees

Practical Problems

1. Practice the resistance band release maneuver with fellow instructors or friends of different heights and weights so that you can learn to perform the release maneuver safely and effectively. Solicit feedback from your helpers to determine whether the amount of tension you applied was sufficient as the lean was initiated and whether your helpers felt safe during the release phase of the maneuver. Practice this technique many, many times before you even consider trying it with your older adult clients, healthy or otherwise.

2. Practice perturbing the same group of fellow instructors and friends by applying quick pushes or pulls to the hips while they are seated on a balance ball or standing on an altered firm support surface. Observe the type of response elicited by the

different levels of force. Now solicit help from 2 to 3 of your most accomplished older adult fitness class members and practice applying force at different levels. You will certainly not be able to apply the same level of force when perturbing your older, albeit very healthy, adult clients, but practicing with your colleagues will help you understand different force levels from a relative perspective.

3. Develop an appropriate set of postural control strategy activities for Larry and Phoebe. Given your knowledge of these individuals, which of the postural control strategies do you think Phoebe and Larry are likely to find the most difficult to acquire? Provide a rationale for your response.

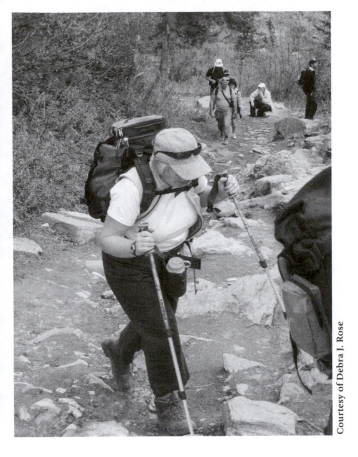

Courtesy of Debra J. Rose

Chapter 7

Gait Pattern Enhancement and Variation Training

Objectives

After completing this chapter, you will be able to

- describe the phases of the gait cycle and the neural mechanisms that control gait,
- identify the changes in the gait cycle that are due to age or pathology,
- describe the characteristics of gait in persons with various medical conditions, and
- develop a set of progressive gait activities designed to help older adults develop a more flexible and efficient gait pattern.

The ability to move about successfully in a variety of environmental contexts that impose different timing (e.g., stepping onto and off of escalators, crossing busy streets) or spatial demands (e.g., stepping over obstacles, walking in crowded malls) requires a gait pattern that is both flexible and adaptable. At its most fundamental level, successful locomotion is contingent on the ability to integrate the control of posture with upper- and lower-body movements. For example, initiating gait, walking, stopping, and turning are all movements that require a change in postural orientation.

> ### Key Point
>
> Successful locomotion is contingent on the ability to integrate postural control with upper- and lower-body movements.

OVERVIEW OF THE GAIT CYCLE

gait cycle—The time from when the heel of one foot first contacts the ground to when the same heel once again contacts the ground.

double-support time—The time during the gait cycle when both feet are in contact with the ground.

Because the act of walking is cyclical, the **gait cycle** is arbitrarily defined as the time between the first contact with the ground by the heel of one foot and the next heel-to-ground contact with the same foot. The gait cycle is measured in seconds. One single-limb cycle usually requires approximately 1 second to complete and is composed of two phases: stance and swing. The stance phase begins when the foot first contacts the ground, and the swing phase begins as the foot leaves the ground. When walking at a preferred speed, adults spend as much as 60 percent of the gait cycle in the stance phase and 40 percent in the swing phase. Figure 7.1 illustrates the complete gait cycle. As you can see in the illustration, both feet are in contact with the ground from the time the right heel contacts the ground to the time the left toe leaves the ground (approximately 10 percent of the gait cycle) and then again from the time when the left heel contacts the ground to the time when the right toe leaves the ground (approximately 10 percent of the gait cycle). The time during the gait cycle when both feet are in contact with the ground is referred to as **double-support time**.

The gait cycle involves three major tasks: weight acceptance, single-limb support, and limb advancement. Weight acceptance (initial contact and loading) is perhaps the most demanding task that must be accomplished during walking. Successful completion requires adequate knee flexion (approximately 15 degrees) so that the shock associated with accepting the body's full weight on impact is absorbed,

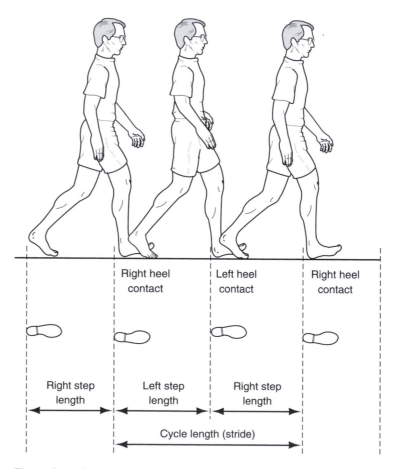

Figure 7.1 The gait cycle.

good limb stability as the foot contacts the ground, and the ability to keep the COM moving forward in preparation for the swing phase. The key muscle groups involved in weight acceptance are the hip extensors (to provide limb stability), quadriceps (to constrain knee flexion), and dorsiflexors (during the heel strike, foot contact with the ground, and preparation for limb loading).

During the single-limb support that occurs during midstance and terminal stance, one limb must assume responsibility for supporting the total body weight, which must also be simultaneously progressed forward in preparation for the swing phase. The key muscle groups activated during this task include the hip abductors (to stabilize the hip), trunk muscles (to maintain an upright position), quadriceps (to assist forward progression of the COG), and plantar flexors (to control the forward movement of the tibia during midstance and terminal stance).

The final task that must be completed during each gait cycle is advancing the limb. This task begins during preswing as the knee starts to flex (approximately 35 degrees) in preparation for the limb being lifted off the floor. During the swing phase, the limb is advanced. The knee continues to flex to approximately 60 degrees to allow for toe clearance (approximately .4 inches, or 1 cm, above the floor) before reaching full extension in preparation for heel contact. How far the limb is advanced during this phase determines the step length. The key muscle groups involved in completing this final task are the hip flexors, knee flexors, dorsiflexors, quadriceps, and ham-strings (during terminal stance). All of the muscle groups involved in each of the tasks associated with gait must remain strong to preserve the quality of the gait pattern and minimize the risk of falls in your older adult clients. In chapter 8 you will find strength and endurance exercises that specifically target each of these major muscle groups.

> ### Key Point
> Three major tasks must be achieved during the gait cycle:
> - Weight acceptance
> - Single-limb support
> - Limb advancement

To achieve a normal gait pattern, a person must have four major attributes: an adequate range of joint mobility; appropriate timing of muscle activation across the gait cycle; sufficient muscle strength to meet the demands involved in each phase of the gait cycle; and unimpaired sensory input from the visual, somatosensory, and vestibular systems. Particularly important muscles for gait are the hip extensors, knee extensors, plantar flexors, and dorsiflexors. A significant weakness in any of these muscle groups will adversely affect the quality of the gait pattern. For lateral stability during walking, the hip abductor muscle groups also must remain strong.

> ### Key Point
> Four major attributes are needed for normal gait:
> - Adequate range of joint mobility
> - Appropriate timing of muscle activation
> - Sufficient muscle strength
> - Unimpaired sensory input

Although many aspects of gait can be measured using sophisticated instrumentation (e.g., force plates, EMG, high-speed videotaping), the variables that are of greatest interest to you as a balance and mobility instructor involve the temporal and distance factors associated with gait. Two variables that you are already familiar with as a result of administering the 30-foot (9 m) walk test are **stride length** (the distance covered from one heel strike to the next heel strike by the same foot) and **cadence** (the number of steps per unit of time). These two variables not only determine walking speed but also influence how much we swing our arms; how far we rotate the hip, knee, and ankle joints; and how long we remain in double-limb

stride length—The distance covered from one heel strike to the next heel strike by the same foot.

cadence—The number of steps per unit of time.

support during each gait cycle. You can also conduct a qualitative analysis of gait as each older adult client completes the 8-foot (2.4 m) up-and-go test and the 30-foot (9 m) walk test at preferred and maximum speeds. As you watch your clients walk, pay particular attention to the swing of the arms, the degree of dorsiflexion at the ankle joint as the heel strikes the floor, the degree of knee flexion before and during the swing phase, the position of the trunk and head during the gait cycle, and the overall symmetry of the gait pattern across the limbs.

MECHANISMS CONTROLLING GAIT

central pattern generators—
Complex sets of neurons located in the spinal cord that control the rhythmic and subconscious coordination of the major muscle groups involved in walking.

avoidance strategy—The momentary modification of the gait cycle to avoid a barrier in the environment.

accommodation strategy— The adaptation of the gait pattern in response to a change in the physical environment.

The act of walking constitutes one of the most complex activities we engage in as humans. Although higher brain centers (e.g., cerebral cortex, basal ganglia, cerebellum, brain stem) play a role in the overall control, variation, and adaptation of the locomotor pattern, complex networks of neurons (often referred to as **central pattern generators**) located in the spinal cord are responsible for the rhythmic and subconscious coordination of the major muscle groups involved in walking. Each of the three sensory systems described in chapter 2 also plays a critical role in locomotion. Vision in particular is important in the control and modulation of gait because it can help us anticipate, rather than just react to, changes in our visual environment.

Patla (1997) has identified two strategies associated with the proactive visual control of locomotion: avoidance and accommodation. An **avoidance strategy** is one that involves the momentary modification of the gait pattern to avoid a barrier within the environment. For example, vision assists us in placing the foot during gait, in avoiding obstacles by lifting the limb higher so that we can successfully step over them, or in changing the direction of the walking pattern if the obstacle is perceived to be too high to clear successfully. Vision is also used in stopping. On the other hand, an **accommodation strategy** is the adaptation of the gait pattern in response to a change in the physical environment (e.g., slope of the ground, type of walking terrain). Characteristics of the gait pattern are altered in this latter scenario. For example, vision helps us accommodate changes in the physical environment by signaling the need to alter stride length (e.g., when walking across an icy surface) or increase the contractile power of certain muscle groups (e.g., when climbing stairs).

Just as the somatosensory system plays a critical role in controlling standing balance, it also plays a reactive role during locomotion. Sensory input received from proprioceptors in the muscles and joints and from cutaneous receptors contributes to the reflexive control and modulation of gait by providing information on limb position during critical phases of the gait cycle. The proprioceptors also inform us about the position of the limbs during the various phases of the gait cycle. Finally, the vestibular system, in conjunction with vision, plays a role in stabilizing the head through the VOR. This reflex allows us to stabilize vision even though the head is moving during locomotion. Specific impairments within the vestibular system lead to increased instability during gait because it becomes more difficult to stabilize the head (Berthoz & Pozzo, 1994).

The musculoskeletal system also contributes to locomotion by providing the muscular force necessary to support the body during the stance phase and move

---

Key Point

The proprioceptors inform us about limb position during the gait cycle, whereas the visual and vestibular systems help us stabilize the head.

the body forward during the swing phase. Because gravity is acting against the body during gait, adequate muscle strength is necessary to minimize energy expenditure while maximizing biomechanical efficiency. Adequate range of motion is also necessary in the joints of the trunk and lower limbs.

AGE-ASSOCIATED CHANGES IN GAIT

Although it is difficult to know whether the changes we observe in the gait pattern of healthy older adults are due to the aging process or some underlying disease process, clear differences exist when healthy older adults are compared with younger adults. The most evident change occurs in gait speed. On average, gait speed declines by 12 to 16 percent per decade in adults aged 70 years and older. Even healthy older adults with no history of falling walk at a preferred speed that is, on average, 20 percent slower than the speed exhibited by younger adults. Conversely, when walking at a fast speed, the difference in gait speed between the two groups is 17 percent (Elble, Thomas, Higgins, & Colliver, 1991). What is most interesting is that the slower gait speed that accompanies age is largely due to a decrease in stride length as opposed to a decrease in cadence. Unfortunately, this reduction in stride length has negative consequences for other aspects of gait, including reduced arm swing; reduced rotation of the hips, knees, and ankles; increased double-support time; and a more flat-footed contact with the ground during the stance phase before toe-off (Elble, 1997).

> **Key Point**
>
> The age-associated reduction in gait speed is due to a decrease in stride length rather than cadence.

Common gait adaptations among older adults are the tendency to load the limb more cautiously during weight acceptance, a flatter foot-to-floor contact, less forward progression of the limb during single-limb support, and reduced knee flexion during the preswing and swing phases. A summary of the changes commonly observed in the temporal and distance variables in the gait pattern of older adults is presented in the feature on page 198. A number of explanations have been advanced to account for the age-related changes in gait. Some researchers propose that the reductions in gait speed constitute a strategy for lowering energy costs (McGibbon, Krebs, & Puniello, 2001), while others cite impaired balance (Gehlson & Whaley, 1990) or muscle weakness (Skelton, Greig, Davies, & Young, 1994; McGibbon & Krebs, 1999) as the primary reason for the observed changes. Finally, the age-associated adaptations are seen as a coping mechanism used by older adults who are beginning to experience more variability in their walking patterns (Wagenaar, Holt, Kubo, & Ho, 2002; Danion, Varraine, Bonnard, & Pailhous, 2003). It has also been demonstrated that when older adults approach obstacles, they further reduce their gait speed and clear the obstacle using a slower, shorter step. This reduction in step length decreases the likelihood of tripping, but it often causes the heel or sole of the foot to contact the obstacle before it returns to the ground on the other side (Chen, Ashton-Miller, Alexander, & Schultz, 1991).

Barak, Wagenaar, and Holt (2006) have found significant kinematic differences in the walking pattern between older adults with and without a history of falling. Older adults with a history of falls demonstrate decreased stride length, ankle plantar flexion, hip extension, and lateral body sway as well as increased stride frequency when compared with older adults with no history of falls. At higher

> ## Summary of Gait Changes
> ## Observed in Older Adults
>
> Alterations in the temporal and distance variables of the gait pattern of older adults include the following:
>
> ◆ Decreased velocity
>
> ◆ Decreased step length
>
> ◆ Decreased step frequency
>
> ◆ Decreased stride length
>
> ◆ Increased stride width
>
> ◆ Increased stance phase
>
> ◆ Increased time in double support
>
> ◆ Decreased time in swing phase

feed-forward role of vision—Using vision to anticipate changes in the environment and prepare the motor system in advance of action.

walking speeds, older adults who have fallen (in the previous 6 months) also demonstrate increased hip flexion and greater kinematic variability from stride to stride.

Age-related changes in each of the sensory systems are also likely to adversely affect gait speed. In addition to providing continuous feedback that is essential for adapting the gait pattern to changes in terrain and the visual display, vision serves a **feed-forward role** by helping us anticipate changes in the environment and thereby preserve a smooth and continuous walking pattern (Rose & Christina, 2007). Age-related decreases that occur in the visual perception of motion are likely to adversely affect the gait pattern, leading to inaccurate responses in some situations or slower movement responses in others. Although some of the age-related changes are inevitable, much can be done to prevent or slow age-associated declines through the careful selection of gait pattern enhancement and variation exercises.

EFFECT OF PATHOLOGY ON THE GAIT PATTERN

Unfortunately, not all changes in the gait patterns observed among older adults can be attributed to the aging process. Certain medical conditions, particularly those of neurological origin, can adversely affect gait. Let's briefly consider five neurological conditions that produce abnormal or pathological changes in the gait pattern: stroke, Parkinson's disease, peripheral neuropathy, cerebellar ataxia, and Alzheimer's disease. Although typical gait patterns are associated with each medical condition, both the type and the severity of the problems observed during gait will vary within the medical condition and among persons who have been diagnosed with a given disorder.

> ## Key Point
>
> The type and severity of problems observed during gait will vary depending on the medical condition and the persons diagnosed with the disorder.

Stroke

Alterations in the gait pattern of older adults who have sustained a stroke are the result of the muscle weakness and **spasticity** that often accompany a stroke. Because a stroke usually affects one side of the body more than the other, the gait pattern typically is asymmetrical. The inability to time the onset and offset of the muscle groups involved in gait will result in an uncoordinated gait pattern—the toe instead of the heel may contact the floor at initial foot contact, the knee may be hyperextended during stance, and the toe may drag on the floor during the swing phase. A step-to gait pattern is often observed wherein the impaired limb steps forward and the unimpaired limb catches up to it on the next swing phase but does not pass it, as it would in a normal gait pattern. Older adults who sustain more serious strokes may also need to use an assistive device (e.g., single-point or three-point cane) on their unimpaired side to help them maintain dynamic balance while walking.

spasticity—Increased muscle tone due to hyper-excitability of the stretch reflex.

Parkinson's Disease

It is estimated that up to 60 percent of older adults with PD who are residing in the community will fall each year (Wood, Bilclough, Bowron, & Walker, 2002). Moreover, approximately 25 percent of those diagnosed with the disease will experience at least one fracture in the first 10 years following their diagnosis (Johnell et al., 1992). In contrast to an older adult who has sustained a stroke, the older adult with PD exhibits a shuffling gait pattern. The foot is often flat at initial contact, the muscles are rigid, the trunk rotation is limited, and the posture is stooped, particularly in the later stages of the disease. Older adults with PD experience difficulty initiating the gait pattern and, once started, have difficulty regulating the length of the step or stopping the gait cycle. These commonly observed impairments are due to the disease affecting the basal ganglia, which play a role in both initiating and scaling (changing the amplitude of a movement) the gait pattern. Older adults with PD also have difficulty adapting their gait pattern and thus experience greater difficulty during turning or stepping over an obstacle. PD also markedly affects the ability of older adults to adapt their posture. In particular, older adults with PD have difficulty shifting their center of mass (COM) forward when attempting to stand up from a chair and tend to fall backward as a result. Because of their shuffling gait pattern, they do not adequately clear the floor with the toe and thus are at risk for tripping during the swing phase. A number of excellent strategies for improving the gait patterns of older adults at various stages of the disease process are described in a recent review by Meg Morris (2006). She emphasizes the need to teach older adults in the early stages of PD to repeatedly practice moving quickly with large amplitude movements and to vary the task and environment in relation to a meaningful set of goals. Verbal cuing (reminding patients to take long strides) and visual cuing (marking lines on the floor to promote steps with larger amplitudes) are also particularly effective when working with individuals with PD.

Peripheral Neuropathy

Because the continuous flow of somatosensory information is critical to knowing where the limbs are positioned during the gait cycle as well as to the ability to adapt the gait cycle to the changing demands of the environment, any disruption in this input results in abnormal gait patterns. In particular, a wider base of support, slower velocity, and decreased floor clearance often occur when the somatosensory information is disrupted. In more severe cases, a foot slap will be evident during initial contact. Older adults experiencing peripheral neuropathy (loss of sensation in the feet or lower limbs) are no longer able to sense where the feet and lower limbs are in space, a loss leading to delays in the initiation of certain phases of the gait cycle (e.g., swing). The ability to adapt the gait pattern is also compromised, particularly when vision is not available (due to visual impairment, low lighting) to anticipate changes occurring in the environment.

Cerebellar Ataxia

ataxia—An inability to coordinate movement.

Any damage to the cerebellum produces an abnormal gait pattern that is referred to as **ataxia.** Recall that the cerebellum plays an important role in maintaining equilibrium or balance during the gait cycle because of its ability to provide continuous error detection and correction information. What you are most likely to observe in older adults with cerebellar dysfunction is a poorly coordinated gait pattern characterized by a wide base of support and irregular or unpredictable step length. Individuals with cerebellar dysfunction may also veer to the right or left when walking and have difficulty stopping, starting, and turning.

Alzheimer's Disease

Alzheimer's disease (AD) also results in adverse changes in the gait pattern. Generally, people with AD adopt a shuffling gait pattern that is nonpurposeful and significantly slower because of the shorter step cycle. The knees are often in excessive flexion throughout the gait cycle, and the individual frequently requires verbal cuing to maintain a walking pattern. Individuals with dementia are at a particularly high risk for falls and should not be included in a group training program unless adequate supervision is available and their judgment skills are good. Although the FallProof program does currently operate in facilities that serve older adults in the early stages of AD, the program has been significantly modified to ensure the safety and success of the clients involved.

Orthopedic Conditions

contracture—The loss of passive range of motion in a joint.

Certain orthopedic conditions may produce abnormal gait patterns. People with soft tissue **contractures** are unable to move the joints through the required range of motion at certain phases of the gait cycle and exhibit restricted movement patterns as a result. Arthritis pain in the joints also leads to abnormal gait patterns as the older adult seeks to limit movement in an effort to reduce pain. Fractures and total joint replacements have also been associated with abnormal gait patterns.

Cardiovascular Disease

orthostatic (postural) hypotension—A drop in systolic or diastolic blood pressure leading to dizziness, light-headedness, or loss of consciousness.

intermittent claudication—Severe pain in the lower extremities that occurs with activity. It results from inadequate arterial blood supply to the exercising muscles. The pain subsides with rest.

A variety of cardiovascular conditions result in abnormal or pathological gait patterns. People with **orthostatic (postural) hypotension,** for example, often experience a fluctuation in blood pressure upon rising that causes dizziness and disequilibrium during the gait cycle. Chronic pain in the calf muscles due to **intermittent claudication** also leads to abnormal adjustments in the gait pattern. In addition, gait speed generally is much slower in older adults with cardiovascular problems as a result of poor aerobic conditioning.

Checking Your Client's Walking Pattern

Here is a quick and easy way to check the quality of your client's walking pattern. All you need is a full-length mirror.

Have your clients walk directly toward the mirror and observe if their body behaves in the following ways:

◆ Their knees are pointing forward.

◆ Their hips are level.

◆ Their arms swing rhythmically as they walk.

◆ Both sides of their body are symmetrical (in the arm swing, step length, and so on).

◆ They are walking tall (e.g., their head is erect and the ears are directly above the shoulders).

Now have your clients walk alongside a wall mirror (a full-length mirror is helpful for this activity) and observe if their body behaves in the following ways:

◆ Their heel makes contact with the floor first on each step.

◆ They can feel the pressure roll up to the toes as they push off from the floor.

◆ Their knee is almost fully extended before the heel contacts the floor.

◆ Their steps are of equal length.

◆ Their ears are directly above their shoulders and their body is upright.

In summary, certain medical conditions produce specific impairments that result in an abnormal or pathological gait pattern. The major impairments that contribute to the development of these abnormal patterns include the following:

• Joint deformity (e.g., contractures)

• Pain (e.g., joint, heel)

• Impaired motor control (e.g., spasticity)

• Muscle weakness (e.g., stroke, cardiovascular disease)

• Sensory system deficits (e.g., peripheral neuropathy)

• Central processing dysfunction (e.g., PD, AD, stroke)

GAIT PATTERN ENHANCEMENT AND VARIATION TRAINING

The activities in this component of the program build on the balance activities already described in earlier chapters and help the older adult achieve a gait pattern that is efficient, flexible, and adaptable to changing task and environmental demands. For example, instructing older adults to start and stop quickly; walk with longer, shorter, or wider strides; and turn in different directions requires them to vary the spatial and temporal characteristics of the gait pattern, making it more flexible in the long term. Other activities designed to enhance or vary the gait pattern include walking on the toes or heels; stopping, starting, and turning on command; and stepping over obstacles, onto and off of different surface types, and up and down inclines.

As your participants become more confident in their balance abilities and demonstrate better overall performance, you can add secondary tasks to force a more subconscious control of balance due to the need to divide attention between two tasks. Incorporate activities that require counting backward by 3s, reaching for or catching objects, or turning the head while walking. These activities will further challenge each individual's abilities while rendering the practice environment more like the everyday performance environment.

LEVEL 1: WALKING WITH DIRECTIONAL CHANGES AND ABRUPT STARTS AND STOPS

a. Instruct participants to start and stop walking abruptly on command (e.g., using your voice, hand clap, music). Provide participants with the opportunity to practice their gaze-stabilization techniques while moving. Verbally cue participants to focus their eyes on a vertical target directly in front of them and walk directly toward it.

b. Have participants change direction on verbal command or when the music is paused. Ask them to make a quarter turn followed by a half turn and, finally, a full turn on command.

c. Repeat the activity but this time have participants use different gait patterns (e.g., side stepping, marching with high knees). Periodically pause the music and announce a new walking pattern.

d. Have participants walk using a variety of directional patterns: zigzag, figure eight, diamond, spiral (walk in progressively smaller circles in a clockwise direction and then reverse and make larger circles in a counterclockwise direction), and participant led.

LEVEL 2: WALKING WITH AN ALTERED BASE OF SUPPORT

a. Have participants walk forward using a narrow step width. To guide participants, mark the floor with lines of masking tape spaced 2 inches (5 cm) apart.

b. Have participants walk forward using a wide step width. This time space the lines of masking tape 8 to 12 inches (20-30 cm) apart.

c. Combine narrow and wide stepping by having participants complete a certain number of narrow steps followed by the same number of wide steps. Increase or decrease the number of steps using each gait pattern to match the coordination abilities of the participants.

d. Have participants practice step-to walking by taking a long step with one leg and bringing the other leg even with it on the next step. Repeat the exercise with the opposite leg leading the action.

e. Repeat the previous exercise but instruct participants to change the leg that is stepping long after a set number of steps.

f. Have participants walk forward on their heels across a firm surface.

g. Have participants walk forward on their toes across a firm surface (see figure 7.2).

h. Combine heel and toe exercises by having participants complete a certain number of steps while walking on the heels followed by the same number of steps while walking on the toes. Increase or decrease the number of steps using each gait pattern to match the coordination abilities of the participants.

LEVEL 3: GAIT PATTERN VARIATIONS— SIDE STEPPING, BRAIDING, AND TANDEM WALKING

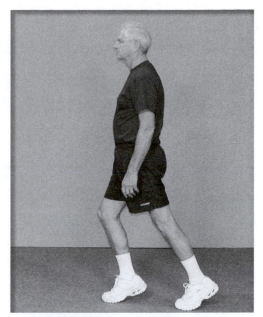

Figure 7.2 Walking with an altered base of support (on the toes) helps the older adult develop a more flexible gait pattern.

a. Have participants move down the room using side stepping. Encourage them to bring their feet together after each step and keep their hips directed forward during each step. Repeat the activity in the opposite direction so that the other leg is now leading the action. As participants become more confident, encourage them to count the number of side steps it takes to reach the end of the room. Ask participants whether they take the same number of steps in each direction or take more steps in one direction than the other. If the latter is the case, have the participants focus on increasing the length of each side step taken in the direction that causes the higher number of steps. Not all participants may be able to achieve the same number of steps in both directions due to preexisting medical conditions (e.g., stroke, arthritis), so direct the challenge appropriately. As practice continues, have the participants try to reduce the number of side steps needed in each direction.

b. Have the participants begin partial braiding across the room by moving the left foot directly behind the right leg on each side step. Then have them repeat the movement in the opposite direction, moving the right foot directly behind the left leg on each side step.

c. Repeat the activity but now step the left foot directly in front of the right foot instead of behind it on each side step. Repeat the movement in the opposite direction, moving the right foot directly in front of the left foot. It is important that participants do not rotate the hips as they move across the room. During all braiding progressions, it is helpful to cue participants to keep their hips facing forward.

If participants are having difficulty placing the foot correctly behind or in front of the other foot as they attempt to move across the room, have them practice placing one foot behind (or in front of) the other while remaining in place and looking in a mirror. This will help them see where they are placing one foot relative to the other. Verbally cue them to allow adequate

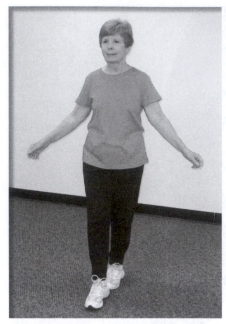

Figure 7.3 Braiding can be used to help older adults vary their gait patterns.

space between the front and rear foot and avoid moving the trailing foot to a position that is past the leading foot. The feet should actually be in a semi-tandem position once the trailing foot contacts the floor. Now have participants practice placing the foot with their eyes closed, then open their eyes to check their foot position once the moving foot has been positioned behind or in front of the other foot. I call this the Low progression, after Margaret Low who shared this wonderful progression with me.

d. Progress to full braiding if participants are able to perform partial braiding without instability or excessive hip rotation. In full braiding, the trailing leg moves forward and directly in front of the leading leg and then behind the leading leg, on alternate steps (see figure 7.3). Full braiding is challenging for many older adults and can lead to tripping if the movement is not coordinated appropriately. To increase the safety of the activity, teach your older adults to bring the trailing leg to a position immediately in front of or behind the other leg (not beyond a centered position as customarily taught). Do *not* progress the activity for clients until they are able to perform the partial braid (front and rear) correctly. Although teaching full braiding to older adults is not always looked upon favorably, I believe the activity should be included in a balance and mobility program because of its relationship to the lateral stepping strategy (introduced in chapter 6). You may recall that one of the lateral stepping strategies commonly observed among older adults is a crossover step. As such, I think it is important to have participants in a balance and mobility class practice this coordination pattern as much as possible. One additional caution is to never have participants practice this activity to music or any other form of external pacing (e.g., hand clap, verbal commands). Do not include it in any warm-up that is paced by music.

> ## Key Point
>
> It is important to teach braiding in a balance and mobility program because a similar pattern of coordination is used to regain balance when the limits of stability are exceeded in a lateral direction. You can maximize participant safety by teaching the partial braid first and by never practicing the full braid in an externally paced practice environment.

e. Repeat full braiding in the opposite direction.

f. Have participants perform semi-tandem walking (e.g., one foot contacts the floor when directly in front of or behind the other foot) in the forward and backward directions. Place a line of masking tape 2 inches (5 cm) wide on the floor and close to a wall to provide a visual path.

g. Have participants repeat the previous exercise (in a forward direction only) while semi-tandem walking on a narrow beam elevated above the floor or on a half-foam roller that is 6 to 12 inches (15-30 cm) wide.

h. Have participants practice walking in a full tandem (sharpened Romberg) position (e.g., one foot contacts the floor when directly in front of and in contact with the toes of the other foot) in a forward and backward direc-

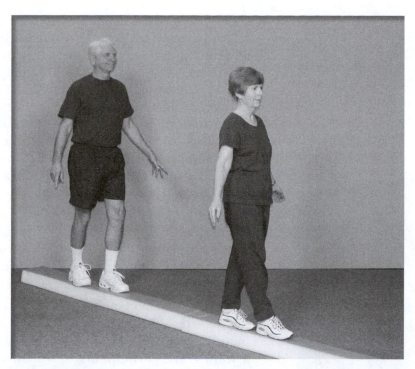

Figure 7.4 Walking along a narrow beam in either a semi-tandem or full tandem position requires participants to alter the gait pattern in order to remain stable.

tion. Provide a visual path by placing a single line of masking tape that is 2 inches (5 cm) wide on the floor and close to a wall.

i. Repeat the previous exercise (in a forward direction only) while tandem walking on a raised narrow beam or half-foam roller (figure 7.4).

Reminders

- When braiding is used as a program activity, participants should move the foot to a midline position only. Minimize the risk of falling by discouraging clients from moving either foot beyond a midline position.
- A participant who complains of discomfort in the hip region should discontinue braiding.
- Never introduce music or any other type of external pacing while participants are practicing braiding.

LEVEL 4: OBSTACLE NEGOTIATION OR AVOIDANCE

The activities presented in this level improve proactive visual control of locomotion by having participants practice avoiding obstacles or barriers within the environment or accommodating their gait pattern in response to changes in the physical environment. Vision will serve a feed-forward function during these activities and make it possible for participants to anticipate the changes in the physical environment based on the demands of the task (i.e., avoidance or negotiation).

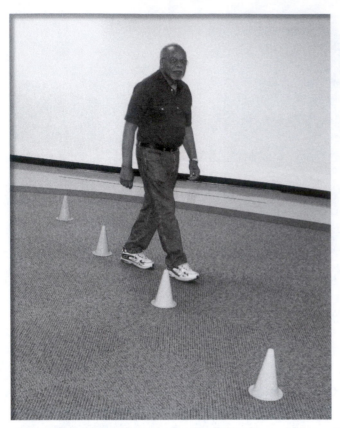

Figure 7.5　Slalom walking can be used to improve obstacle negotiation skills.

a. Have participants negotiate a walking course comprising 8 to 10 cones that are set apart at different distances. Begin with the cones approximately 5 to 10 feet (1.5-3 m) apart and at a 45-degree angle to one another. Gradually reduce the distance between the cones so that the turning radius is reduced. Encourage participants to look forward to the next cone and try and maintain a consistent cadence (speed) and stride length as they move through the course.

b. Have participants negotiate a slalom walking course. Place the cones approximately 5 feet (1.5 m) apart in a straight line and have each participant move through the course while maintaining the same cadence and stride length (see figure 7.5).

c. Place small barriers such as half-foam rollers or low benches (2 inches, or 5 cm, tall) approximately 3 to 5 feet (.9-1.5 m) apart and close to a wall. Have participants move through the course, stepping over each object. The goal is to move through the course using a continuous gait. Encourage participants to anticipate their approach to the objects and maintain the same gait speed throughout the course. It may take some participants several tries to achieve a smooth and continuous gait pattern. Substitute new barriers after a few trials so that the participants must accommodate their gait pattern to a new course. During the early practice trials, start with fewer objects on the course, and place the objects farther apart. Progressively reduce the distance between objects as practice continues and your clients develop a more consistent gait. If you have an assistant you might consider setting up two courses—one easier and one more challenging—along the walls on either side of the room so that you can better individualize the challenge for clients.

d. To help participants practice obstacle negotiation, set up a walking course (close to a wall) that is made up of obstacles such as benches of different heights, foam pads, and half-foam rollers that participants must step onto and off of as they move through the course. Initially, allow the participants to choose how they wish to interact with each object (e.g., step up and over the bench or step up onto and then off of the bench), and then later direct them to use a particular coordination pattern as they become more comfortable with the course. You can reinforce many of the level 7 COG training activities during this activity.

LEVEL 5: GAIT PATTERN ENHANCEMENT AND VARIATION OBSTACLE COURSE

One of the best ways to practice the gait patterns introduced in levels 1 through 4 is to set up different types of obstacle courses that combine the different gait pattern activities presented earlier. Just be sure that you do not introduce any objects into an obstacle course that are unfamiliar to your clients. For example, you should not introduce benches of different heights into an obstacle course until your clients have had an opportunity to practice using them in a previous COG module.

The following are obstacle courses that reinforce the various gait pattern activities:

a. Walk this way—place masking tape on the floor to mark different walking paths around the outside of the room: tape two lines spaced 2 inches (5 cm) apart for narrow walking, make a single line of masking tape for semi-tandem or tandem walking (use the short side of the room), tape two lines spaced 8 to 12 inches (20-30 cm) apart for wide walking, and put down a single line of masking tape for side stepping. If the room is large enough you could place a second course within the first course (the second course will be a little shorter because it is closer to the center of the room). Have participants alternate the type of walking patterns on each of the shorter, single lines of masking tape to add variety to the course. You could also designate a leader on each course who chooses the gait pattern (from a list provided by the instructor) that the participants following must attempt to copy.

b. Over, onto, around, and through—set up an obstacle course that requires participants to step over obstacles of appropriate height, step onto and off of objects (benches, half-foam rollers), walk around objects (cones, chairs), and move through objects (cones or chairs set at different distances apart). This type of obstacle course requires participants to alter their gait pattern to suit the type of obstacles encountered. Post large signs at the beginning of each new section to reinforce the type of gait pattern you want participants to use (e.g., step over, step on and off, go around, go through).

c. Altered surfaces—set up an obstacle course that is composed of different surfaces (e.g., foam pieces of different thicknesses, a firm surface). Such a course requires participants to accommodate their gait pattern to the different surfaces encountered. Consider using natural outdoor surfaces if they are available or try conducting this activity in a nearby park or arboretum that has gravel paths, grassy areas, inclines, declines, and lots of uneven surfaces. This final activity makes for an excellent transfer task and really prepares your participants for moving about in the outside world. Just make sure that they are ready for this challenging activity by having them practice all of the lead-up progressions presented in this chapter.

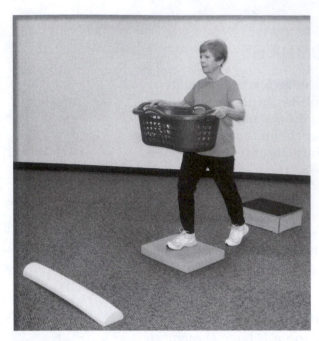

Figure 7.6 Requiring participants to carry an object along an obstacle course divides their attention between walking and carrying. It also prevents them from looking at their feet.

The level of balance challenge associated with each activity can be progressively increased by manipulating the task or environmental demands. Ways in which you can increase the task or environmental demands when designing obstacle courses include the following:

Task Demands

- Increase the number of obstacle types that must be negotiated along the course.
- Introduce an object (e.g., laundry basket) to be carried through the course (see figure 7.6).
- Introduce a cognitive task (e.g., counting by 3s) that participants must perform while negotiating the course.
- Require each participant to perform an activity after stepping onto each piece of equipment in the obstacle course (e.g., march in place 10 times on a foam pad, perform swing-through steps on a bench, balance for 10 seconds on a half-foam roller with the eyes closed, step onto and off of a Dyna-Disc). Having to remember what has to be done at each obstacle makes this an excellent memory game for participants. Progressively increase the number of activities participants need to remember each time they move through the course. You can also engage the participants who are waiting to move through the course by asking them to think of a new activity that could be done at each object or having them prompt the participants going through the course if they forget what has to be done at a particular object.
- Require participants moving through the course to retrieve objects of different shapes from the floor.
- Introduce an external timing demand. For example, require that the course be completed in a given amount of time. Indicate that time will be added if the activities are not performed correctly or with control. This added constraint tends to minimize unsafe behavior.

Environmental Demands

- Have participants negotiate the obstacle course while wearing dark glasses.
- Vary the support surfaces placed along the course. For example, intersperse foam of different densities with Dyna-Discs, half-foam rollers, and balance beams.
- Introduce a busy background or floor surface (a length of material with a busy visual pattern) from which participants are required to retrieve various objects.
- Have 2 to 4 class participants negotiate the same obstacle course at the same time—start 2 participants at one end of the course and 2 participants

at the opposite end. Start the second participant at each end after the first participant has gone about a third of the way through. This activity creates a more complex visual environment as participants pass each other on the course.

CULMINATING ACTIVITIES

Now that your clients have had an opportunity to practice the various gait pattern progressions it is time to have them engage in some culminating activities that will involve the group and simulate the types of walking environments they are likely to encounter during their daily lives. Including culminating activities at various times during your gait pattern enhancement and variation modules also provides an excellent way to engage the clients socially and create a game-like atmosphere in the class. I have always found that clients find the culminating activities to be the highlight of any class.

Busy Street

Have participants form at least two lines at each end of the room, with no more than three or four participants in each line. The lines formed at each end of the room should be alternately spaced so that participants are aligned in the space between the lines formed at the other end of the room. There should be enough space between the lines to allow each line to turn at the opposite end of the room and walk back to the starting position (see figure 7.7). Have each row of participants begin walking toward the opposite end of the room. The goal of this activity is for each row to walk continuously, turning to the right or left (as you determine) at each end of the room and then walking back to the other end of the room until you instruct them to stop. Participants will pass each other as they move between the two ends of the room, creating the type of visual flow encountered when passing people on a busy city street. Participants will need to accommodate their gait to the speed of the person in front and ignore the visual flow created by the movement of the lines to the right and left.

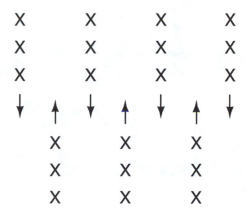

Figure 7.7   Formation for busy street.

Walk the Gauntlet

This activity was introduced during multisensory training (chapter 5) but is an appropriate culminating activity for this section of the program also. Review the description of this activity on pages 171 to 172.

Memory Walk

Participants are given a set of activities (no more than 3 to 4 in the first few classes) that are associated with a number (e.g., turn 180 degrees and continue walking when the number 1 is called). Have participants begin walking around the room, making sure to keep sufficient space between themselves and other class participants. Call out a number and watch to see that participants perform the correct activity associated with the number. Increase the number of activities they must remember as class progresses. Do not ask participants to keep more than seven activities in memory. Add partner activities (e.g., partner circle, do-si-do) to keep things interesting.

Emily Post Relay

Divide the class into two teams of 5 to 6 members, with half the members of each team standing at the opposite side of the room. The first person in line places a beanbag (or other suitable object) on the top of the head and begins walking across the room after the instructor calls *go* (see figure 7.8). The goal is to walk across the room without letting the beanbag slip off the head. The beanbag is given to the next person on the team, who then walks to the opposite end of the room. If the beanbag falls off the head while the participant walks across the room, the participant must stop, pick up the beanbag, and put it back on the head before proceeding. This is an excellent activity to reinforce postural alignment and gaze stabilization.

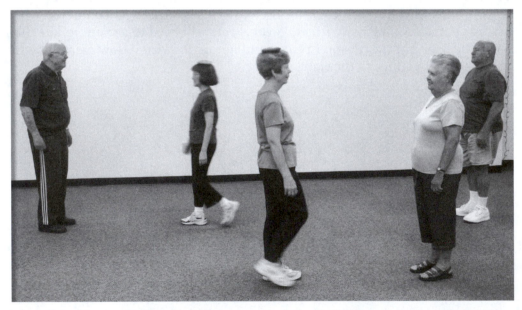

Figure 7.8   The goal of the Emily Post relay is to keep the object on the head while walking toward the next person in line.

Waiter's Relay

Divide the class into two teams of 5 to 6 members, with half the members of each team standing at the opposite end of the room. Give a tray holding a set of items to the first person in each team. On the signal to go, the person holding the tray (with two hands) must walk across the room without spilling any of the contents on the tray. The tray is handed to the next person in line, who then returns to the other end of the room with the tray. As participants get more adept at carrying the tray of contents, you can encourage them to carry the tray with one hand along side of the head as a waiter does in a fine restaurant. Consider giving bonus points by subtracting seconds off the team's time if a team member carries the tray with one hand. This dual-task activity requires participants to divide their attention between walking and carrying and so should not be introduced until participants have practiced dual-task activities during COG training. Be sure to disallow running during this activity in order to maximize client safety.

SUMMARY

The gait pattern enhancement and variation activities presented in this chapter help the older adult develop a gait pattern that is more efficient, flexible, and adaptable. As you learned earlier in the chapter, the aging process results in a number of changes in the walking pattern. The most observable change is a decrease in gait velocity caused by a reduction in stride length. This change negatively affects other aspects of gait, including the arm swing; the hip, knee, and ankle rotation; and the quality of foot-to-floor contact. A reduction in stride length also results in longer double-support times during the gait cycle. When required to negotiate obstacles, older adults further reduce their gait speed and take slower, shorter steps as they approach the obstacles. Having your class participants negotiate several different obstacle courses that include obstacles of various heights and varying support surfaces will do much to improve their confidence and their ability to adapt their gait pattern to changing environmental demands. Although you can expect to see much smaller changes in the gait patterns of older adults who are experiencing medical conditions that have affected different areas of the neurological system (e.g., stroke, PD, dementia), it is nevertheless important to have them practice the lower-level progressions described in this chapter so they can maintain their functional independence for as long as possible.

Test Your Understanding

1. The stance phase
   a. occupies 20 percent of the gait cycle
   b. occupies 40 percent of the gait cycle
   c. occupies 50 percent of the gait cycle
   d. occupies 60 percent of the gait cycle
   e. occupies 70 percent of the gait cycle

2. The gait cycle is arbitrarily defined as
   a. the distance between the heel strike of one foot and the next heel strike with the same foot
   b. the time between the heel strike of the right foot and the heel strike of the left foot
   c. the time between the heel strike of one foot on first contact and the subsequent heel-to-floor contact with the same foot
   d. the distance between the heel strike of one foot and the heel strike of the other foot
   e. any point you wish to start timing from within the gait cycle

3. Which of the following is a common alteration observed in the walking pattern of someone who has experienced a stroke?
   a. stooped posture
   b. reduced foot clearance
   c. shuffling
   d. asymmetrical gait pattern
   e. lateral veering

4. All of the following are normal age-related changes that adversely affect the gait pattern except
   a. muscle weakness
   b. poor depth perception
   c. impaired ankle proprioception
   d. spasticity
   e. decreased stride length

5. Which of the following key muscle groups are activated during the single-limb support phase of gait?
   a. trunk muscles, quadriceps, and dorsiflexors
   b. quadriceps, hip abductors, plantar flexors, and trunk muscles
   c. hip extensors, quadriceps, and dorsiflexors
   d. hip flexors, hamstrings, and plantar flexors
   e. hip flexors, knee flexors, dorsiflexors, quadriceps, and hamstrings

6. A person with Parkinson's disease would most commonly demonstrate the following type of gait pattern:
   a. shuffling with decreased step length, forward trunk, decreased trunk movement with lack of arm swing
   b. wide base; unsteadiness, lateral veering; difficulty turning, starting, stopping
   c. knee hyperextension with foot slap
   d. excessive knee flexion, lateral veering, wide base, foot slap
   e. retracted pelvis, toe drag, step-to gait pattern

7. The purpose of gait variation and enhancement training is to improve all of the following except
   a. the strength of the lower limbs for walking
   b. dynamic balance for walking
   c. flexibility of the gait pattern
   d. gait in different environmental contexts
   e. speed of walking

8. Which of the following culminating activities is *not* an effective way to challenge an individual's ability to adapt the gait pattern?
   a. walking within a crowded room
   b. negotiating an obstacle course
   c. slalom walking
   d. marching in place
   e. braiding

9. Which of the following is an example of multitasking during gait pattern variation and enhancement training?
   a. walking while counting backward
   b. walking on heels followed by walking on toes followed by walking on heels
   c. going up and down stairs
   d. stepping over obstacles of various heights
   e. side stepping

10. A person who becomes unsteady during the turn of the 8-foot up-and-go test would benefit from
   a. marching in place
   b. stepping over obstacles
   c. walking with head turns
   d. going up and down stairs
   e. walking backward

Practical Problems

1. Review the health and activity questionnaires completed by Phoebe and Larry and the results of their 30-foot (9 m) walk tests at preferred and maximum speeds. What can you glean from a review of their questionnaires and test results that might lead you to believe they have an abnormal or pathological gait pattern? If you conclude that either Larry or Phoebe does have an abnormal gait pattern, list the impairments you believe are contributing to it.

2. Design three obstacle courses for Larry or Phoebe that progress from easy to more difficult to most difficult to negotiate. Describe what you have changed about each course to make it more difficult to negotiate and why the types of obstacles you included in one person's course might differ from the obstacles in the other person's course. Be sure to review either Phoebe's or Larry's test results once more to ensure that the surfaces and activities you have selected will challenge balance appropriately without exceeding the individual's capabilities.

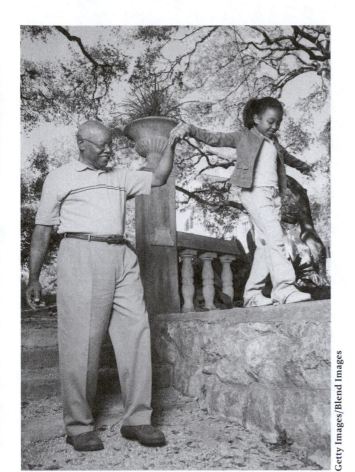

Getty Images/Blend Images

Chapter **8**

Strength and Endurance Training

Objectives

After completing this chapter, you will be able to

- understand the contribution of muscle strength to the multiple dimensions of balance and mobility,
- develop a set of exercise progressions designed to improve upper- and lower-body muscle strength, and
- incorporate strength exercises into a balance environment.

Age-associated declines in muscle mass and strength have been well documented in literature (Landers, Hunter, Wetzstein, Bamman, & Wiensier, 2001; Akima et al., 2001). Men and women over the age of 60 years lose muscle mass at a rate of .5 to 1.0 percent per year, whereas muscle strength declines as much as 20 to 40 percent between the third and eighth decades of life (Aloia, McGowan, Vaswani, Ross, & Cohn, 1991). In the United States, 28 percent of men and 66 percent of women above the age of 74 years cannot lift objects that weigh more than 10 pounds (4.5 kg), the average weight of a bag of groceries (Rhodes et al., 2000). More recently, researchers have begun to study age-related changes in muscle power, or the velocity with which a muscle can generate force, so as to better understand its effect on the older adult's functional independence (American College of Sports Medicine, 2002; Foldvari et al., 2000).

Given that many activities of daily living (ADLs) (e.g., climbing stairs, rising from a chair, walking) require different levels of leg muscle power and that

215

declines in power are much greater than the declines in absolute strength, activities that increase both absolute strength *and* power should be included in a balance and mobility training program.

This chapter describes numerous upper-body and lower-body strength training activities. Some of the strength activities, particularly those that include a balance component, are recommended for the class session, whereas others should be assigned for homework. The strength activities that have been included exercise the key muscle groups involved in balance and gait (e.g., hip flexors and extensors, hip abductors, knee flexors and extensors, dorsiflexors and plantar flexors), described in chapters 1 and 7, respectively. Activities designed to strengthen the musculature of the feet, an often underexercised area of the body, have also been included.

Many of the strength activities described can be performed seated or standing (with or without support). In some cases, alternative methods of performing the strength activity are described to accommodate the greatest number of older adults in your class. Once a participant is able to demonstrate correct form consistently and performance improves, you can add a balance component by having participants perform the strength activity while seated on a compliant surface (e.g., Dyna-Disc, balance ball) and then while standing on a compliant or moving surface (e.g., foam pad, rocker board). Limit strength activities performed on a moving surface to only those class members who are higher functioning or performing the more advanced COG balance progressions.

Before introducing strength activities into your program, consider the following guidelines related to intensity, progression, and safety:

- Always have participants complete the warm-up and dynamic flexibility exercises before engaging in any strength exercises.

- Have participants select a hand or ankle weight or resistance band that allows them to perform 10 to 15 repetitions before fatiguing (American College of Sports Medicine, 2007). Review the results of the two strength-related test items on the Senior Fitness Test to help you decide on the proper weight and resistance.

- Once participants can complete 15 repetitions of an exercise, encourage them to increase the amount of weight or resistance.

- Encourage participants to perform at least one upper-body and one lower-body strength exercise while waiting to perform a balance activity.

- Recommend exercises that target the muscles identified as weak during your initial assessment. A review of each individual's performance on the 30-second chair stand (measure of lower-body strength) and arm curl (upper-body strength) during the Senior Fitness Test will inform you as to whether individuals are below average, average, or above average in terms of their upper- and lower-body muscle strength.

- Instruct more unstable or weak participants to perform the strength exercises in a seated position to minimize the stability requirements.

- If participants are fatigued, do not ask them to perform any strength or power exercises.

- Remind participants to avoid or stop performing any exercise that they feel is unsafe or causes pain.

Choosing the Appropriate Amount of Resistance

The amount of resistance provided by elastic tubing or resistance band is color coded. Although manufacturers do not all use the same color-coding system, the following is an example of the color coding used by Thera-Band®:

◆ Yellow—light
◆ Red—medium
◆ Green—heavy
◆ Blue—extra heavy
◆ Black—special heavy

Handles and extremity straps are also available. These accessories are useful for class participants with weak hand muscles or arthritis.

- Remind participants to never hold their breath during an exercise. In fact, instruct them to exhale during the exertion phase of the exercise.
- Correct form is important, so take the time to teach the appropriate form to participants. Also instruct program assistants to carefully monitor participants during the performance of each exercise.

SELECTED UPPER-BODY STRENGTH EXERCISES

The strength exercises described in this section address the muscle groups of the upper body and are organized from the head to the hand, with the exercises involving the larger muscle groups described before those involving the smaller muscle groups. Table 8.1 on page 225 summarizes these upper-body exercises.

Shoulder Shrug With Hand Weights

Shoulder shrugs target muscles in the upper back and neck.

a. Sit tall with the lower back pressed firmly against the backrest of a sturdy chair.

b. Relax the shoulders and keep the arms down at the sides while holding the hand weights.

c. Keep the head erect and the chin pulled back toward the chest so that the ears are directly above the shoulders and the eyes are directed forward. Inhale.

d. Raise both shoulders simultaneously in a shrugging action during the exhale (figure 8.1).

e. Inhale and lower the shoulders to the original starting position.

f. Perform two sets of 10 to 15 repetitions with the appropriate hand weights.

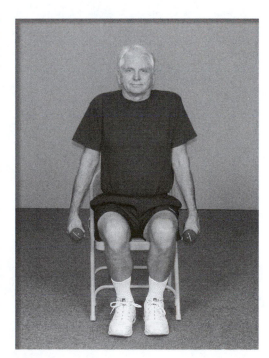

Figure 8.1 Shoulder shrug with hand weights.

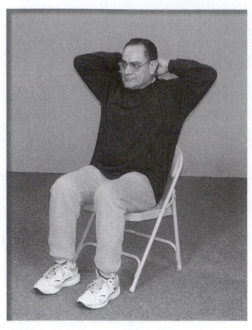

Figure 8.2 Back extension.

Back Extension

Back extensions target muscles in the upper back and shoulders.

a. Stand or sit tall with the lower back pressed firmly against the backrest of a sturdy chair.

b. Keep the shoulders relaxed and level, the chin tucked in so that the ears are directly above the shoulders, the head erect, and the eyes focused on a target directly ahead and at eye level. Keep the abdomen tucked in.

c. Position the hands behind the head; the fingers should be interlocked and the elbows pointing out (figure 8.2). Inhale.

d. Push the elbows back and pinch the shoulder blades together, exhaling as you do so. Hold the position for 10 seconds before returning the arms to the starting position. Breathe evenly during the hold phase.

e. Stand behind participants as they perform the exercise to see that they are actually pinching the shoulder blades together.

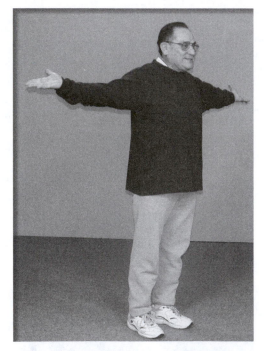

Figure 8.3 Back and arm extension.

Back and Arm Extension

Back and arm extensions target muscles in the upper back and shoulders.

a. Sit tall with the lower back pressed firmly against the backrest of a sturdy chair or stand with the knees slightly flexed and the feet hip-width apart. Raise the arms to shoulder level with the palms facing up toward the ceiling (figure 8.3).

b. Check postural alignment, position of head, and eyes. Inhale.

c. Pull both arms back with the thumbs leading; pinch the shoulder blades together, exhaling. Hold the position for 10 seconds while breathing evenly.

d. Return the arms slowly to the starting position.

e. Repeat the exercise 5 to 10 times.

Side Bend With Hand Weights

Side bends target muscles in the upper and middle back, shoulders, and arms.

a. Sit tall with the lower back pressed firmly against the backrest of a sturdy chair or stand with feet hip-width apart, knees slightly flexed, and weights held in the hands at hip level.

b. Sit or stand tall, tuck in the abdomen and chin, and look directly ahead. Inhale.

c. Slowly bend the trunk to one side as the weight on the other side is raised to hip level (figure 8.4). Exhale during the side bend. Inhale during the return to the starting position.

d. Repeat the exercise on the opposite side.

e. Repeat on both sides 5 to 10 times.

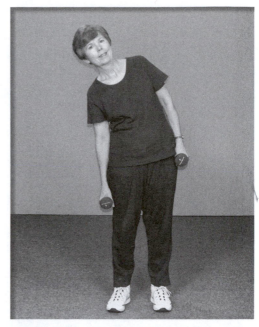

Figure 8.4 Side bend with hand weights.

Chest Press (Resistance Band)

The chest press targets muscles in the chest, shoulders, and arms.

a. Sit or stand tall with the feet hip-width apart, the abdomen and chin tucked in, and the eyes focused on a target directly ahead and at eye level. Place the resistance band around the back and under the armpits. Make sure the band is flat against the back (figure 8.5).

b. Hold onto the ends of the band, adjusting the length by wrapping the band around the hands to increase tension. Inhale.

c. Push the arms directly forward and press the chest muscles together. Exhale during the pushing phase.

d. Pause, then slowly return to the starting position, releasing the tension on the band. Inhale during this phase of the movement.

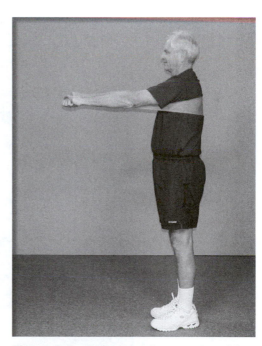

Figure 8.5 Standing chest press with resistance band.

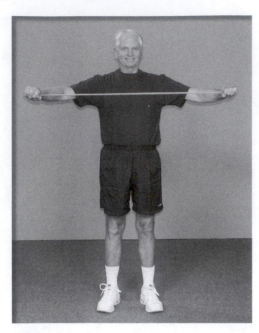

Figure 8.6 Horizontal pull with resistance band.

Horizontal Pull (Resistance Band)

Horizontal pulls target muscles in the upper and middle back, shoulders, and arms.

a. Sit or stand in an upright position, feet hip-width apart, abdomen and chin tucked in, eyes directed forward.

b. Wrap the excess portion of the band around the hands for shoulder-width positioning (figure 8.6).

c. Keep the arms at chest level and the elbows slightly bent.

d. Pull the arms out horizontally to the sides of the body while squeezing the shoulder blades together and exhaling.

e. Pause, then slowly return to the starting position.

f. Repeat the exercise 5 to 10 times.

Ball Lift With Added Balance Challenge

Ball lifts target muscles in the upper, middle, and lower back; shoulders; arms; and abdomen.

a. Sit tall and in the middle of a chair (with or without a Dyna-Disc below the buttocks) or a balance ball (for more advanced participants) with the feet positioned shoulder-width apart.

b. Hold a weighted ball (2-5 pounds, or 1-2 kg) directly in front of the body at waist height. Inhale.

c. Extend the arms and raise the ball directly above the head (figure 8.7a). Exhale while lifting the ball.

d. Bend forward at the hips and lower the ball toward the floor (figure 8.7b). Bring the ball back up to the waist.

e. Continue moving the ball in various directions, but always bring it back to the waist after each movement away from the body.

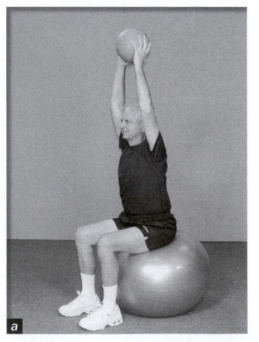
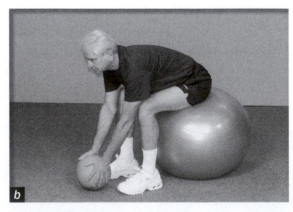

Figure 8.7 Ball lifts on a balance ball. (a) Highest point. (b) Lowest point.

Diagonal Arm Extension (Resistance Band)

Diagonal arm extensions target muscles in the shoulders, upper and middle back, and abdomen.

a. Tie a loop knot at one end of the band and place the left foot inside the loop. Alternatively, wrap one end of the band around the instep of the foot at least 1.5 times to ensure that it does not slip out from under the foot during the exercise.

b. Hold the other end of the band with the right hand.

c. Sit tall and in the middle of a chair (with or without a Dyna-Disc under the buttocks) or balance ball (to add a higher level of balance challenge) with both feet flat on the floor and hip-width apart.

d. Slowly extend the right arm across the body, forming a diagonal line from the left hip to the outstretched right hand, head and eyes following the movement of the resistance band to create a small amount of trunk rotation.

e. Pause, then slowly return the band to the starting position.

f. Repeat the exercise 5 to 10 times.

g. Repeat using the opposite foot and arm.

Partner Push-Pull (Resistance Band)

Partner push-pulls target muscles in the shoulders, upper and middle back, chest, and abdomen.

a. Sit on a chair (with or without a Dyna-Disc below the buttocks) or balance ball (with or without a ball holder) and face a partner seated on a chair or ball approximately 4 feet (1.2 m) away (see figure 8.8).

b. Use two lengths of resistance band, with each partner holding onto one end of each band.

c. Sit tall and in the middle of the balance ball with the feet hip-width apart and flat on the floor. Inhale.

d. Pull on one length of band while the partner pulls on the other length of band in a push-and-pull motion. Exhale on each pulling motion.

e. Keep the body erect during each phase of the push-and-pull movement.

f. Repeat the exercise 10 times.

g. Make sure that partners are of similar height and strength for this activity.

h. Perform this activity in a standing position as standing balance abilities improve.

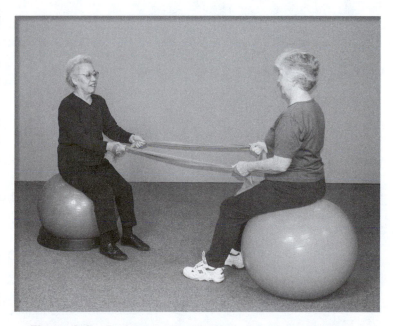

Figure 8.8 Partner push-pull with resistance bands.

Standing Triceps Extension (Hand Weight)

Triceps extensions with hand weights target muscles in the elbows, arms, and back.

a. Stand with one knee resting on a sturdy chair with no armrests. The other leg should be to the side of the chair with the knee slightly flexed.

b. Bend the body slightly forward and support the body by resting the forearm on the back of the chair on the same side as the flexed knee.

c. Hold the weight in the other hand at waist level and point the elbow backward at or above shoulder height and toward the ceiling. Inhale.

d. Slowly straighten the arm holding the weight while keeping the elbow, as well as the knee on that side, slightly flexed. Exhale as the arm is extended. Maintain a stable trunk position throughout the extension phase of the movement—the trunk should not sway or arch during the exercise. Reduce the weight if the trunk cannot be maintained in a stable position throughout the exercise.

e. Pause, then inhale and slowly bend the arm holding the weight back to the starting position.

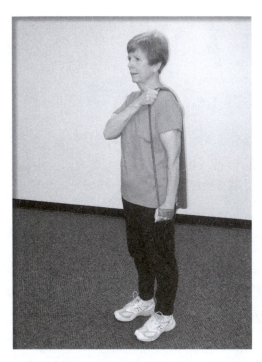

Figure 8.9 Standing triceps extension with resistance band.

Seated or Standing Triceps Extension With Resistance Band

Triceps extensions with the resistance band target muscles in the back of the upper arms.

a. Place the resistance band over the left shoulder and hold it in place at shoulder height with the right hand.

b. Grasp the band with the left hand about waist level (figure 8.9).

c. Slowly extend the left arm, keeping the elbow close to the side of the body and palm facing into the body. Exhale as the arm is extended just behind the body.

d. Pause, then slowly bend the left upper arm at the elbow until the hand is just below the hand remaining at shoulder height. Inhale as the arm returns to the starting position.

e. Move the band to the right shoulder and repeat the exercise with the right arm.

Manipulating the Level of Challenge

You can manipulate the level of challenge associated with any of the strength and endurance exercises by adjusting any of the following variables:

◆ Performance position (seated or standing)
◆ Type of seated (e.g., Dyna-Disc, balance ball) or standing (e.g., foam) surface
◆ Level of resistance or amount of weight
◆ Plane of motion (e.g., below or above the shoulder)
◆ Number of repetitions (not to exceed 15) or sets (not to exceed three)

Seated Biceps Curl With Hand Weight

The seated biceps curl targets muscles in the front of the upper arms (the biceps) and wrists.

a. Sit tall on a balance ball (advanced participants) or with the lower back pressed firmly against the backrest of a sturdy chair. Position the side of the body on which the exercise will begin close to the edge of the side of the chair. Tuck in the abdomen and chin, and direct the eyes forward.

b. Position the feet flat on the floor and hip-width apart. Hold the weight in one hand, with the arm hanging down beside the thigh and the palm facing inward. Inhale.

c. Slowly lift the weight by bending the lower arm up toward the chest, turning the palm of the hand toward the chest as the weight is lifted (figure 8.10). Exhale during the lifting phase.

d. Slowly lower the weight to the starting position with the palm facing inward again. Inhale during the lowering phase.

e. Complete 5 to 10 repetitions and repeat the exercise with the opposite arm.

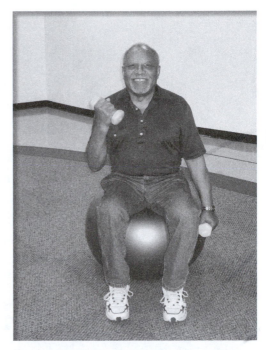

Figure 8.10   Seated biceps curl with hand weight.

Double Biceps Curl With Added Balance Component

The double biceps curl targets the biceps and abdominal muscles.

a. Sit tall and in the middle of a chair (with a Dyna-Disc under buttocks) or balance ball (with or without a ball holder) with the feet flat on the floor and hip-width apart. The resistance band should be positioned beneath the feet. Wrap equal lengths of the band around each hand or grip the band's handles (figure 8.11).

b. Begin with the arms in an extended position and the palms facing the sides of the body. Inhale.

c. Slowly bend the forearms toward the shoulders, turning the palms upward without bending the wrists. Keep the elbows tight against the body throughout the lifting phase. Exhale as the band is lifted.

d. Pause, then slowly return the band to the starting position. Inhale as the band is lowered.

e. Complete 5 to 10 repetitions.

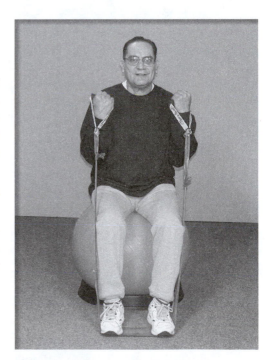

Figure 8.11   Seated double biceps curl with resistance band.

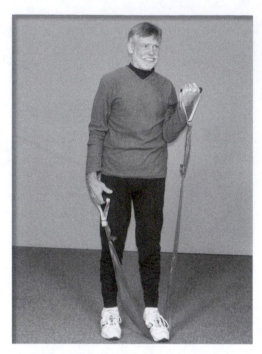

Figure 8.12 Standing biceps curl with resistance band.

Standing Biceps Curl With Resistance Band

The standing biceps curl targets muscles in the front of the arms and wrists.

  a. Secure one end of the resistance band with the foot (figure 8.12).

  b. Wrap the other end of the band around the hand or grip the handle and let the arm hang loosely at the side. Inhale.

  c. Slowly bend the forearm toward the shoulder, turning the palm upward without bending the wrist. Keep the elbow tucked against the body as the band is raised. Exhale during this phase.

  d. Pause, then slowly return the band to the starting position.

  e. Complete 5 to 10 repetitions and then repeat the exercise with the opposite arm.

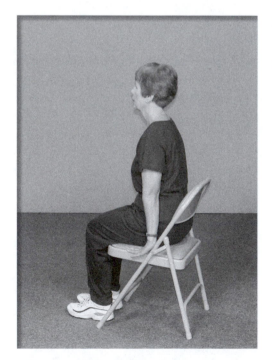

Figure 8.13 Seated press-up.

Seated Press-Up

Seated press-ups target muscles in the elbows, arms, chest, and back.

  a. Sit tall with the lower back pressed firmly against the backrest of a sturdy chair (figure 8.13). The shoulders should be relaxed and level.

  b. Tuck in the abdomen and chin and focus the eyes on a target directly ahead and at eye level.

  c. Grasp the sides of the chair next to the hips. Inhale.

  d. Slowly lift the body while keeping the back straight. Exhale as the body is lifted.

  e. Hold the position for 5 to 10 seconds, breathing evenly.

  f. Slowly return to a seated position.

Palm Squeeze

Palm squeezes target muscles in the hands and wrists.

a. Perform this exercise in a seated or standing position. The elbows should be at the sides and flexed to 90 degrees.

b. Grasp a soft ball or object (figure 8.14). Inhale. Begin squeezing the object firmly. Exhale during the squeezing motion.

c. Maintain the squeeze for 5 seconds. Repeat the exercise with the other hand.

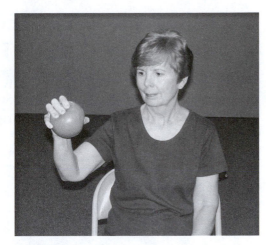

Figure 8.14   Palm squeeze.

Table 8.1   Upper-Body Strength and Endurance Exercises at a Glance

Exercise	Muscles targeted	Position	Accessories
Shoulder shrug	Upper back and neck	Seated or standing	Hand weights
Back extension	Upper back and shoulders	Seated or standing	
Back and arm extension	Upper back and shoulders	Seated or standing	Wrist weights
Side bend	Upper and middle back, shoulders, arms	Seated or standing	Hand weights
Chest press	Chest, shoulders, arms	Seated or standing	Resistance band
Horizontal pull	Upper and middle back, shoulders, arms	Seated or standing	Resistance band
Ball lift	Upper, middle, and lower back, shoulders, arms, abdomen	Seated	Weighted ball, Dyna-Disc, balance ball
Diagonal arm extension	Shoulders, upper and middle back, abdomen	Seated or standing	Resistance band
Partner push-pull	Shoulders, upper and middle back, chest, abdomen	Seated	Resistance bands (2)
Standing triceps extension	Elbows, arms, upper back	Standing	Chair, hand weight
Triceps extension	Elbows, arms	Seated or standing	Chair, resistance band
Single biceps curl	Fronts of upper arms, wrists	Seated or standing	Hand weight or resistance band, chair
Double biceps curl	Fronts of upper arms, abdomen	Seated or standing	Resistance band, chair
Standing biceps curl	Fronts of upper arms, abdomen	Standing	Hand weight or resistance band
Seated press-up	Elbows, arms, chest, back	Seated	Chair
Palm squeeze	Hands and wrists	Seated or standing	Soft ball or object, chair

Many of the strength and endurance exercises can be performed with an added balance component such as a Dyna-Disc or stability ball (with or without holder) for seated exercises or a foam balance pad or rocker board for standing exercises.

SELECTED LOWER-BODY STRENGTH EXERCISES

The lower-body strength exercises described in this section focus on the muscle groups that are important for good standing balance and mobility. Exercises that involve the larger muscle groups are described first, followed by exercises that involve smaller muscle groups. Table 8.2 on page 235 summarizes these lower-body exercises.

Wall Squat

Wall squats target the quadriceps and the muscles in the hips, back, and abdomen. This exercise can be performed with or without a balance ball.

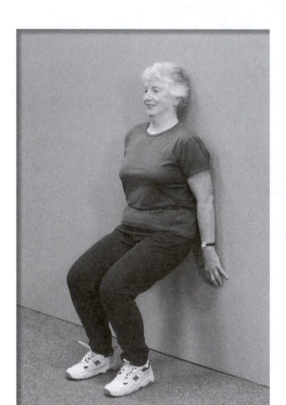

   a. Start in a standing position with the back against a wall, or against a small (55 to 65 cm) balance ball positioned against the wall, with the feet placed 12 to 24 inches (30-61 cm) from the wall and hip-width apart. Make sure the floor beneath the feet has a nonslip surface.

   b. Stand with the hips and buttocks slightly tucked and the shoulders relaxed.

   c. Slowly slide the back down the wall (or roll the ball down the wall) to lower almost to a sitting position (figure 8.15). The knees should be behind or directly above the ankles. Exhale as the body is lowered.

   d. Hold the position for 5 to 10 seconds while breathing evenly, then slowly return to the starting position.

   e. Repeat the exercise 5 to 10 times.

Caution: Keep the knee angle of the squat greater than 90 degrees if the participant has particularly weak quadriceps or pain in the knees. Placing a small balance ball behind the back can help the client move up and down the wall with greater ease.

Figure 8.15 Wall squat.

Sit-to-Standing Squat

Sit-to-standing squats target the quadriceps and the muscles in the hips, back, and abdomen.

a. Sit tall and toward the front of a chair. Tuck in the abdomen and chin and hold the head erect with the eyes directed forward. The feet should be flat on the floor and hip-width apart. Inhale.

b. Stand up from the chair, lifting the body about two-thirds of the way up (figure 8.16). Exhale as the body is lifted.

c. Keep the back straight and the knees slightly behind or directly above the ankles.

d. Hold the position for 3 to 5 seconds and then slowly return to the original seated position.

e. Repeat the exercise 5 to 10 times.

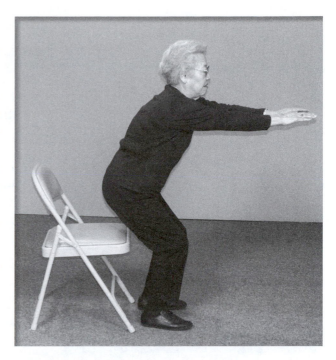

Figure 8.16 Sit-to-standing squat.

Dyna-Disc Thigh Squeeze

Thigh squeezes target the quadriceps and hip adductors and the muscles in the hips, back, and abdomen.

a. Perform the sit-to-standing squat exercise described earlier but place a Dyna-Disc between the knees.

b. Rise from the chair while squeezing the Dyna-Disc between the knees (figure 8.17). Exhale during the rising phase of the squat. Hold the position for 3 to 5 seconds.

c. Return to a seated position while keeping the Dyna-Disc between the knees. Inhale.

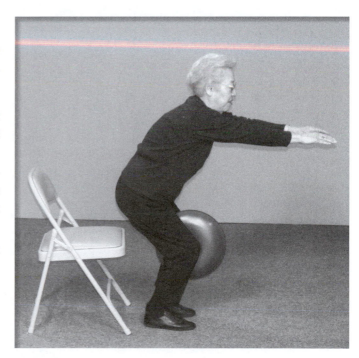

Figure 8.17 Dyna-Disc thigh squeeze.

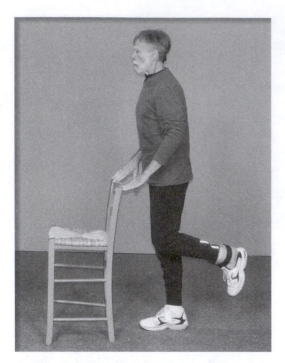

Figure 8.18 Standing leg curl.

Standing Leg Curl With or Without Ankle Weights

Standing leg curls target the hamstrings and calf muscles.

a. Stand with the feet shoulder-width apart. Hold onto the back of a chair and stand tall. Inhale.

b. Shift body weight over to one side and slowly bend the other knee, lifting the lower leg backward to form a 90-degree angle at the knee (see figure 8.18). Do not allow the thigh of the leg with the knee being flexed to move behind the other thigh. Maintain a slightly flexed (i.e., soft) knee on the standing leg during each leg curl. Exhale as the knee is flexed.

c. Return the leg slowly to the starting position.

d. Repeat the exercise with the other leg.

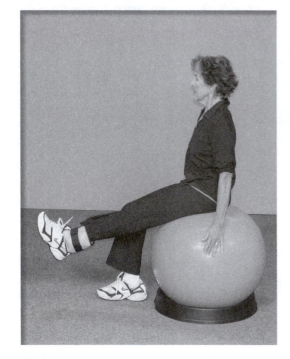

Figure 8.19 Seated leg extension with ankle weight.

Seated Leg Extension

Seated leg extensions target the muscles in the abdomen, hips, and legs.

a. Sit tall on a ball or chair. If sitting on a chair, press the lower back firmly against the backrest. The abdomen and chin should be tucked in, the head erect, and the eyes directed forward. Inhale.

b. Hold onto the side of the ball and tighten the muscles in the leg.

c. Extend one leg and raise it into a 90-degree angle with the floor (figure 8.19). Flex the ankle and point the toes toward the ceiling as the leg is raised. Exhale during the lifting phase.

d. Slowly lower the leg to the starting position. Inhale as the leg is lowered.

e. Repeat the exercise with the opposite leg.

f. Add an ankle weight to increase resistance once the movement can be performed correctly and each leg can complete 10 repetitions successfully.

Standing Flexion and Extension

Standing flexion and extension target muscles in the hips and legs.

a. Stand upright with the feet hip-width apart and hold onto the side of a chair or a wall for support. Inhale.

b. Shift weight onto one side and slowly raise and extend the other leg in a forward direction (see figure 8.20). The knee of the standing leg should be slightly flexed throughout the exercise. Exhale as the leg is raised.

c. Inhale and lower the leg back to the floor; pause momentarily before extending the leg in a backward direction. Exhale as the leg is moved backward.

d. Return the leg to the starting position. Inhale as the leg is lowered.

e. Avoid bending at the hips by not raising the leg too high in either direction.

f. Repeat the exercise with the other leg.

g. Add ankle weights to increase resistance if correct form is being used during the exercise.

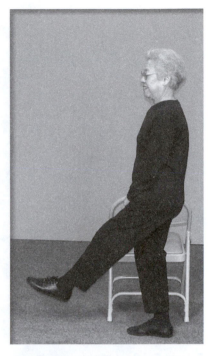

Figure 8.20 Standing flexion and extension.

Seated Hip Abduction

Seated hip abduction targets the hip abductors.

a. Sit tall in the center of a chair with the feet flat on the floor and hip-width apart.

b. Wrap a resistance band once or twice around the thighs of both legs and hold the ends firmly against the thighs (see figure 8.21). Inhale.

c. Exhale and push the outside of the thighs against the band.

d. Inhale and slowly move the thighs back to the starting position.

e. Complete 5 to 8 repetitions. Increase the resistance as practice progresses.

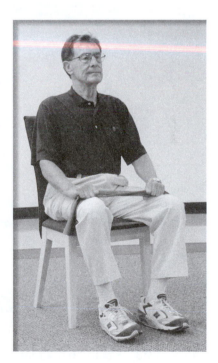

Figure 8.21 Seated hip abduction.

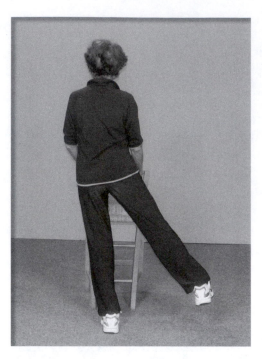

Figure 8.22 Lateral leg lift.

Lateral Leg Lift

Lateral leg lifts target the hip abductors and adductors and the leg muscles.

a. Stand with the feet together and hold onto a wall or chair for support. Shift weight onto one leg. Inhale.

b. Slowly raise the other leg out to the side, leading with the heel (figure 8.22). Maintain an upright posture and exhale as the leg is raised.

c. Slowly return the leg to the floor. Inhale as the leg is lowered.

d. Repeat the exercise with the opposite leg.

e. Add ankle weights to increase resistance if correct form can be maintained during the exercise.

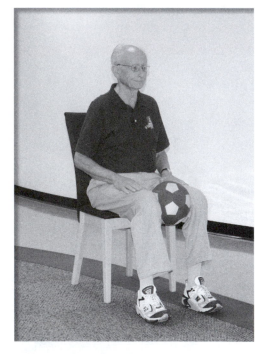

Figure 8.23 Seated hip adduction.

Seated Hip Adduction

Seated hip adduction targets the hip adductors.

a. Sit tall in the center of a chair with the feet flat on the floor.

b. Place 4- to 8-inch (10-20 cm) ball between the thighs and inhale.

c. Exhale and slowly squeeze the ball by moving the insides of the thighs toward each other (figure 8.23).

d. Slowly release the pressure on the ball by moving the thighs back to the starting position.

e. Perform 5 to 8 repetitions.

f. Increase the ball size as strength increases.

Standing Forward Lunge

The standing forward lunge targets the quadriceps and the muscles in the hips, legs, and ankles.

a. Stand with the feet shoulder-width apart and hold onto a chair. Tuck in the abdomen and chin, and keep the head erect and the eyes directed forward. The knees should be slightly flexed. Inhale.

b. Position one foot slightly behind the other and raise the heel (figure 8.24).

c. Slowly flex the back knee toward the floor while also flexing the forward knee. Exhale as the knees are flexed.

d. Pause, then slowly return to the starting position.

e. Repeat the exercise with the opposite leg.

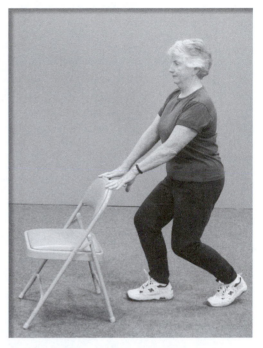

Figure 8.24   Standing forward lunge.

Seated Hip Flexion

Seated hip flexion targets the hip muscles.

a. Sit with the knees shoulder-width apart.

b. Slowly lift one knee, keeping the upper body erect (figure 8.25).

c. Pause, then slowly lower the leg.

d. Complete 5 to 10 repetitions with the same leg, then repeat the exercise using the other leg.

e. Sit on a Dyna-Disc or balance ball to further challenge balance.

f. Perform this exercise with or without ankle weights.

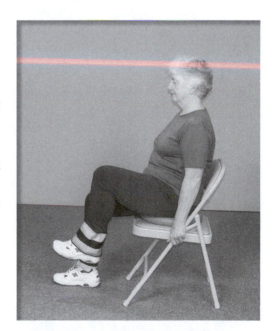

Figure 8.25   Seated hip flexion with ankle weights and added balance component.

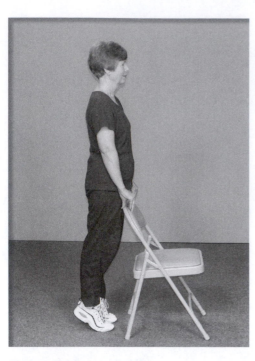

Figure 8.26 Heel raise.

Heel Raise

Heel raises target the calf muscles.

   a. Stand tall with the feet flat on the floor and hip-width apart. Hold onto the back of a chair or a wall for additional support. The head should be erect with the eyes directed forward. Inhale.

   b. Slowly lift both heels off the floor (figure 8.26). Exhale as the heels lift.

   c. Hold the position for 5 to 10 seconds, breathing evenly, and then slowly lower the heels to the floor.

   d. Repeat the exercise 10 times.

   e. Add ankle weights for greater resistance.

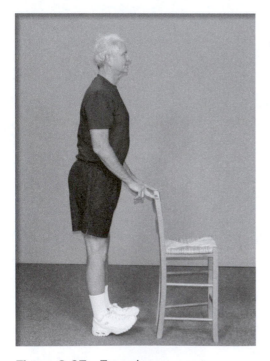

Figure 8.27 Toe raise.

Toe Raise

Toe raises target the shin muscles.

   a. Stand tall with the feet flat on the floor and hip-width apart. Hold onto a chair or wall for extra support. Inhale.

   b. Slowly raise the toes off the floor until weight is on the heels only (figure 8.27). Exhale as the toes rise from the floor.

   c. Hold the position for 5 to 10 seconds, breathing evenly, and then slowly lower the toes to the floor.

Foot Press

Foot presses target the muscles in the shins, ankles, and feet.

a. In a seated position, flex the ankle of one foot and place the heel of the other foot on top of the flexed foot (see figure 8.28). Inhale.

b. Slowly push the flexed foot down toward the floor with the heel of the opposite foot. Resist lowering of the flexed foot by continuing to pull the toes of that foot back toward the shin. Exhale.

c. Complete five repetitions before performing the exercise with the other foot.

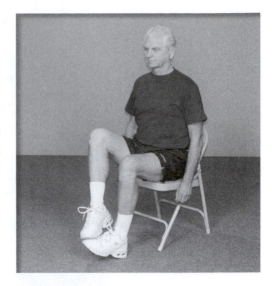

Figure 8.28   Foot press.

SELECTED EXERCISES FOR THE FOOT AND TOES

This final set of exercises is best performed in a seated position with the shoes and socks removed. Table 8.2 on page 235 summarizes these exercises.

Toe Pointing and Flexion

Toe pointing and flexion targets the plantar flexors and dorsiflexors.

a. Sit upright toward the front edge of a chair, keeping the trunk erect.

b. Wrap a resistance band once around the right foot, keeping the left knee flexed and the right knee extended.

c. Maintaining the tension on the band, slowly point and flex the toes (figure 8.29).

d. Complete 5 to 10 repetitions before performing the exercise with the opposite leg.

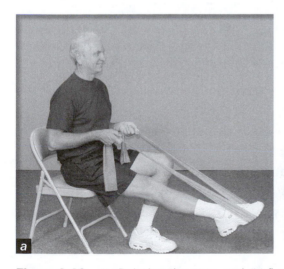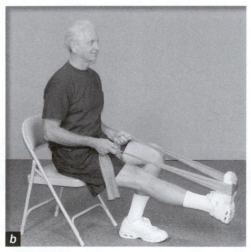

Figure 8.29   *(a)* Pointing the toes and *(b)* flexing the toes.

Heel Raise, Toe Point, and Curl

The heel raise, toe point, and curl target the muscles of the feet and toes.

    a. In a seated position, slowly raise the heel of one foot and hold for 5 seconds (see figure 8.30*a*).

    b. Continue lifting the heel until the tips of the toes are touching the floor (figure 8.30*b*).

    c. Hold the position for 5 seconds.

    d. Gently curl the toes under and hold for 5 seconds (figure 8.30*c*).

    e. Reverse the movement sequence and repeat.

    f. This is a good exercise for individuals with hammertoes or toe cramps.

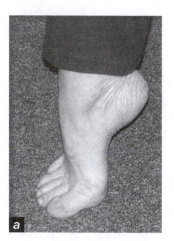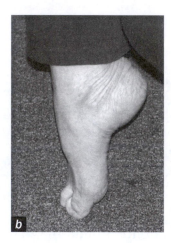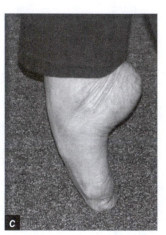

Figure 8.30 *(a)* Heel raise, *(b)* toe point, and *(c)* toe curl.

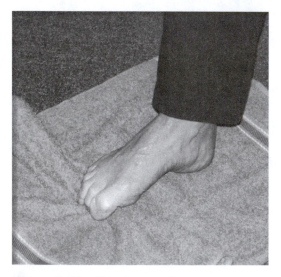

Figure 8.31 Towel scrunch.

Towel Scrunch

Towel scrunches target the muscles of the ankles, feet, and toes.

    a. Place a small towel on the floor and pull it toward the body, using only the toes (figure 8.31).

    b. Increase the resistance by putting a weight on the end of the towel.

    c. Relax and repeat the exercise three times before repeating it with the opposite foot.

    d. This is a good exercise for individuals with hammertoes, toe cramps, or pain in the balls of the feet.

Marble Pick-Up

The marble pick-up targets the muscles of the feet and toes.

a. Place 10 marbles on the floor. Use the toes to pick up one marble at a time and place it in a small bowl (figure 8.32).

b. Continue until all marbles have been retrieved.

c. This is a good exercise for individuals with hammertoes, toe cramps, or pain in the balls of the feet.

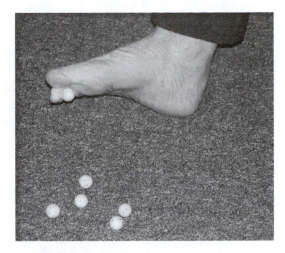

Figure 8.32 Marble pick-up.

Table 8.2 Lower-Body Strength and Endurance Exercises at a Glance

Exercise	Muscles targeted	Position	Accessories
Wall squat	Fronts of thighs, hips, back, abdomen	Standing	Small balance ball
Sit-to-standing squat	Fronts of thighs, hips, back, abdomen	Seated	Chair
Dyna-Disc thigh squeeze	Fronts of thighs, hip adductors, back, abdominal muscles	Seated	Chair, Dyna-Disc
Standing leg curl	Backs of thighs, calves	Standing	Ankle weights, chair
Seated leg extension	Abdomen, hips, and legs	Seated	Ankle weights
Standing flexion and extension	Hips and legs	Standing	Ankle weights, chair
Seated hip abduction	Hip abductors	Seated	Resistance band
Lateral leg lift	Hip abductors and adductors, legs	Standing	Ankle weights, chair
Seated hip adduction	Hip adductors	Seated	4-8 in. (10-20 cm) ball that can be compressed
Standing forward lunge	Fronts of thighs, hips, legs, ankles	Standing	Hand weights
Seated hip flexion	Hip muscles	Seated	Ankle weights
Heel raise	Calves, feet, toes	Standing	Ankle weights, chair
Toe raise	Shins	Standing	Chair
Foot press	Shins, ankles, feet	Seated	Chair
Toe pointing and flexion	Ankle muscles	Seated	Resistance band
Heel raise, toe point, and curl	Feet and toes	Seated	Chair
Towel scrunch	Feet and toes	Seated or standing	Towel, weighted object, chair
Marble pick-up	Feet and toes	Seated	Marbles, bowl

Many of the strength and endurance exercises can be performed with an added balance component such as a Dyna-Disc or stability ball (with or without holder) for seated exercises or a foam balance pad or rocker board for standing exercises.

SUMMARY

Maintaining adequate muscle strength and endurance is important for good postural alignment, balance, and mobility. Despite the age-related declines observed in absolute muscle strength and power, much can be done to offset the losses by having your clients engage in strength and endurance activities of increasing difficulty. As performance improves, the amount of resistance and the number of repetitions performed per set can be increased. In addition, many of the strength and endurance activities introduced in this chapter can be performed in a balance environment to further increase the challenge associated with the activity and also simulate the challenges that may be encountered in ADLs.

Test Your Understanding

1. Men and women over the age of 60 years lose muscle mass
   a. more slowly than younger adults lose muscle mass
   b. at a rate of .5 to 1.0 percent per decade
   c. at a rate of .5 to 1.0 percent per year
   d. more quickly than they lose muscle power
   e. at a rate of 2 percent per year

2. Strength exercises should be introduced into the class
   a. during the warm-up and before any flexibility exercises are performed
   b. during the cool-down when the muscles are warm
   c. after the dynamic flexibility component of the warm-up has been completed
   d. when a sufficient amount of postural stability has been achieved
   e. when class participants have reached a level of fatigue that will facilitate better attention to the strength and endurance activities

3. The level of resistance should be increased once class participants are able to
   a. complete three sets of 15 repetitions at a given weight
   b. complete one set of 15 repetitions at a given weight
   c. perform the activity in both seated and standing positions
   d. complete 10 repetitions successfully
   e. perform the activity using correct form

4. Which of the following strength activities would be most appropriate if the goal is to improve the older adult's lateral stability during gait?
   a. wall squats
   b. standing leg curls
   c. standing flexion and extension
   d. lateral leg lifts with ankle weights
   e. heel raises

5. Which of the following activities would be best suited to improving core stability as well as strength in a given muscle group?
   a. standing biceps curls
   b. ball lifts while seated on a balance ball
   c. forward lunge
   d. heel raises while seated on a balance ball
   e. leg extensions while seated on a chair with a backrest and a Dyna-Disc under the buttocks

6. During which phase of a strength activity should you encourage the participant to exhale?

    a. during the exertion phase

    b. before the start of the movement

    c. after the movement has been completed

    d. before, during, and after the movement

    e. at any time during the activity

7. It is most appropriate to adjust the knee angle while performing the wall squat if

    a. the client has weak hamstrings

    b. the client is very tall

    c. the client has weak quadriceps

    d. the client is experiencing pain in the knees when performing the task

    e. both c and d

8. Which additional muscle group is recruited when a client performs a sit-to-standing squat while holding a Dyna-Disc between the thighs?

    a. hamstrings

    b. hip adductors

    c. hip abductors

    d. quadriceps

    e. rectus femoris

9. Which one of the following exercises would you select to improve quadriceps strength with the goal of improving walking?

    a. forward lunge

    b. standing leg curls with ankle weights

    c. standing flexion and extension

    d. standing lateral leg lifts

10. Which of the following exercises specifically targets the dorsiflexors and plantar flexors of the feet?

    a. towel scrunches

    b. marble pick-up

    c. pointing and flexing toes

    d. heel raises

Practical Problems

1. Develop a set of progressive strength and endurance activities for either Phoebe or Larry after a review of their baseline test results. List the muscle groups you think should be prioritized during this component of the program and provide a rationale for their selection.

2. Describe five strength and endurance activities you would add to the repertoire of activities already provided.

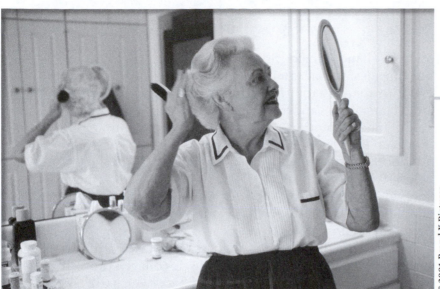
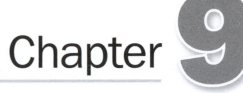

Chapter 9

Flexibility Training

Objectives

After completing this chapter, you will be able to

- understand the contribution of joint and muscle flexibility to the multiple dimensions of balance and mobility,
- describe the age-associated changes in joint and muscle flexibility,
- develop a set of exercise progressions to improve upper- and lower-body joint and muscle flexibility, and
- incorporate flexibility exercises into a balance environment.

Like strength, joint range of motion and muscle flexibility gradually decline with age. Specific losses of joint range of motion and muscle strength have been directly linked to the progression of various disabilities among older adults and a declining ability to perform basic and instrumental activities of daily living (ADLs) (Jette, Branch, & Berlin, 1990). More recently, Morey, Pieper, and Cornoni-Huntley (1998) have shown that loss of flexibility in shoulder rotation and cervical and spinal rotation is directly related to functional limitations and increased susceptibility to falls among older adults in their 70s. Although declines in joint range of motion and muscle flexibility are inevitable, the rate at which the decline occurs is joint specific (Bell & Hoshizaki, 1981). For example, the loss of flexibility is more evident in the lower-extremity as opposed to upper-extremity joints. The reduced flexibility observed in the lower-body joints has particularly important implications for dynamic balance and functional mobility.

The aging process results in increased stiffness in all joints and surrounding muscle tissues. Stiffness is defined by the force required to move a joint through

> ### Key Point
>
> The rate at which joint range of motion and muscle flexibility decline is joint specific.

a specified range of motion (Holland, Tanaka, Shigematsu, & Nakagaichi, 2002). Tendons, ligaments, joint capsules, fasciae, and slow-twitch muscle fibers are all affected. Even muscles that are used on a routine basis (e.g., calf muscles) show an increase in stiffness (Lung, Hartsell, & Vandervoort, 1996). Of particular importance is the significant loss of range of motion at the ankle joint, especially among older women. Women between the ages of 55 and 85 lose as much as 50 percent of their ankle range of motion, whereas men lose approximately 35 percent of their ankle range of motion (Bandy & Sanders, 2001). Reductions in ankle range of motion place the older adult at heightened risk for falling, especially while walking. Special attention should therefore be given to improving ankle flexibility during the balance and mobility training program.

Age-related changes in muscle structure also lead to increased muscle stiffness and reduced tensile strength. The age-related increase in muscle collagen (known to be very resistant to stretch) and degeneration of elastin fibers (which are less resistant to stretch) contribute to this increased muscle stiffness (Holland et al., 2002). As a result, ballistic stretching routines should be avoided at all costs because of the likelihood of injuring muscle. It is also recommended that older adults perform their stretching activities more slowly and maintain a given stretch for a longer duration (i.e., 30-60 seconds) once the internal temperature of the body and muscle tissue is sufficiently warm (Asp, 2000). Remember that the most effective stretching program will be one that is not only based on the individual needs of your participants but also performed regularly. Thus, you should encourage your participants to incorporate a stretching routine into their daily lives. Flexibility exercises should also be assigned as homework once correct form has been taught during class. Incorporating stretching activities into your classes will also benefit older adults who are experiencing reduced range of motion as a result of musculoskeletal or neuromuscular diseases (e.g., arthritis, PD, multiple sclerosis). A gentle stretching routine has also been shown to be beneficial for older adults who are experiencing chronic pain.

> ### Key Point
>
> Ballistic stretching routines should be avoided at all costs due to the likelihood of injury to muscle tissue in older adults.

Be sure to review selected test results obtained during the preprogram assessment to determine which areas of a participant's body are less flexible and therefore in need of additional attention. The results of the sit-and-reach test and scratch test of the Senior Fitness Test (Rikli & Jones, 2001), which test lower- and upper-body flexibility, respectively, will be particularly helpful to you in deciding how to proceed with the flexibility component of your program. You should also note the joint flexibility demonstrated at the hip, knee, and ankle joints during performance of the 30-foot walk test. In addition to reviewing the test results of your participants, also review each client's medical history to determine whether you need to modify or delete certain exercises due to predisposing medical conditions or client concerns (e.g., joint contractures, osteoporosis).

When incorporating flexibility activities into your balance and mobility training program, consider the following guidelines, some of which have been established by the American College of Sports Medicine (1998, 2007):

- Avoid ballistic (bouncing) stretching exercises.
- Incorporate more multijoint, dynamic stretches during the warm-up phase of the class. The continuous contraction of muscles helps warm the muscle tissue and prepare it for subsequent exercise.

- Introduce movements and joint actions that mimic those to be performed later in the class, and progressively increase the range of motion with each repetition.
- Have participants perform flexibility exercises 2 (for maintenance) to 7 (for increased range of motion) days per week based on individual needs.
- During static stretches, have participants hold the stretched position for 5 to 40 seconds (depending on which muscles are being stretched). A hold time of 60 seconds may be preferable for certain muscle groups (e.g., hamstrings).
- Repeat a stretch 1 to 5 times (depending on which muscles are being stretched).
- Gradually increase the range through which the muscle is stretched as tolerance increases.
- In later classes, have clients perform selected flexibility exercises while seated on a Dyna-Disc or balance ball to increase the balance challenge.
- Approach flexibility exercises systematically. Work from top to toe, or stretch the lower body during warm-up and the upper body during cool-down.

Table 9.1 (on page 253) summarizes the flexibility exercises presented in this chapter.

SELECTED NECK AND UPPER-BODY FLEXIBILITY EXERCISES

The exercises presented in this section are designed to help your clients maintain the flexibility needed to perform many basic and instrumental activities of daily living. Just a few examples of the types of daily activities that require good levels of flexibility in the neck, shoulders, and trunk include combing or brushing one's hair, reaching for objects on the upper shelves of a closet, and turning to check that a lane is clear when driving.

Seated Chin-to-Chest Stretch

The chin-to-chest stretch targets the muscles in the back of the neck.

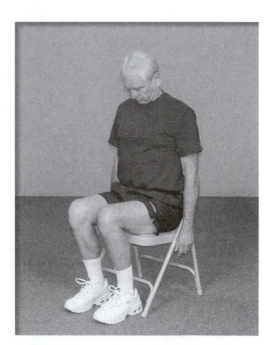

a. Sit tall with the lower back pressed firmly against the backrest of a chair. Keep the shoulders relaxed and the chin tucked in so that the ears are directly above the shoulders. The eyes should be focused on a target directly ahead and at eye level. Inhale.

b. Slowly tuck the chin toward the chest while exhaling (figure 9.1).

c. Hold the position for 5 to 10 seconds while breathing evenly.

d. Inhale and raise the head back to the starting position, one vertebra at a time.

e. For an added balance challenge, perform the exercise while seated on a Dyna-Disc or balance ball.

Figure 9.1 Seated chin-to-chest stretch.

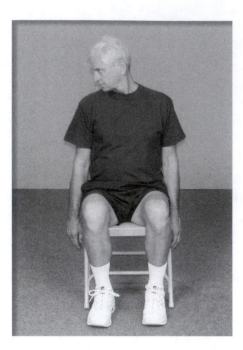

Figure 9.2 Seated neck rotation.

Neck Rotation

Neck rotations target the muscles in the back and sides of the neck.

 a. Sit tall with the lower back pressed firmly against the backrest of a chair. Keep the shoulders relaxed and the chin tucked in and gently resting on the chest. The eyes should be focused on a target directly ahead and at eye level. Inhale.

 b. With the head in a comfortable position and the chin gently tucked in, slowly turn the chin up toward the right shoulder (figure 9.2), then back across the chest and up toward the left shoulder. Exhale during the rotation.

 c. Keep the chin in contact with the chest throughout the rotation.

 d. Repeat the exercise 3 to 5 times.

 e. For an added balance challenge, perform the exercise while seated on a Dyna-Disc or balance ball or while standing behind a chair.

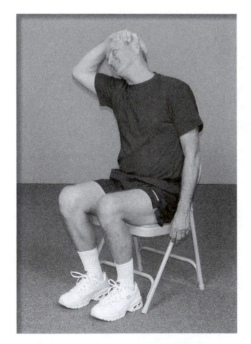

Figure 9.3 Assisted neck side stretch.

Assisted Neck Side Stretch

The assisted neck side stretch targets the muscles in the sides of the neck.

 a. Sit tall with the lower back pressed firmly against the backrest of a chair. Keep the shoulders relaxed and the head erect, with the eyes focused on a target directly ahead and at eye level. Inhale.

 b. Slowly bend the head so the right earlobe moves toward the right shoulder. Bend the head as far down as is comfortable while reaching the left hand down toward the floor.

 c. Reach the right hand up and over the head until it is resting on the left side of the head (see figure 9.3). Use the weight of the hand to increase the stretch to the right side. Exhale as the head bends toward the shoulder.

 d. Hold the position for 5 to 10 seconds, breathing evenly.

 e. Inhale as the head moves back to the starting position. Repeat the stretch to the left side.

 f. Perform the exercise three times to each side.

Assisted Neck Flexion

Assisted neck flexion targets the muscles in the back of the neck, the upper back, and the shoulders.

a. Sit tall with the lower back pressed firmly against the backrest of a chair. Keep the shoulders relaxed and the head erect, with the eyes focused on a target directly in front and at eye level.

b. Position the fingers behind the head. Inhale.

c. Gently move the chin toward the chest as the shoulders remain level, allowing the weight of the hands to increase the amount of stretch (see figure 9.4). Exhale during this phase of the stretch.

d. Do not allow the upper back or spine to lean forward during the stretch. The action must be isolated to the neck.

e. Hold the stretch for 5 to 10 seconds, breathing evenly.

f. Inhale as the head returns to the starting position.

g. Repeat the exercise 3 to 5 times.

Turtle Stretch

The turtle stretch targets the muscles in the front and back of the neck.

a. Perform this exercise while seated or standing.

b. Place the thumb side of the hands next to the ears, palms facing forward. Inhale.

c. Gently bring the head backward and behind the thumbs (figure 9.5a). Be sure to keep the chin level during the movement. Have participants imagine that they are sliding the chin along a tray.

d. Without pausing, move the head forward until it has passed the thumbs again (figure 9.5b).

e. Repeat 5 to 10 times in the forward and backward directions, breathing evenly throughout the exercise.

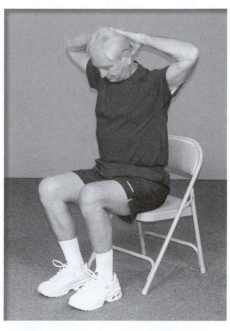

Figure 9.4 Assisted neck flexion.

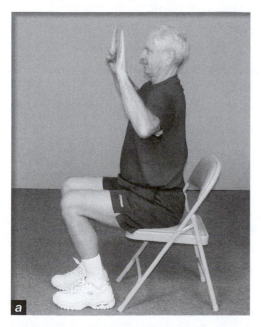 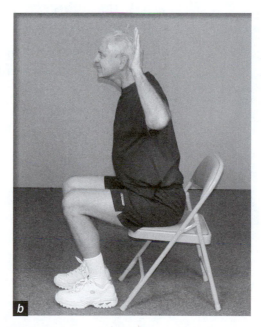

Figure 9.5 Turtle stretch: (a) backward and (b) forward movements.

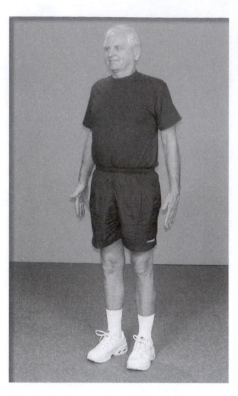

Figure 9.6 Shoulder roll.

Shoulder Roll

The shoulder roll targets the muscles in the shoulders, upper back, and chest.

a. Perform this exercise in a seated or standing position. Inhale before beginning the action.

b. Roll the shoulders up toward the ears and then backward and down as the shoulder blades are squeezed together (figure 9.6). Exhale during the downward phase of the movement.

c. Inhale as the shoulders move back up toward the ears for the start of the second repetition.

d. Repeat five times and then reverse the direction of the shoulder movement for an additional five repetitions.

e. For an added balance challenge, perform the exercise while seated on a Dyna-Disc or balance ball or while standing on a foam or moving surface (i.e., rocker board).

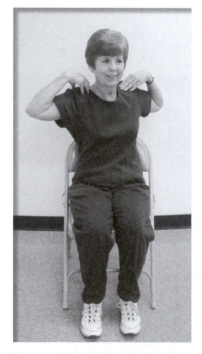

Figure 9.7 Elbow circle.

Elbow Circle

Elbow circles target the muscles in the scapulae and shoulders.

a. Perform this exercise in a seated or standing position.

b. Place the hands on the shoulders (see figure 9.7). Inhale.

c. Circle both arms in a wide arc, first in a backward direction and then in a forward direction Breathe evenly throughout the exercise.

d. For an added balance challenge, perform the exercise while seated on a Dyna-Disc or balance ball.

Finger Walking

Finger walking targets muscles in the chest and shoulders.

a. Stand tall and face a wall such that the toes are almost touching it. Keep the head erect and the eyes directed forward throughout the exercise.

b. Place the hands at waist level with the palms facing the wall and the fingertips in contact with the wall. Inhale.

c. Walk both arms up the wall, leading with the fingertips, until the arms are as far above the head as is comfortable (figure 9.8). Exhale as the fingers are walked up the wall.

d. Inhale and walk the fingers back down the wall without pausing at the top.

e. Repeat the finger walking 10 times.

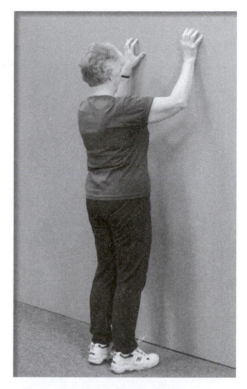

Figure 9.8   Finger walking.

Full-Body Stretch

The full-body stretch targets the muscles in the fingers, arms, shoulders, back, and abdomen.

a. Stand tall with the feet shoulder-width apart. The abdomen and chin should be tucked in, with the head erect and the eyes directed forward. The shoulders should be relaxed. Inhale.

b. Slowly extend the arms up over the head to a comfortable height (figure 9.9). Exhale as the arms are lifted; inhale when the arms reach the highest point.

c. Stretch the right arm farther toward the ceiling than the left arm is stretched. Exhale during the upward stretch.

d. Pause and inhale, then stretch the left arm farther toward the ceiling than the right arm is stretched.

e. Repeat the exercise five times with each arm.

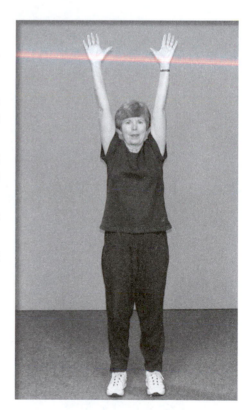

Figure 9.9   Full-body stretch.

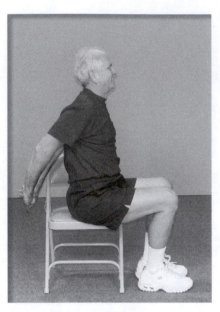

Figure 9.10 Chest stretch.

Chest Stretch

The chest stretch targets muscles in the front of the shoulders and upper chest.

  a. Perform this exercise while standing or while sitting sideways on a chair with no armrests.
  b. Clasp the hands behind the back while maintaining a straight back (do not arch the back; see figure 9.10). Inhale.
  c. Exhale as the arms are slowly raised upward as far as is comfortable.
  d. Hold the stretch for 15 to 30 seconds, breathing evenly throughout the hold.
  e. Repeat the stretch twice.

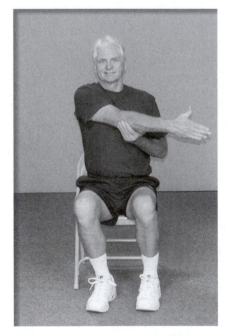

Figure 9.11 Lateral shoulder stretch.

Lateral Shoulder Stretch

The lateral shoulder stretch targets the muscles in the shoulders.

  a. Perform this exercise while seated or standing.
  b. Reach one arm across the front of the body and as close to shoulder height as is comfortable. Do not allow the shoulders to lift as the arm reaches across the body.
  c. Reach the opposite arm under the outstretched arm and grasp it above the elbow (figure 9.11).
  d. Slowly pull the elbow toward the body and slightly in the direction of the outstretched arm to increase the stretch. Exhale during the stretch.
  e. Feel the tension across the shoulders and back.
  f. Hold the stretch for 15 to 30 seconds, then repeat the stretch to the opposite side.
  g. Repeat the stretch twice to each side.

Roll-Down

The roll-down targets the muscles in the lower back.

a. Sit tall in a chair or stand with the feet hip-width apart (if balance is good).

b. Slowly roll the upper body down toward the floor with the arms hanging loosely by the sides (see figure 9.12).

c. Gently roll back up to the starting position, keeping the head and chin tucked in until the trunk has returned to an upright position.

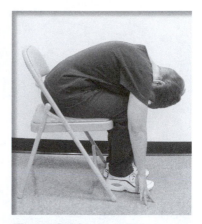

Figure 9.12 Roll-down.

Wrist Circle

Wrist circles target the muscles in the wrists and hands.

a. Sit tall with the lower back pressed firmly against the backrest of a chair.

b. Extend and raise the arms to shoulder height (figure 9.13).

c. Begin slowly circling both wrists in a clockwise direction 5 to 10 times, and then reverse the direction and repeat the exercise 5 to 10 times.

Palm-Up and Palm-Down Wrist and Finger Extensions

The wrist and finger extensions target the muscles in the wrists, hands, and forearms.

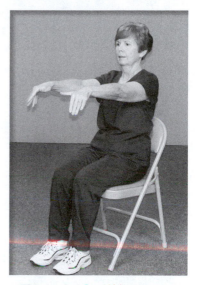

Figure 9.13 Wrist circle.

a. Sit tall with the lower back pressed firmly against the backrest of a chair. The shoulders should be relaxed, with the head erect and the eyes directed forward.

b. Extend and raise one arm to shoulder height and flex the wrist so the palm is pointing up toward the ceiling (figure 9.14a).

c. With the other hand, gently press the back of the hand toward the body.

d. Hold the position for 5 to 15 seconds, breathing evenly throughout the exercise.

e. Repeat the exercise with the other hand.

f. Repeat this exercise with the palms facing down (extend and raise each arm to shoulder height with the palm facing down and the fingertips pointing up toward the ceiling; see figure 9.14b).

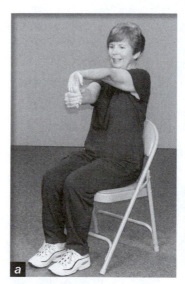 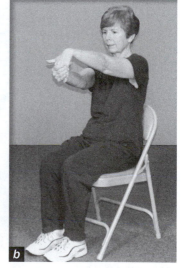

Figure 9.14 Wrist and finger extensions with (a) the palm up and (b) the palm down.

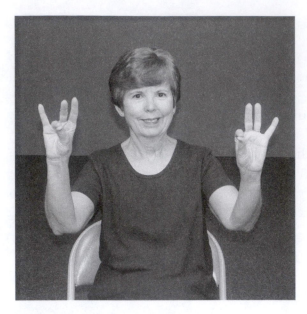

Figure 9.15 Thumb-to-finger touches.

Thumb-to-Finger Touch

Thumb-to-finger touches target the muscles in the thumb and fingers.

a. Sit tall with the lower back pressed firmly against the backrest of a chair. The shoulders should be relaxed, with the head erect and the eyes directed forward.

b. Open the palms of one or both hands and extend and spread the fingers.

c. Exaggerating each move, touch the tip of the thumb to each finger in sequential order (i.e., thumb to index finger, middle finger, ring finger, little finger; see figure 9.15).

d. Return the thumb and finger to the original starting position before proceeding to the next finger.

e. Repeat the entire sequence five times with each hand.

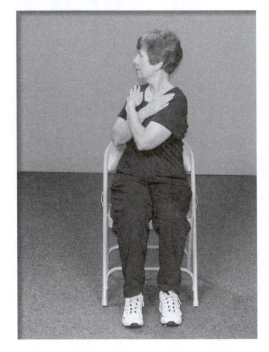

Figure 9.16 Seated trunk rotation.

Seated Trunk Rotation

The seated trunk rotation targets the muscles on the side of the trunk.

a. Sit tall with the lower back pressed firmly against the backrest of a chair. The shoulders should be relaxed, with the head erect and the eyes directed forward.

b. Fold the arms across the chest. Inhale.

c. Gently rotate the trunk to one side as far as is comfortable (figure 9.16). Exhale during the twisting motion. Hold the end position for 5 to 10 seconds, breathing evenly throughout the hold.

d. Slowly rotate the trunk as far to the opposite side as is comfortable. Exhale during the twisting motion.

e. Keep the hips facing forward throughout the exercise.

f. Repeat the exercise five times to each side.

g. For an added balance challenge, perform the exercise while seated on a Dyna-Disc or balance ball.

Side Stretch

The side stretch targets the muscles on the side of the trunk.

a. Sit tall with the lower back pressed firmly against the backrest of a sturdy chair or stand tall with the feet hip-width apart and the knees slightly bent. The abdomen and chin should be tucked in, the head erect, and the eyes directed forward. The arms should be hanging loosely at the sides. Inhale.

b. Gradually slide the right arm down toward the knee as far as is comfortable (figure 9.17). Keep the head aligned with the trunk during the downward stretch. Exhale as the arm slides down the leg.

c. Slowly return to the starting position, pause momentarily, and then repeat the exercise to the left side.

d. Repeat the exercise 3 to 5 times to each side.

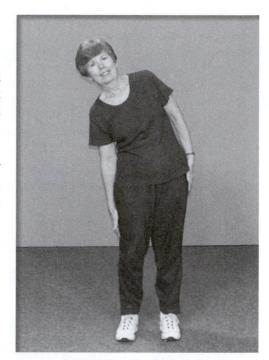

Figure 9.17 Side stretch in standing position.

Bowing to the Gods

Bowing targets the muscles in the shoulders, upper back, and arms.

a. Holding onto the top of a chair, step backward until the back and arms are extended (figure 9.18). Position the feet shoulder-width apart. Inhale.

b. Gradually tuck the head between the arms and push downward until tension is felt in the shoulders and upper back. Exhale during the stretch.

c. Hold the end position for 10 to 15 seconds, breathing evenly throughout the hold.

d. Relax and walk the feet back toward the chair and roll up slowly.

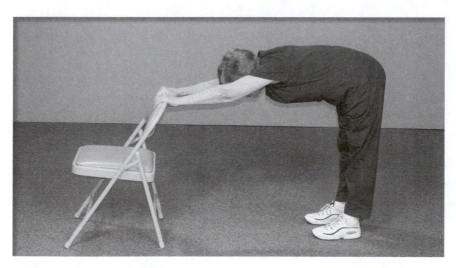

Figure 9.18 Bowing to the gods.

SELECTED LOWER-BODY FLEXIBILITY EXERCISES

The exercises described in this section are intended to improve flexibility in the hip, knee, and ankle joints as well as improve the flexibility of the musculature and smaller joints in the feet. Just as strength influences how well an older adult is able to move through space so too does the level of flexibility. For example, daily activities such as stepping up onto curbs or over obstacles, climbing stairs, getting into and out of a vehicle, and avoiding tripping when walking are dependent on having a sufficient level of flexibility in the joints and muscles of the lower body.

Hip Abductor Stretch

The hip abductor stretch targets the hip abductors and the muscles in the thighs, sides of the trunk, and upper arms.

    a. Stand tall and face sideways to a wall. Keep the abdomen and chin tucked in, the head erect, and the eyes directed forward.

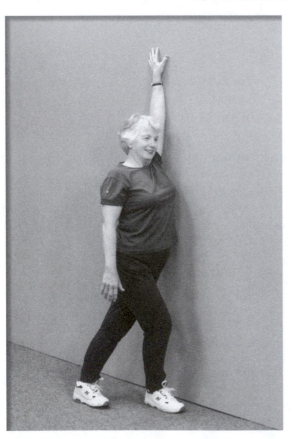

    b. Raise the arm closest to the wall above the head and rest it against the wall. The opposite arm should also be extended and resting against the body. Inhale.

    c. Cross the foot closest to the wall behind the ankle of the opposite foot (figure 9.19). The knee of the opposite leg should be slightly bent.

    d. Slowly lean into the wall, keeping the leg closest to the wall extended during the lean.

    e. The stretch should be felt on the outside of the thigh closest to the wall. Exhale during the lean.

    f. Hold the stretch for 15 to 30 seconds, breathing evenly throughout the hold. Uncross the leg and turn to face the opposite side. Repeat the stretch.

    g. Repeat the exercise 3 to 5 times on each side.

Figure 9.19 Hip abductor stretch.

Forward Lunge

The forward lunge targets the muscles in the front of the thigh.

a. Stand tall with the feet parallel and hip-width apart. Step forward (i.e., lunge) as far as feels comfortable and stable with one foot and bend the knee so that it is aligned with the ankle joint. Use a chair if needed (figure 9.20).

b. Lower the knee of the back leg slowly to the floor. Inhale.

c. Straighten the back leg and slowly lean forward, maintaining a straight back throughout the stretch.

d. Hold the position for 15 to 30 seconds before returning to the starting position. Repeat the stretch with the opposite leg.

e. Repeat the exercise three times on each side.

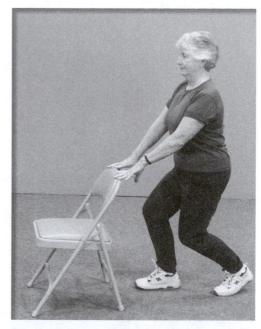

Figure 9.20 Forward lunge.

Hamstrings Stretch

The hamstrings stretch targets the muscles in the back of the thighs (the hamstrings).

a. Perform this exercise in a seated or standing position (figure 9.21). If performed in a standing position, the back of a chair positioned against a wall can be used for added support.

b. Stand tall with the abdomen and chin tucked in, the head erect, and the eyes directed forward. The feet should be parallel and positioned hip-width apart.

c. Extend the right leg forward, maintaining a slight bend in the knee, and place the heel on the floor with the toes pointing up toward the ceiling.

d. Bend the left knee and place the hands on the thigh (or on the back of the chair), and slowly lean forward from the hips. Keep the back straight during the forward lean.

e. Continue leaning forward until gentle tension is felt in the back of the extended leg.

f. Hold the position for 15 to 30 seconds and repeat with the opposite leg forward.

g. Be sure to keep your back straight rather than rounded.

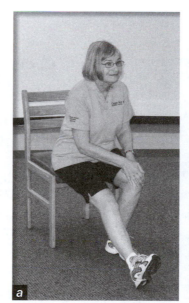
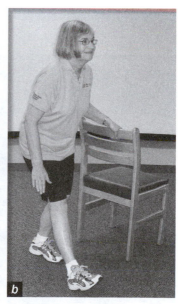

Figure 9.21 Hamstrings stretch in (a) seated and (b) standing positions.

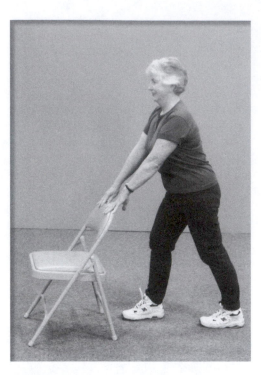

Figure 9.22 Standing calf stretch.

Standing Calf Stretch

The calf stretch targets the muscles in the back of the lower leg.

a. Stand tall at approximately an arm's length away from a chair or wall. Place both hands on the back of the chair or on the wall with the palms at shoulder height. Position one leg forward with the knee bent and aligned with the ankle of the same leg. The heel should be in contact with the floor.

b. Extend the other leg as far behind the body as possible, with the heel in contact with the floor (figure 9.22). Inhale.

c. Lean slowly into the chair, increasing the angle of knee flexion of the front leg. Keep the heel of the back foot in contact with the floor throughout the forward lean.

d. Hold the stretch for 15 to 30 seconds, breathing evenly throughout the hold.

e. Relax and return the front leg to the starting position before repeating the exercise on the other side.

f. Repeat the exercise three times on each side.

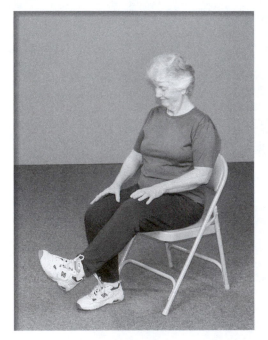

Figure 9.23 Ankle circle.

Ankle Circle

Ankle circles target the muscles of the ankle and foot.

a. Sit tall with the lower back pressed firmly against the back of a chair. The head should be erect, with the eyes directed forward.

b. Raise one leg off the floor and begin slowly circling the ankle in a clockwise direction (figure 9.23). Make five increasingly larger circles with the ankle before reversing the direction for the same number of circles.

c. Lower the leg to the floor and repeat the exercise with the opposite leg raised off the floor.

d. Repeat the exercise three times on each side.

Golf Ball Roll

The golf ball roll targets the muscles of the foot, particularly the arch.

a. Sit tall with the lower back pressed firmly against the backrest of a chair.

b. Place a golf ball under the ball of the right foot and begin rolling it forward and backward for 2 minutes (figure 9.24). Breathe evenly throughout the exercise.

c. Repeat with the other foot for the same amount of time.

d. This is a good exercise for individuals with plantar fasciitis (heel pain), arch strain, or toe cramps.

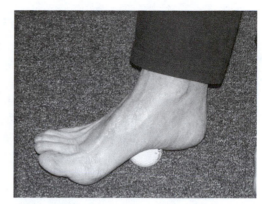

Figure 9.24 Golf ball roll.

Table 9.1 Flexibility Exercises at a Glance

Exercise	Muscles targeted	Type of stretch
Seated chin-to-chest stretch	Back of neck	Static
Neck rotation	Back and side of neck	Dynamic
Assisted neck side stretch	Side of neck	Static
Assisted neck flexion	Back of neck, upper back, shoulders	Static
Turtle stretch	Back and front of neck, upper back	Dynamic
Shoulder roll	Shoulders, upper back, chest	Dynamic
Elbow circle	Scapulae, shoulders	Dynamic
Finger walking	Chest, shoulders	Dynamic
Full-body stretch	Fingers, arms, shoulders, back, abdomen	Dynamic
Chest stretch	Fronts of shoulders, upper chest	Static
Lateral shoulder stretch	Shoulders	Static
Roll-down	Lower back	Dynamic
Wrist circle	Wrists, hands	Dynamic
Palm-down wrist and finger extension	Wrists, hands, forearms	Static
Palm-up wrist and finger extension	Wrists, hands, forearms	Static
Thumb-to-finger touch	Thumbs, fingers	Dynamic
Seated trunk rotation	Side of torso	Static
Side stretch	Side of torso	Dynamic
Bowing to the gods	Shoulders, upper back, arms	Static
Hip abductor stretch	Hips, thighs, side of torso, upper arms	Static
Forward lunge	Thigh	Static
Hamstrings stretch	Backs of thighs	Static
Standing calf stretch	Backs of lower legs	Static
Ankle circle	Ankles, feet	Dynamic
Golf ball roll	Feet	Dynamic

Dynamic stretches are best suited to the warm-up, whereas static stretches should be incorporated into the cool-down.

SUMMARY

Each of the exercises presented in this chapter is designed to improve the range of motion in joints and muscles that are required for balance and mobility. Despite the decline in flexibility that occurs with age, much can be done to improve overall flexibility in older adults. Whereas the dynamic stretching activities presented in this chapter are appropriate for the class warm-up, the static stretching activities are better suited to the cool-down, when the internal temperature of the body and muscles are at their warmest. During the performance of each flexibility exercise, emphasize correct form as well as the need to avoid stretching to the point of discomfort or pain. The regular inclusion of flexibility exercises in each class session, combined with daily home exercise, will help your older adult clients improve their flexibility so they can continue to perform essential ADLs as well as other recreational activities.

Test Your Understanding

1. Age-associated declines in flexibility are more evident in
   a. upper-body joints and muscles
   b. lower-body joints and muscles
   c. muscles in the cervical region
   d. the shoulders

2. Increased muscle stiffness with age is the result of
   a. an increase in muscle collagen and elastin fibers
   b. reduced muscle mass
   c. reduced muscle collagen and an increase in elastin fibers
   d. degeneration of elastin fibers and increased muscle collagen
   e. no known reason

3. How much does ankle range of motion decline in women between 55 and 85 years of age?
   a. 10 percent
   b. 35 percent
   c. 50 percent
   d. 65 percent
   e. 75 percent

4. Which of the following preprogram assessments is most helpful in deciding what type of flexibility exercises to use to improve range of motion in the upper body?
   a. FAB scale
   b. chair stand
   c. scratch test
   d. sit-and-reach test
   e. 8-foot up-and-go test

5. Which types of flexibility exercises are best suited for the warm-up?
   a. static stretches
   b. ballistic stretches
   c. dynamic stretches
   d. a combination of static and dynamic stretches
   e. a combination of ballistic and dynamic stretches

6. Which of the following flexibility exercises targets muscles in the side of the neck?
   a. seated chin-to-chest stretch
   b. neck rotations
   c. assisted neck flexion
   d. assisted neck side stretch
   e. turtle stretch

7. Which of the following flexibility exercises is most appropriate for improving stride length during gait?
   a. bowing to the gods
   b. hip abductor stretch
   c. forward lunge
   d. ankle circles
   e. golf ball roll

8. The flexibility exercise called *bowing to the gods* is designed to improve flexibility in which of the following?
   a. upper back and arms
   b. hamstrings
   c. quadriceps and calves
   d. chest and shoulder
   e. hip and ankle

9. Which of the following exercises is designed to increase range of motion in the ankles and feet?
   a. calf stretch
   b. ankle circles
   c. bowing to the gods
   d. forward lunge
   e. golf ball roll

10. How often should flexibility exercises be performed if the goal is to maintain the gains made in range of motion?
    a. 3 to 5 times per week
    b. twice a week
    c. every day
    d. twice a day
    e. once per week

Practical Problems

1. Develop a list of the flexibility exercises you would select for Phoebe and Larry based on the results of their sit-and-reach and back scratch tests performed during the Senior Fitness Test. Identify the flexibility exercises you would select that specifically target the key joints and muscles required for good functional mobility.

2. Design a home exercise program for Phoebe or Larry that targets the joints and muscles most in need of improved range of motion. List the order of exercises, how long each stretch position should be held, and the number of repetitions to be performed.

Part III

Implementing the FallProof Program

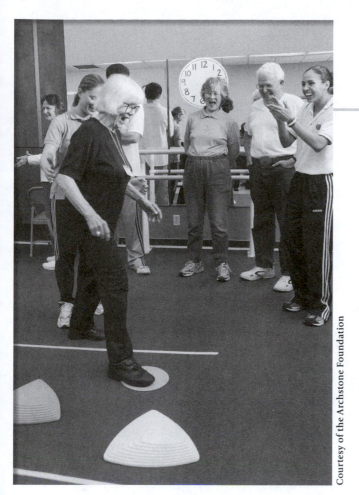

Courtesy of the Archstone Foundation

Chapter 10

Setting the Stage for Learning

Objectives

After completing this chapter, you will be able to

- identify and apply basic principles of motor learning for optimal participant learning and retention,

- understand when and how to apply basic motor learning principles based on each participant's stage of learning,

- design tasks and practice environments that progress participants from a more conscious to a less conscious control of balance, and

- understand what type of feedback to present at each stage of learning and how often it should be presented for optimal learning and transfer.

Now that you are familiar with each of the major components of the Fall-Proof program, it's time to introduce three motor learning principles that should guide you as you implement each of the exercise components associated with this program. The judicious application of each of the motor learning principles described in this chapter will set the stage for optimal learning and transfer. Although many more principles of motor learning are relevant to effective implementation of the FallProof program, any discussion of them is beyond the scope of this book. Several excellent textbooks on motor learning can be consulted if you wish to learn more about this area of study (Magill, 2007; Rose & Christina, 2007; Schmidt & Wrisberg, 2008). The three topics discussed in this chapter include how to introduce new skills to your participants, how to organize the practice environment, and how to provide feedback to your clients in a meaningful way.

UNDERSTANDING THE STAGES OF LEARNING

Several models of motor learning have been developed in an attempt to describe the cognitive and behavioral changes occurring in the learner at each hypothetical stage of learning (Fitts & Posner, 1967; Vereijken, 1991; Gentile, 1972). Although each of these models provides a unique perspective on the learning process, the model presented in this chapter is one specifically designed to help the practitioner better understand not only what the learner is attempting to do in each of the learning stages but also how the practitioner can manipulate the practice environment to facilitate that learning (Gentile, 1972, 1987, 2000). This model, developed by Gentile, describes two stages of learning. The primary focus of the learner during the first stage is to develop an understanding of the goal of the movement, whereas in the second stage, the learner focuses on determining how best to adapt the movement pattern acquired in the first learning stage to the specific demands of the environment in which the skill will ultimately be performed. Let's consider each learning stage in more detail.

> ### Key Point
>
> According to Gentile, the learner's focus during the first stage of learning is to develop an understanding of the goal of the movement, whereas in the second stage, the focus shifts to determining how best to adapt the acquired movement pattern to the demands of the performance environment.

Getting the idea of the movement is the first task that confronts learners who are seeing a new motor skill modeled or hearing a new motor skill described for the first time. To do that, they must begin to explore how the various parts of the movement pattern are coordinated to achieve the goal. As a result of trial and error, learners begin to acquire the basic movement pattern by discriminating between those performance characteristics that determine how the movement is to be performed and those characteristics that are present but do not influence how the skill is to be performed. Gentile described the characteristics of the performance environment that directly influence how a skill is to be performed as the **regulatory conditions,** whereas he called those characteristics of the performance environment that do not or should not influence how a skill is performed the **nonregulatory conditions.**

For example, an older adult who is attempting to reach for an object while standing on a half-foam roller must learn how to coordinate the movements of the body and the arms in order to retrieve the object successfully while standing on a surface that is narrower than the length of the feet. The regulatory features associated with this task include such things as the size and shape of the object, the distance and height of the object's position relative to the body, and the width and compliance of the raised surface on which the individual is standing (figure 10.1). Conversely, the nonregulatory conditions might include things such as the color of the object to be retrieved, the color of the clothing worn by the person

regulatory conditions— Characteristics of the performance environment that directly influence how a skill is performed.

nonregulatory conditions—Characteristics of the performance environment that do not or should not influence how a skill is performed.

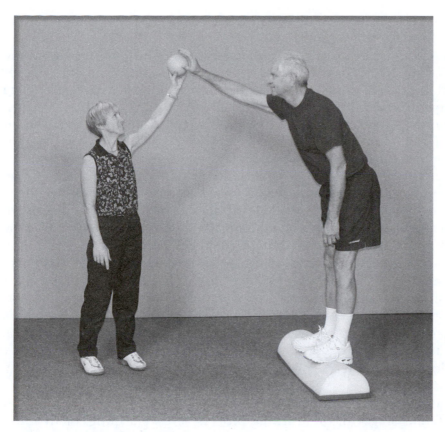

Figure 10.1 The regulatory conditions associated with this task include the size and shape of the object, the distance and height of the object's position relative to the body, and the width and compliance of the support surface.

holding the object, or, if the task is taking place in a group setting, the positions or movements of other people in the room.

As practice continues, the learner begins to develop a movement pattern that often leads to successful completion of the task but still requires a great deal of effort to be expended. At a cognitive level, the learner clearly understands the idea of the movement despite being unable to perform the task consistently and efficiently on all practice attempts. In the second stage of learning, the learner's goal shifts to adapting the acquired movement pattern to the specific demands of the environment in which the task is to be performed. Depending on the type of motor skill being learned, the goal may be one of either **fixating** or **diversifying the movement pattern.** For example, if the skill being learned is to be performed in a closed or unchanging environment, then the learner's goal is to fine-tune the movement pattern so it is performed with the highest degree of consistency and efficiency.

Conversely, if the performance environment in which the skill is ultimately to be performed is open or frequently changing, then the goal is one of learning how to modify the movement pattern to meet a constantly changing set of temporal or spatial conditions. Consider the reaching example. We could actually design the environment to be more open or closed depending on how we structure the task

fixating the movement pattern—The goal of performing the same movement pattern as consistently as possible on each subsequent practice attempt.

diversifying the movement pattern—The goal of varying how the movement pattern is performed on subsequent practice attempts so that the movement pattern becomes more flexible.

demands. For example, if the object is placed on a shelf at the same distance and height from the learner, and the surface on which the learner is standing remains unchanged in terms of its surface characteristics or height from the ground, then the goal for the learner would be to fixate the skill. On the other hand, if the spatial location of the object and its distance from the body are changed on each subsequent trial or the characteristics of the surface on which the learner is standing are frequently altered (e.g., changed from half-foam roller to rocker board to Dyna-Disc), then the goal for the learner would be to diversify the movement pattern to meet the changing task demands and environmental constraints.

Given that in real-life circumstances, the older adult must reach for objects of different weights and shapes that are often located at different heights (e.g., in cupboards, washing machines, or wardrobes or on the floor) and the surface on which the older adult stands often changes (e.g., tiled floor, step stool, carpet), the skill of reaching while maintaining upright balance is probably most conducive to being diversified. In fact, as an instructor you must constantly vary the practice environment by manipulating the regulatory conditions directly associated with the task. For example, in each of the chapters describing the program components, the regulatory conditions associated with the balance activities were constantly being manipulated as the level of difficulty increased. These regulatory conditions related to task demands (e.g., weight or shape of objects being retrieved, timing of task, distance of reach) or environmental constraints (e.g., surface type, lighting, visual flow).

As an instructor, you must understand that your participants will often be at different stages in the learning process as they acquire, or in some cases reacquire, the skills necessary to improve their overall balance and mobility. Those of you who are already teaching balance and mobility classes most likely can readily identify some participants who are in the first stage of learning a particular balance skill and other participants who have already moved into the second stage. What is most helpful about Gentile's model is that it not only describes the learning process from the learner's perspective but also provides the instructor with insight into how to shape the learning environment or alter the task demands in each of the learning stages. These ideas are summarized in the feature on page 263.

UNDERSTANDING DIFFERENT LEARNING STYLES

In addition to understanding the different stages of learning, it is important that you become familiar with different styles of learning. A learning style is defined as the way in which people would choose to learn a new movement skill if they were in charge of the learning process (Rose & Christina, 2007). McCarthy (1987) described four basic learning styles that will be discussed in this section: (1) dynamic, (2) innovative, (3) common sense, and (4) analytical.

- **Dynamic.** This style of learner prefers to learn by trial and error and self-discovery. These learners tend to take risks and ignore authority. They are adventurous, intuitive, or insightful thinkers, and they are synthesizers of information. They prefer a varied and flexible learning environment and are at ease with others, so group environments should work well for them.

Practical Implications
of Gentile's Stages-of-Learning Model
for Instruction

Stage 1: Getting the Idea of the Movement Being Learned

Learner's goal: Develop a basic movement pattern that will accomplish the goal of the task. Performance is characterized by inconsistency and lack of efficiency.

Instructor's goal: Provide ample opportunity for the learner to practice and explore different ways of performing the skill. Regulatory conditions are not altered until some level of performance consistency is achieved (e.g., 3 of 6 practice attempts are successful).

Stage 2: Diversification or Fixation of the Movement Pattern

Learner's goal if the skill being learned will be performed in a closed or unchanging environment: Fine-tune the movement pattern so that it can be performed with a high level of consistency and little cognitive or physical effort.

Learner's goal if the skill being learned will be performed in an open and frequently changing environment: Learn how to modify the movement pattern to meet the changing demands of the performance environment.

Instructor's goal if the skill being learned will be performed in a closed or unchanging environment: Manipulate the nonregulatory conditions while holding the regulatory conditions relatively constant. Certain parameters of the task (e.g., weight or shape of objects) can be manipulated as long as the timing features of the movement pattern remain relatively the same.

Instructor's goal if the skill being learned will be performed in open or changing environments: Manipulate the regulatory conditions (task demands or environmental constraints) so that the movement pattern must be altered on subsequent practice attempts. At first only the parameters of the task (e.g., weight, shape, height, and distance of object) are varied, and then the actual pattern of coordination (e.g., one-hand versus two-hand reach) are varied. Characteristics of the surface on which the learner is standing (e.g., foam of different densities and height, rocker board, Dyna-Disc) or environmental conditions (e.g., lighting, amount of visual flow, complexity of visual scene) can also be varied. As practice progresses, the nonregulatory conditions (e.g., the proximity of other learners practicing similar tasks, background music) are varied so that the learner practices focusing on the task being performed despite external distractions.

- **Innovative.** This style of learner tends to be a divergent thinker. Innovative learners are imaginative, cooperative, and sociable. They prefer to learn through social interaction, discussion, and personal involvement and so are also well suited to group learning environments.

- **Common sense.** This style of learner prefers to learn by doing and therefore welcomes opportunities for hands-on experience. These learners enjoy a learning environment that promotes problem solving and makes a strong connection with real-life applications. They also tend to be judicious and prudent thinkers.

- **Analytical.** This fourth style of learner prefers traditional instructional environments. These learners enjoy being recognized for their efforts. They tend to be intellectual and logical and place great emphasis on personal control when learning new movement skills. They seek facts, collect data, and are likely to separate new movement skills into their component parts. They are also very systematic in their approach to learning.

When instructing a class, you will likely find each of these learning styles among your group members, and in some cases you will see a combination of learning styles. While clients with a dynamic and common sense style learn best from doing, innovative and reflective learners prefer watching. It is therefore important to provide multiple opportunities to observe a new movement skill being performed as well as lots of opportunities to physically practice the new skill. Good class management skills are needed to ensure that both of these motor learning techniques are optimized in each session.

INTRODUCING THE SKILL BEING LEARNED

When instructors decide to introduce a new motor skill to a class of learners, they invariably begin with a brief verbal description of the skill followed by one or more visual demonstrations of the correct movement pattern. Instructors prefer this mode of instruction because they believe it will convey the greatest amount of information in its most meaningful form. Although the use of visual demonstration has been well supported in the literature on motor learning, researchers have recently engaged in a debate as to whether visual demonstrations are always the most effective method of introducing different types of skills. They have also begun addressing issues such as who should demonstrate the skill, when and how often to demonstrate the skill, and how to supplement the skill to promote optimal learning (McCullagh & Meyer, 1997; Pollock & Lee, 1992; Weir & Leavitt, 1990).

First, demonstrations appear to be most effective when a new pattern of coordination is to be learned (figure 10.2). Conversely, when the goal is to fine-tune

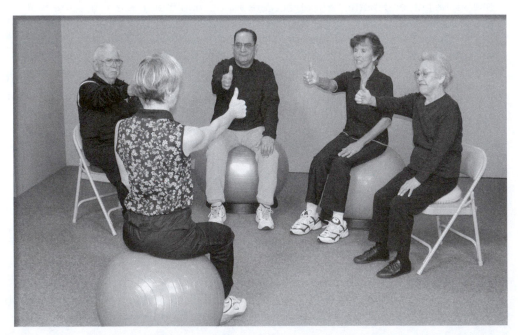

Figure 10.2 Visual demonstrations appear to be most effective when learning new motor skills.

a previously learned skill, other techniques such as verbal cuing may prove more effective (Magill, 2007). Although it is customary to have someone who is highly skilled demonstrate a new motor skill, recent studies have shown that observing unskilled performers can also be beneficial to novice performers. Two probable advantages are associated with this type of model. First, the observer is less likely to try to imitate the action of the unskilled performer, and instead will engage in more problem-solving activities. Second, it is easier to observe the underlying strategy being used to accomplish the goal of the movement when it is demonstrated by someone who is less skilled, particularly when the demonstration is supplemented with corrective feedback delivered by the instructor. The observer can

> ### Key Point
>
> Demonstrations appear to be most effective when a new pattern of coordination is to be learned.

then watch how the strategy is altered on subsequent practice trials. Perhaps the most interesting outcome noted by researchers who have investigated the learning benefits associated with watching unskilled models is that once the observers begin practicing that skill, they perform it at a significantly higher level than the person who first demonstrated it (McCullagh & Meyer, 1997; Pollock & Lee, 1992; Weir & Leavitt, 1990).

Practical Implications

A balance and mobility class provides many opportunities to incorporate demonstrations by unskilled models. These demonstrations can be done in small groups, with one member serving as the learning model while several other participants watch the model demonstrate the skill, receive corrective feedback from the instructor, and subsequently reattempt the skill. Although this technique is not always appropriate for teaching young learners, it is extremely effective when teaching older adults. An alternative strategy is to develop performance checklists that describe the key elements of movement skills. Form 10.1 on page 266 is an example of a performance checklist.

Having your participants work as partners, with one serving as the teacher while the other attempts to perform the skill, is an effective way to use these checklists. The job of the teacher is to look for performance errors by comparing the learner's movements to those described on the checklist. As soon as an error is noticed, the teacher provides corrective feedback and then watches how the learner uses it to improve performance on the next practice attempt. This teaching technique not only provides a valuable learning experience for both the teacher and the learner by fostering a better understanding of the skill to be performed but also makes it easier to manage a large class.

Even though visual demonstrations are highly effective in learning how to perform a new pattern of coordination, an alternative strategy you can employ as an instructor is to allow participants to learn the desired movement by self- or guided discovery. This is a particularly valuable teaching technique to use in the FallProof program because many of the skills you would like your participants to acquire are not amenable to demonstration or explicit verbal instructions. They are best learned **implicitly.**

A good example of using an implicit approach to teach a new movement technique associated with the FallProof program is attempting to help older adults learn to transition from one postural strategy to another (e.g., from an ankle strategy to a hip strategy) to control postural sway. Rather than telling or showing them how and when to switch from an ankle to a hip strategy, the instructor

implicit learning— Improving the performance of a skill subconsciously. The learner is unaware of how improvements are achieved. Implicit teaching techniques foster self- or guided discovery of a movement solution through manipulation of task and environmental demands.

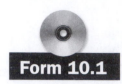

Form 10.1

Performance Checklist
for Multidirectional Weight Shifts
in a Seated Position

Body Alignment

_____ Performer is sitting tall and eyes are focused on a target at eye level.

_____ Shoulders are level.

_____ Feet are no more than hip-width apart and pointed forward.

_____ Hands are positioned on ball, chair, or thighs or folded across chest.

Weight Shift

_____ Movement is initiated without hesitation in the correct direction following the cue to move.

_____ Good body alignment is maintained as the hips are moved in the cued direction.

_____ Shoulders remain level and relaxed when weight shifts are performed to the right or left side.

_____ Feet remain in place during the weight shift.

_____ Eyes are fixed on a target at eye level during each weight shift.

_____ Performer returns to a centered position after each weight shift.

From D. Rose, 2010, FallProof! 2nd ed. (Champaign, IL: Human Kinetics).

---

in-phase movement—The upper and lower body move in the same direction.

out-of-phase movement—The upper body and lower body move in opposite directions.

manipulates the task demands in such a way that the transition becomes inevitable. For example, if you ask an older adult to stand between two chairs and sway forward and backward to the slow beat of a metronome, you will generally observe a pattern of movement that is controlled by the ankle joint as the upper and lower body move in the same direction, or **in phase.** As you increase the speed of the metronome or the distance through which the sway occurs, however, you will observe a relatively spontaneous shift in the movement pattern from one that is in phase to one that is **out of phase** as use of the larger hip muscles becomes necessary for controlling the sway (figure 10.3). Voila! The learner has discovered the hip strategy and not a word has been spoken.

Just as using unskilled models to demonstrate new skills minimizes the tendency of the observers to mimic the action, verbally posing a movement problem to a group of learners or manipulating the task demands or environmental constraints in such a way that the learner is guided to the solution fosters greater problem solving and a range of solutions that better reflect the individual's unique capabilities. Although a picture is worth a thousand words, there are

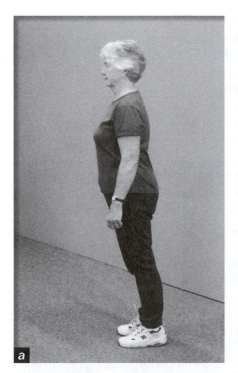 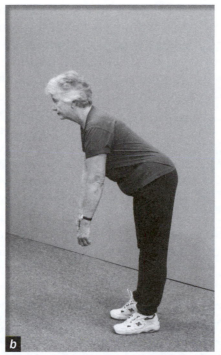 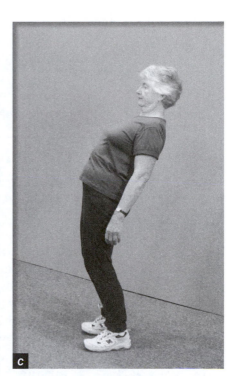

Figure 10.3 An ankle strategy requires that the body move (a) in phase, whereas a hip strategy results in a (b) forward or (c) backward out-of-phase movement.

many ways to introduce a new skill to a learner, particularly one who is older and wiser. While **explicit** teaching techniques, whether verbal instructions or visual demonstrations, are those most often used to introduce a new skill, there are many opportunities to use more implicit teaching techniques, particularly when teaching several different balance and mobility activities. These may be invoked simply by having the learner discover a given pattern of coordination by manipulating either the demands of the task or the environment in which the task is being performed. At other times, it is sufficient to pose a movement problem to be solved while manipulating either the task or the environment in such a way that the solution emerges without the learner ever being consciously aware of how it was achieved.

explicit learning—Consciously improving the performance of a skill. The learner is aware of how improvements were achieved. Explicit teaching techniques include verbal instructions and visual demonstrations.

Practicing the Skill

Once participants have acquired a good understanding of how to perform a particular movement pattern, begin varying the practice environment so that it better prepares them for performing the skill in a variety of environments and in response to a range of task demands. As you learned in chapter 4, the challenge associated with performing a particular task can be manipulated by altering the task demands or the environmental constraints. Manipulating either or both of these variables results in a more varied

> ### Key Point
>
> Manipulating either the task demands or the environmental constraints will result in a more varied practice environment.

practice environment that benefits the learning of not only the skills being practiced currently but also the skills to be learned at a later time.

In deciding how to vary the practice environment, you as an instructor need to consider the learner's current skill level, the characteristics of the skill to be learned, and the type of environment in which the skill ultimately will be performed. As discussed earlier, skills that will be performed the same way every time or in an environment that does not change should be fixated, whereas skills that will be performed differently on consecutive attempts or in changing environments should be diversified. Although varying the practice environment is the best way to help learners diversify a skill, it can be argued that varying the practice environment is valuable even when the learner's goal is to fixate a skill. The practice environment can be varied simply by manipulating the regulatory and nonregulatory conditions described in Gentile's two-stage learning model. Although both the regulatory and the nonregulatory conditions should be manipulated when a skill needs to be diversified, manipulating only the nonregulatory conditions is appropriate when the goal is to fixate a skill.

> ### Key Point
>
> Varying the practice environment is still valuable even when the learner's goal is to fixate the skill.

In addition to varying the regulatory and nonregulatory conditions associated with a movement skill, an instructor can vary the practice environment by manipulating how variations of one skill or different skills are practiced. For example, varying the practice schedule can help learners practice variations of a single skill or multiple skills. This technique increases the **contextual interference,** or the variety, introduced into a practice setting and has been shown to be an effective method of improving both the learning and the transfer of motor skills among novice and skilled performers alike (Hall, Domingues, & Cavazos, 1994; Magill & Hall, 1990; Shea & Morgan, 1979; Wrisberg & Lui, 1991).

The level of contextual variety can be further manipulated by varying the practice environment according to a blocked or random practice schedule. In the case of a **blocked practice schedule,** a particular skill is practiced for a given number of repetitions before a new variation of the same skill or a different movement skill is practiced. Conversely, in a **random practice schedule,** the learner performs a skill or a variation of a skill only once before practicing a different skill or skill variation. The practice order is randomized so that the learner does not know what skill will be practiced on the subsequent trial. Although the latter practice schedule is believed to require much greater cognitive effort on the part of learners and results in more errors during practice, it has been shown to significantly benefit skill learning.

Perhaps the best way to progressively increase the level of cognitive effort required of learners is to have them practice different variations of a single skill first according to a blocked schedule and then according to a random schedule. The practice environment can be made even more difficult by having the participant follow the same practice schedule progression (blocked to random) while practicing 2 to 3 different skills in the same practice session. One skill that is particularly well suited to variable practice techniques is obstacle negotiation. During the course of a day, the older adult is likely to encounter curbs, stairs, and other obstacles that vary in height, width, and surface characteristics. A section of the center of gravity (COG) control training that addresses obstacle negotiation is devoted to performing a variety of stepping movements on benches. These movements progress from alternating toe touches to step-ups and step-downs on the same and then opposite sides of the bench to step swing-through sequences.

contextual interference— A practice method that involves practicing multiple variations of a single skill or multiple skills in a single practice session. It is used to increase the variability of a practice session.

blocked practice schedule—A schedule in which the same skill or skill variation is practiced for a given number of practice trials before a new skill or variation is introduced.

random practice schedule—A schedule in which a new variation or skill is practiced on each subsequent practice trial.

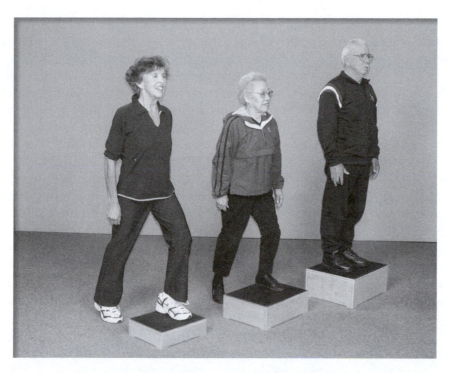

Figure 10.4   Class participants performing stepping sequences on benches of different heights.

A good starting point in varying the practice of these different skills is to vary only the height of the bench on which the participant is performing. For example, a participant might begin practicing toe touches on a bench that is 2 inches (5 cm) high for a set number of repetitions before moving to a bench that is 4 inches (10 cm) high and then to one that is 6 inches (15 cm) high (figure 10.4). Practicing the same skill for a set number of repetitions before moving to the next bench height is an example of varying the practice according to a blocked schedule. Conversely, you could have the participant perform only one toe touch with each foot before moving to a new bench height. Not allowing multiple repetitions of a skill at the same bench height results in a more random practice schedule. The latter practice schedule is considered to be more cognitively challenging because it requires learners to change how they perform the skill each time a new bench height is encountered. The belief is that a skill is learned better this way because the movement must be repeatedly reconstructed and modified to accommodate the changing bench height. This is not the case in a blocked practice schedule because participants are able to practice the same skill variation multiple times before moving on. They can therefore use the same action plan from the previous repetition with little or no modification. Thus, less cognitive effort is expended.

To further increase the level of cognitive effort required of the learner, you can increase the number of different movement skills being practiced on different bench heights within the same practice session. For example, you might have participants practice toe touches, step-ups

> **Key Point**
>
> A random practice schedule is considered to require more cognitive effort.

and step-downs, and step swing-through sequences according to either a blocked or a random practice schedule. When following a blocked schedule, participants would practice one of the three movement skills for a set number of trials before practicing the next movement sequence on the same bench height. When following a random schedule, they would practice each movement sequence only once before switching to a different movement skill according to a randomly presented order.

The final practice variation you could introduce is a change in not only the type of movement sequence being performed but also the height, width, and surface characteristics of the bench. An advantage of this practice technique is that the practice difficulty can easily be matched to the capabilities of the learner. For participants who are in the early stages of learning or who lack confidence, the practice can be varied, but only one skill is practiced for a given number of repetitions before the height of the bench is altered. At the same time, participants who are more skilled can practice different movement sequences in a random order on the same or different bench heights after one or more repetitions.

Previous research has demonstrated that varying the practice environment not only leads to better learning of movement skills but also improves a learner's ability to transfer what has been learned in one environment to a different environment and from one skill to another (Goode & Magill, 1986; Magill & Hall, 1990). In addition, introducing practice variability results in a more enjoyable, albeit a more cognitively challenging, practice environment for the participants.

IDENTIFYING AND CORRECTING ERRORS IN PERFORMANCE

augmented feedback— Information provided to a learner from an external source.

knowledge of results (KR)— Information provided to a learner about the outcome of a movement pattern.

knowledge of performance (KP)— Information provided to a learner about the quality of the movement.

One of the most effective ways to help learners identify and correct their errors is to supplement the feedback they derive from their own internal sensory systems with external information (provided by you as the instructor). This externally provided feedback is often referred to as **augmented feedback** in the literature on motor learning. The information can be provided in different forms (e.g., verbal, visual, auditory) either during or after a given performance. It is used to supply learners with information about the outcome of their performance, often referred to as **knowledge of results (KR)**, as well as information about the quality of their performance, known as **knowledge of performance (KP)**.

During the first stage of learning, as participants struggle to understand the goal of the movement and how best to achieve that goal, they will derive the greatest learning benefit from receiving a more prescriptive feedback that describes not only what they are doing incorrectly but also what they need to do to correct their errors on subsequent practice attempts (KP). Once the learners enter Gentile's second stage of learning and have a better understanding of how to perform the movement pattern necessary to achieve the goal, the type of feedback provided should shift from being prescriptive to descriptive (KR). That is, the feedback should describe the nature of the error (if the learner has not already identified it) but not how to correct the error.

Previous research also suggests that some time should elapse between the completion of the movement attempt and the delivery of the feedback. Moreover, learners should be encouraged to estimate the accuracy of their own performance during the delay between the completion of the movement attempt and the delivery of feedback from the instructor (Lui & Wrisberg, 1997; Swinnen, 1990). To further encourage learners to engage in error estimation, consider delivering the augmented feedback in the form of a question rather than a statement. By posing one or more questions to the learner about the accuracy of the previous performance, you encourage the learner to identify not only what went wrong but also what could be done differently to correct the problem. This process nurtures the problem-solving abilities of the learner and over time will result in a more independent learner.

Which of the two types of augmented feedback, KR or KP, is likely to be most meaningful to a learner? Should the feedback focus only on the outcome of a particular skill performance (KR) and whether it was consistent with the intended goal, or should the feedback focus more on the characteristics of the movement that led to the observed outcome (KP)? According to Magill (2007), both types of augmented feedback are beneficial to learners, but they are beneficial for different reasons. KR is beneficial for skill learning because (a) learners can use it to confirm their own assessment of the internal sensory feedback they received about the skill, even though this information may be redundant; (b) learners may not be able to determine the actual outcome of their performance based on the intrinsic sensory feedback alone; (c) learners are often motivated by KR to continue practicing a skill; and (d) learners are encouraged to figure out how to achieve the desired outcome through self-discovery when the feedback being provided is limited to KR. Magill also believes that providing KP can be very beneficial to learners, particularly when the skill being learned must be performed in a particular way (e.g., for gymnastics or diving). KP also becomes important when certain movement components of a skill that require complex coordination need to be corrected (figure 10.5).

Irrespective of what type of augmented feedback you provide during the learning of a new motor skill, you must remember that more is not better. In fact, research has shown that providing too much feedback actually hinders learning. One reason for this finding is that learners become overly dependent on external feedback if it is provided too often. Conversely, learners who receive feedback less often are forced to rely on their internal sensory feedback for making the necessary corrections on subsequent practice attempts. This helps them better recall what needs to be done when the external feedback is no longer available. As an instructor, you will not be there to correct errors that your program participants make during their everyday activities, so you must provide them with the skills needed to become proficient not only at detecting but also at correcting the errors they are making. Developing these error detection and correction skills is what is most likely to improve their ability to perform daily activities that require good balance and mobility as well as reduce their risk for falling.

> ## Key Point
>
> Time should elapse between the completed practice attempt and the feedback being provided. Learners should also be encouraged to estimate the accuracy of their performance before feedback is provided.

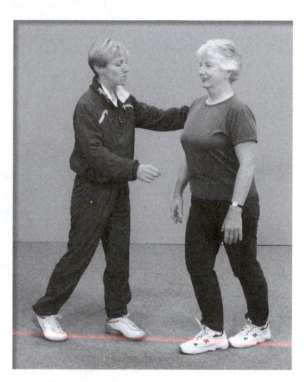

Figure 10.5 Providing knowledge of performance is important when teaching skills that require complex coordination.

> ## Key Point
>
> More is not better: Learners become overly dependent on augmented feedback when it is provided too often.

> ## Guidelines to Follow
> ## When Providing Augmented Feedback
>
> ◆ The augmented feedback must direct the learner's attention to the pivotal error or skill component that, when corrected, will result in an appreciable improvement in performance.
>
> ◆ Augmented feedback should not only inform the learner about the elements of a skill that are being performed incorrectly but also inform the learner about the components of the skill that are being performed correctly. This second type of feedback serves to motivate the learner.
>
> ◆ Providing too much feedback too often is detrimental to learning. Although learners need more feedback during the early stages of learning, the frequency should be reduced as their error-detection abilities improve.
>
> ◆ Learners need sufficient time to evaluate the accuracy and quality of their own performance before feedback is provided.
>
> ◆ Error-correcting feedback should be interspersed with other feedback that reinforces what the learner is already doing correctly, such as, "You are clearing the obstacle much better with your rear foot," or motivates the learner to continue practicing, such as, "Good effort on that last practice attempt."

SUMMARY

Applying each of the principles of motor learning described in this chapter will significantly enhance the quality of your program and the outcomes achieved by your participants. The application of each of these principles, however, will be influenced by the participants' current stage of learning, previous motor skill experience, and particular style of learning. Whereas the principles underlying the presentation of a new motor skill should be applied during the first stage of motor learning, the application of other principles (e.g., variability of practice) should be deferred to the second stage, when the learner better understands the goal of the movement being learned.

How much augmented feedback is provided to learners is also influenced by the stage of learning. Although providing more augmented feedback during the early stages of learning is beneficial to the learner, the frequency with which augmented feedback is provided should be reduced as the learner moves into the second stage. The nature of the feedback provided should also change from information that helps learners detect *and* correct their errors to information that only helps them identify the error, if they have not already identified it for themselves.

Always remember that your goal as an instructor is to provide your older adult learners with the skills and strategies needed to accomplish a variety of daily tasks that impose varying demands and must be performed across a variety of sensory environments. Given that you cannot always be there to guide your program participants through each of these tasks, you need to structure your class sessions in a manner that fosters their problem-solving abilities. Although the learning environment you create as a result will require much more cognitive effort on the part of your learners, it will lead to optimal learning and the ability to transfer what is learned in the classroom into daily life.

Test Your Understanding

1. According to Gentile (1972), during the first stage of motor learning, the learner's primary goal is to
    a. fixate the movement pattern being learned
    b. understand the goal of the movement pattern
    c. diversify the movement pattern so it becomes more flexible
    d. learn how to perform the skill correctly
    e. learn how to identify errors in performance

2. A higher level of cognitive effort is introduced into a practice setting when a learner practices
    a. the same pattern of coordination according to a blocked practice schedule
    b. multiple patterns of coordination in a defined order during a practice session
    c. multiple patterns of coordination in a random order during a practice session
    d. one pattern of coordination for a given time before practicing a second pattern of coordination
    e. multiple movement skills in a game setting

3. One advantage of using initially unskilled models to demonstrate a new movement pattern to learners is that
    a. they make it much more difficult to learn a motor skill
    b. they prevent learners from imitating the movement to be learned
    c. learners are able to devote all of their attention to the critical components of the skill being modeled
    d. the instructor does not need to be able to perform the skill to teach it
    e. it results in an easier learning environment

4. The term *augmented feedback* is defined as
    a. information provided to a learner from an external source either during or following the completion of a movement
    b. outcome information provided to a learner from an external source
    c. process information provided to a learner from an external source
    d. information provided to a learner from an external source at any time before, during, or after the completion of a movement
    e. external information provided to a learner about internal physiological events

5. Information provided to a learner that emphasizes the quality of the form used to perform a skill is called
    a. knowledge of form
    b. augmented sensory feedback
    c. knowledge of results
    d. knowledge of performance
    e. biofeedback

6. Feedback should be provided to a learner
    a. immediately after completion of each practice attempt
    b. immediately after completion of at least five practice attempts
    c. following a short temporal delay after a practice attempt
    d. only during the performance of the skill
    e. following a short temporal delay and preferably in the form of a question

7. Presenting a skilled model is more effective when
    a. the learner is able to correctly reproduce the skill being presented
    b. the skill involves learning a new pattern of coordination
    c. the model also performs the skill incorrectly on some occasions
    d. the learner is attempting to rescale an already familiar movement pattern
    e. the learner is not confident in having the ability to perform the skill

8. The regulatory conditions associated with a learning environment include
    a. all the irrelevant aspects associated with the performance of a skill
    b. all the errors that occur during the performance of a skill
    c. both the relevant and the irrelevant aspects associated with performance of the skill
    d. the trajectory of the ball and the spatial orientation of the glove in the case of attempting to catch a fly ball in baseball or softball
    e. all those factors that determine whether the learner is motivated to learn a particular motor skill

9. According to Gentile (1972), during the second stage of learning,
    a. the primary goal for the learner is to develop a consistent movement pattern
    b. the regulatory conditions associated with the skill to be learned should be manipulated
    c. the primary goal for the learner is to match the movement pattern to the environment in which it is ultimately performed
    d. the nonregulatory conditions associated with the skill to be learned should be manipulated
    e. the learner should begin to vary the type of movement pattern being used to perform the skill

10. Augmented feedback that is prescriptive in nature should be provided
    a. during all stages of learning
    b. during the early stages of learning
    c. during the later stages of learning
    d. only to older adults
    e. after every practice attempt during the early stages of learning

Practical Problems

1. Given your knowledge of Phoebe and Larry and their beginning skill levels, how would you apply each of the following principles of motor learning?
    a. Introducing the skill to be learned
    b. Practicing the skill
    c. Identifying and correcting errors in performance

2. Design a performance checklist for two balance exercises that program participants could use during a class session.

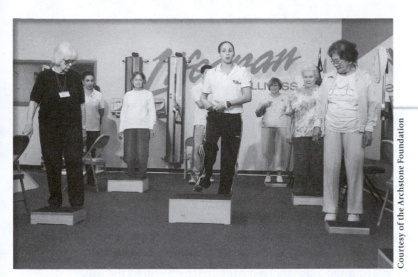

Courtesy of the Archstone Foundation

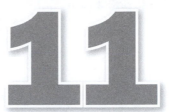

Chapter 11

Program Planning and Class Management Techniques

Objectives

After completing this chapter, you will be able to

- plan and implement group-based lessons,
- manage participants in group-based programs to ensure optimal activity levels and safety, and
- communicate effectively with participants.

The focus of this final chapter is to review essential program planning and class management techniques needed to ensure your success as a balance and mobility instructor. Some readers may have many years of experience working with older adults in a group setting, whereas others may have only one-to-one experience through working as a clinician or personal trainer. Although many of the leadership and communication skills used in the two settings are similar, you will find that preparing for and managing group classes require a different approach from the one you use when instructing individuals. This chapter discusses the various activities you will need to perform (a) after the completion of your assessment and before the program begins, (b) before the start of each class session, (c) during each class session, (d) between class sessions, and finally (e) after each follow-up assessment.

FOLLOWING THE INITIAL ASSESSMENT

As you complete each assessment associated with the FallProof program, you need to begin identifying and listing the balance and mobility problems observed. The test interpretation tables provided in chapter 3 will greatly assist you with this task as well as provide you with ideas as to the exercises that address each of the problems identified. The next step in this process is to separate the problems you believe to be temporary or amenable to change with targeted exercise progressions from those that you know to be more permanent. For example, if lower-body muscle weakness, which is a temporary problem in most cases, is common among the group tested, you can begin to develop a set of progressive strength exercises to address the problem.

Although there is nothing you can do as an instructor to change the more permanent balance problems an individual is experiencing, you may be able to select several exercises that will help the participant better compensate for the permanent loss. For example, selecting exercises that focus on improving a participant's use of ground cues for balance control will do much to offset permanent changes in the visual system that are associated with eye diseases such as age-related macular degeneration and glaucoma. Categorizing each of the observed balance and mobility problems in this way not only will assist you in choosing an instructional focus during the early stages of the program but also will help you select the appropriate program components and exercise progressions for each identified balance or mobility problem.

> ## Key Point
>
> Following the initial assessment, you should make a list of all the temporary balance and mobility problems and a second list of all the permanent balance and mobility problems identified among your participants.

During your program planning, you need to remember that because multiple systems within the body contribute to good balance and mobility, not all of your program participants will begin at the same starting point in each program component. Although some older adults in your class may be experiencing sensory problems, others may be experiencing greater decline in the motor system. Some adults will move through the exercise progressions more quickly than others do because their balance problem is a temporary one (e.g., muscle weakness, reduced range of motion) and therefore easier to resolve. You will also find that your clients' previous motor skill experience and current level of physical activity influence how quickly they progress during the program. You therefore need to individualize your lesson plans by selecting a range of exercise progressions that can be presented to the same group. This requires a careful review of each participant's test results followed by thoughtful lesson planning.

> ## Key Point
>
> Your clients' previous motor skill experience and current level of physical activity will influence how quickly they progress during the program.

The programming triad that was presented in chapter 1 should guide the process of individualizing the exercises presented within a group setting. By manipulating the demands associated with a given exercise or the environment in which the exercise is performed, you can increase or decrease the challenge associated with any activity in your balance and mobility program (figure 11.1). In fact, this core ingredient of the FallProof program is what makes it possible to cater to a broad continuum of functional levels—from the very healthy to the very frail—within the same classroom.

SETTING INDIVIDUAL PROGRAM GOALS

Before the start of the program or during the very first class, take the time to have your clients write down 3 to 4 goals that they would like to accomplish as an outcome of being in your balance and mobility program. These goals should meet four requirements: They should be measurable, specific, realistic, and behavioral. For a goal to be measurable, the client should be able to ascertain whether it was or was not achieved at some point during the program. A specific goal specifies when the behavior will take place (e.g., on specified days of the week or times during any given day), while a realistic goal is one that can actually be achieved. Many clients will be quite unrealistic in their expectations when they first begin your program, so it will be your job to make sure that

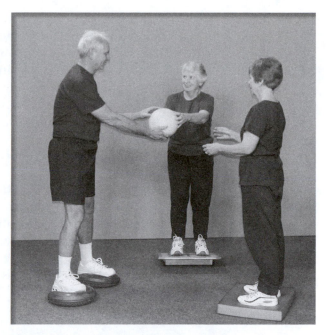

Figure 11.1 Different support surfaces can be used to increase or decrease the challenge of a group exercise.

the goals they establish are small enough that you can be certain that they will be successful. You are going to do little to enhance their self-efficacy if they do not experience success in the program. Finally, your clients should set goals that are more behavioral than outcome oriented because they have more control over their behavior than they have over a particular outcome. For example, a goal of climbing a set of 10 stairs without holding onto the handrail is an outcome-oriented goal. Conversely, a behavioral goal of attending your balance and mobility class two times a week and performing a home exercise program (that includes strength, balance, and flexibility exercises) at least three times a week for the next month is one that is likely to be achieved much more quickly and will lead to less frustration caused by progress that appears to be slow. Of course, a goal of climbing the stairs without holding onto a handrail is probably not a good idea in the first place because it encourages a potentially unsafe behavior.

Your clients should set both short- and long-term goals, with the short-term goals constituting the stepping stones to achieving the long-term ones. Just as the short-term goals should be behavioral, so too should the long-term goals that you ask your clients to set. For example, the short-term goal of attending class two times a week and performing a home exercise program at least three times a week might, in the long-term, increase to attending your balance class two times a week and performing the home exercise program five times a week.

Although it is important to set goals with your clients, it is equally important to review their progress toward those goals on a regular basis (every week or two during the early stages of a program and monthly or bimonthly as success with achieving goals occurs). In some cases, you may have to adjust some goals based on your participants' progress, health status, and long-term objectives. Always be prepared to discuss participants' successes as well as struggles toward achieving a certain goal. In that way you can identify what factors help your participants meet their goals and then point out these factors during the times your clients are struggling. Finally, help your clients develop their self-monitoring skills by having them keep logs in which they record their activities that are related to the goals they set. Making your clients responsible for their own behavior is crucial if you want them to continue engaging in the behaviors and activities that will lower their risk for falls.

BEFORE EACH CLASS SESSION

To be a successful instructor and achieve the program outcomes you desire, you will need to spend an adequate amount of time selecting the exercises you intend to present during the class. When preparing for the early classes in a program, you do not need to select as many exercises as you will need to select for later classes because in early classes it takes more time to determine where in the exercise progression each participant should begin. In addition, more practice time should be allotted to each exercise so the participants can become familiar with it.

Planning the Lesson

Once you have selected the exercises, you need to develop a lesson plan using a format similar to the one presented in figure 11.2. (Figure 11.2 includes only the first page of the lesson plan, showing the basic lesson plan outline, the warm-up, and the cool-down; the complete sample lesson plan can be viewed on the DVD.) The lesson plan should include a warm-up of no less than 10 minutes, a skills section lasting approximately 40 minutes, and a 10-minute cool-down. In addition to listing the exercises to be presented during the skills portion of the class, you should determine which activities you plan to present to the entire class and which activities you will have participants practice in small groups. Your lesson plan should also list all the equipment you plan to use during the class. Some instructors also find it helpful to include a column that lists the verbal cues associated with each exercise.

You or your program assistants should retrieve the equipment you plan to use during a particular class from its storage area and place it in different areas of the room in preparation for the activities you have included in your lesson plan. For example, if you are planning to have participants work on seated balance activities, you should have the necessary number of chairs, Dyna-Discs, balance balls, and ball holders available to accommodate the different ability levels of your participants. An illustration of a possible classroom setup is provided in figure 11.3 on page 280.

As a standard practice, you should develop a master list that indicates whether a participant generally performs the seated balance activities on a Dyna-Disc, ball with ball holder, or ball alone. The size of the ball that each participant uses should also be recorded. This list will be particularly helpful in the early stages of the program so that your assistants can get the proper equipment assigned to participants efficiently. Even though the surface a client sits on is likely to change as skill improves, it will still be helpful to maintain your master list, particularly if you teach multiple classes. Similarly, if you are planning to practice standing activities on altered surfaces, it will be helpful to arrange a station in the room with chairs and the surfaces to be used positioned beneath or behind the chairs.

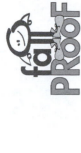

Figure 11.2

Sample Lesson Plan

Outline

10 min	Warm-up
10 min	MST somatosensory
	• Seated balance with voluntary arm movements
	• Seated balance with voluntary trunk movements
10 min	GPEV
	• Introduction to walking pattern
	• Walking with directional changes and abrupt starts and stops
	• Walking with altered base of support
10 min	PST
	• Voluntary ankle strategy
10 min	Strength
	• Seated lower body
10 min	Cool-down

Warm-up

Select appropriate warm-up exercises that can be performed while seated and standing. Emphasize large body movements that are rhythmical and continuous.

Cool-down

Upper-body flexibility
- Chin-to-chest stretch
- Neck rotation
- Neck side stretch
- Shoulder roll
- Chest stretch
- Lateral shoulder stretch
- Trunk rotation

Lower-body flexibility
- Ankle circle
- Calf stretch
- Hamstrings stretch

Breathing and relaxation

Homework assignment

Figure 11.2 The first page of a sample lesson plan. The entire lesson plan is included in the DVD-ROM that accompanies this book.

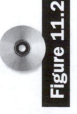

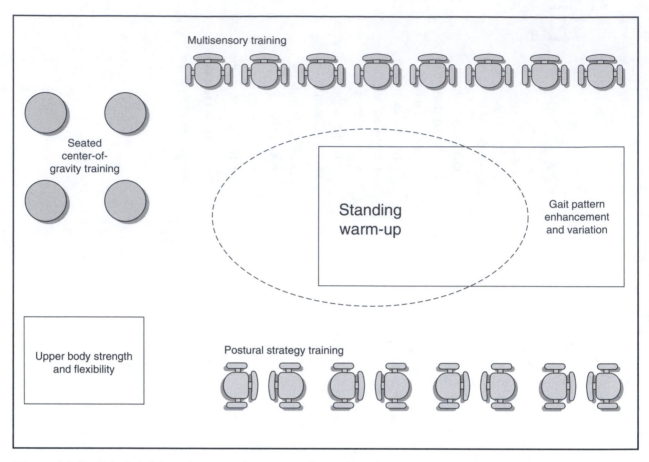

Figure 11.3 It is helpful to diagram where you will conduct each component of a class and the placement of the equipment you plan to use.

Then participants can move between stations and start the next set of activities immediately. This preclass preparation will save you valuable time during class and will facilitate group transitions between exercise stations. Group transition skills are discussed later in this chapter.

Warm-Up

The warm-up of a balance and mobility class tends to be a little shorter than the warm-up in a more traditional fitness class. Its primary purpose of elevating the heart rate and preparing the muscles and joints for activity can usually be accomplished within a 10-minute time frame. Because your clients are likely to be more deconditioned as a result of their balance and mobility problems, the warm-up should adequately prepare them for the balance activities to follow but should not lead to undue fatigue that will affect the quality of their physical performance as well as diminish their ability to focus their attention.

Many of the activities described in the COG control, gait pattern enhancement and variation, and strength and flexibility components of the program are well suited to the warm-up (figure 11.4). Fun warm-up activities include starts and stops

> ### Key Point
>
> The warm-up should adequately prepare clients for the balance activities to follow but should not lead to undue fatigue.

to music, seated balance ball activities, and progressive aerobic exercise sequences combining upper- and lower-body coordination. Do not be concerned about developing a new warm-up for every class because older adults often enjoy performing the same set of activities on a regular basis. Repeating the same set of warm-up activities will also allow participants to focus on physically performing the activity rather than on what they have to do. Simply adding one or two new movements to a repeating aerobic sequence or adding arm or leg movements to a balance ball movement sequence can create sufficient variety. Progressively adding new movements also challenges the working memory skills of your program participants.

Skills Section

The skills section of the class is when you introduce the various balance exercises you have selected based on the results of your initial assessments. During the 40 minutes that have been planned for this section, you will be able to present three or four program components. Depending on the size of your class and the availability of equipment, you may choose to present certain activities to the class as a whole or to divide the class into smaller groups according to a station format. Although teaching an activity to the whole class allows you to monitor the progress of your participants more directly, it requires greater attention to creating a safe practice environment, particularly if the exercise being practiced is one of the more challenging progressions. How well you match the demands of the exercise to the capabilities of each participant will significantly affect the level of safety. For example, teaching seated center of gravity (COG) activities to a larger group can be easily and safely accomplished by making sure that the participants who are less stable are seated on Dyna-Discs on chairs with a back and armrests while the participants who are more stable are seated on balance balls with or without a ball holder for added stability.

Allowing for adequate space between participants or placing a chair next to a participant seated on a balance ball also enhances the safety of an activity. Similarly, positioning the group close to a wall and placing chairs directly in front of each participant maximizes safety when your clients are standing on altered surfaces (e.g., half-foam roller, foam pad, rocker board). Again, safety can be increased by matching the difficulty of the support surface to the participant's abilities. The challenge of an exercise can be manipulated just by altering the height and width of the half-foam rollers, the height and density of the foam pads, or the degree of tilt associated with the rocker boards being used during the exercise.

Creating exercise stations can be an effective means of implementing the skills section of a class. Organizing the class into smaller groups helps you individualize the program a little more by allowing participants to work at a specific exercise station or spend more time at a station that addresses their particular balance

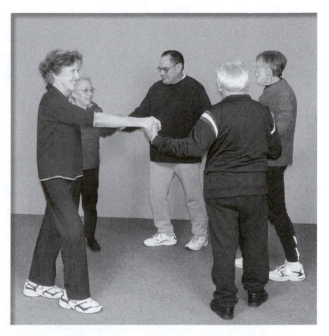

Figure 11.4 Using circle formations during a warm-up allows the instructor to observe all participants easily and increases the safety and confidence of the clients by having them hold hands.

> ### Key Point
>
> How well you match the demands of an exercise to the capabilities of each participant will significantly affect the level of safety achieved in your class.

problems. The use of multiple exercise stations also allows you to better distribute your available equipment. While one group is working on seated balance activities requiring Dyna-Discs, balance balls, and ball holders, a second group can be practicing standing transfer activities on benches of various heights, and a third group can be engaged in strength or flexibility exercises using resistance bands, hand weights, or no equipment at all.

In your planning, allocate an appropriate length of time for practice at each station (i.e., 8-10 minutes at each of four stations). Organize the exercise stations so that the activities designed for one station logically follow from those assigned at the previous station (i.e., seated to standing) and vary in terms of their balance challenge or aerobic intensity. As the program progresses, the activities planned for each station also need to increase in difficulty.

Cool-Down

Just as the warm-up creates a clear beginning to a class, the cool-down brings closure to a class. The activities planned for this section should lower both the heart rate and the anxiety level of the participants. Remember that a large number of the activities you present in the skills section of the class will induce anxiety because they are unfamiliar or push participants beyond a certain comfort level and increase fear of falling on occasion. Relaxation exercises should be incorporated regularly into the cool-down. These exercises can take the form of gentle stretching activities performed in a comfortable seated position, rhythmic breathing to music, inspirational readings, self- or partner massage, and postural awareness activities. Planning cool-down activities that involve lying on mats on the floor will also provide you with an excellent opportunity to review the floor-to-standing transition strategies (described at the end of chapter 4) following completion of the cool-down. Do not precede this activity with the relaxation exercises, however, because for many older adults, getting up from the floor is anything but relaxing.

> ### Key Point
>
> The activities presented during the cool-down should lower both the heart rate and the anxiety level of participants.

In addition to lowering the heart rate and anxiety level of your participants, the cool-down provides an opportunity to review what has taken place during the class, solicit feedback from class participants, recognize the efforts of individual participants and the class as a whole, and assign homework to be done before the next class. Your goal is to prepare your participants to leave the class and transition back into their daily lives in a relaxed and satisfied state. If you have planned your lessons carefully, they will leave each class with a sense of accomplishment as well as an eagerness to attend the next class.

Before beginning any relaxation exercises you have planned for the cool-down, create a conducive atmosphere by dimming the lights, closing any doors to outside noise, and playing soft instrumental music. Lower the volume of your voice and speak more slowly so that it has a calming effect on your participants as you present each exercise, read an inspirational poem, or verbally guide your participants through a series of visual images (e.g., floating down a river, stepping onto a cloud). Avoid ending the cool-down abruptly. Allow the participants to take additional time as needed before you brighten the lights or open the doors to the outside world. Be mindful that any abrupt movements or change in voice volume can quickly reverse the relaxed state you have helped your participants achieve.

DURING EACH CLASS SESSION

By taking the time to develop a clear lesson plan before the start of each class, you have already done much to ensure that each session will be successful. Going into a class with a clear idea of what you plan to do will minimize the time wasted in transitioning between activities and maximize the amount of time each participant is engaged in activity. By knowing the order of activities to be presented in each section of the class, you will not only teach with greater confidence but also be perceived by your class participants as a well-organized and knowledgeable instructor.

Begin your class promptly with the warm-up so that you set the tone for the entire session. Be positive in your presentation style and provide clear verbal instructions before starting each new exercise in the warm-up or moving on to a new movement in your aerobic sequence. Ensure that all participants are positioned so that they can see what you are doing and hear what you are saying. Encourage participants with particularly poor vision or impaired hearing to stand closer to you during the warm-up. If you use music during your warm-up, which many older adults

> ### Key Point
> Be sure that your participants are positioned so that they can see what you are doing and hear what you are saying.

enjoy, remember to choose music that is age appropriate, has a moderate tempo (e.g., 100-120 beats per minute) and a strong beat, and is played at a volume that allows for verbal instructions to be heard.

Where you position yourself relative to your class members when leading the warm-up, introducing a new exercise, monitoring group activities, or making skill corrections is particularly important in group settings. When leading the warm-up or introducing a new exercise or skill, position yourself where all students can see you clearly. For example, if you choose to incorporate seated activities into your warm-up, have your class sit in a semicircle, with you seated directly in front of them. Be sure to position individuals with hearing or visual impairments on the edges of the semicircle (see figure 11.5). When leading standing warm-up

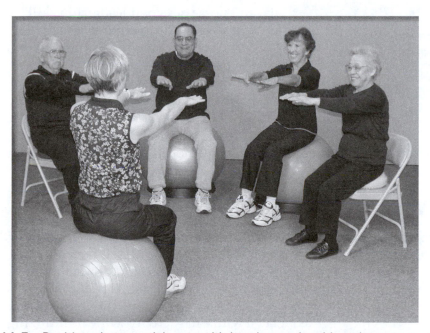

Figure 11.5 Position class participants with hearing or visual impairments on the edges of a semicircle so they are closer to you.

exercises, organize your class into staggered rows, with the shorter people toward the front. Position yourself in front of the class and facing the group. Although it is often more difficult for older adults to mirror your movements when you are facing them, it is more important that you be able to watch closely to ensure that they are being monitored by program assistants or holding onto a chair if extra support is needed. You can minimize any confusion that might arise by verbalizing and pointing in the direction you want them to go just before changing the movement sequence.

If you are using several exercise stations during the skills section of the class, the two major difficulties you are likely to encounter as an instructor are (1) where to position yourself in the room so you can monitor the activities of each group and (2) how to move efficiently among the groups so you can provide additional instruction and corrective feedback. Certainly, if you have program assistants to help you during each class, this problem is easier to solve. How many assistants you require will depend greatly on the functional levels of your participants. If clients are only moderately impaired, you may need only one assistant per every 4 to 6 participants, whereas if participants are more severely impaired, as is likely to be the case in programs operating in residential care facilities, you may need as many as one assistant for every 2 to 3 clients. Knowing how many assistants are available for each class lesson will also guide you in determining your class size. Although it is not always possible to set a class maximum, particularly if you are employed by a community college district or other state-funded organization, it may be possible to divide the class into two smaller groups and shorten the lesson to 30 minutes to better ensure the safety of your clients while providing a sufficient level of challenge that will lead to observable improvements in balance and mobility.

A program assistant can be given a list of appropriate activities to present and then assigned to lead a small group. Alternatively, you might appoint a participant in each group to lead the activities. If you have established your groups in planning the class, you can identify an appropriate participant who is at a higher level of function and possesses good leadership skills. However you decide to organize the activities within each group, remember to position yourself on the perimeter of the group you are instructing so you can easily view the other groups in the room. In addition, assess which group activities require expert instruction or involve the greatest challenge and lead those yourself. As mentioned earlier, taking the time to plan your lesson and prepare your classroom in advance will result in smooth transitions between activities and exercise stations.

> ### Key Point
>
> Position yourself on the perimeter of the group you are instructing so you can easily view other groups in the room.

BETWEEN CLASS SESSIONS

As soon as possible after each class, evaluate what went well and what did not. If you determine that there are problems associated with the exercises you selected, make any changes to the lesson plan you think are appropriate to resolve them. Also evaluate how effectively you matched the difficulty of the exercise progression to each participant's individual capabilities. Remember that your goal is to maximize the challenge associated with each activity while minimizing the risk to participants. You also want participants to experience success when performing the various exercises. Being successful, at least part of the time, raises each participant's balance-related self-confidence. Carefully review the exercise progressions presented in this book and decide how to adjust the difficulty level if you plan to present the same set of exercises in the next class.

> ### Key Point
> Being successful, at least a good portion of the time, improves the participant's balance-related self-confidence.

In addition to evaluating how effectively you selected and progressed the exercises, evaluate your class management skills by estimating how much time your participants were engaged in actual exercise during the hour they spent in your class. For example, how much time elapsed between the completion of one set of exercises and the start of the next set? How long did it take to get the exercises started at each station or to move the groups between stations? Did all members of a group appear to be actively engaged in the exercise for the allotted time? Although you need to provide sufficient rest between activities to avoid undue fatigue among your participants, you can often do so simply by sequencing the activities effectively. For example, following a

> ### Key Point
> Evaluate your class management skills by estimating how much time your class participants were engaged in exercise during the time they spent in class.

more vigorous set of gait pattern activities with a set of seated exercises coordinating head and eye movements will allow your participants to rest the muscles of their legs while still engaging in balance activities. You can also make use of the time participants spend waiting to move through an obstacle course or perform an activity that requires individualized attention by having them complete a set of exercises they can perform safely while unsupervised. Good waiting exercises include upper-body strength and flexibility exercises that can be performed in a seated position with or without a partner.

As the program progresses, you should maintain a log of the exercise components and progressions you present in each class session. This log will help you (1) select exercises from each of the five program components so that each dimension of balance is addressed regularly and (2) remember which level in the exercise progression of each component your class has reached at any point during the program. These two elements of the program will be particularly important to monitor if you teach multiple classes a week.

AFTER EACH FOLLOW-UP ASSESSMENT

Regularly assessing the performance of your class participants is essential for several reasons. In addition to providing your participants with information about their progress, it will assist you in evaluating your own effectiveness as an instructor. From a programming perspective, the collective results of each individual test, once compared with previous test outcomes, can be used to identify which dimensions of balance are beginning to improve and which might require more attention in the coming weeks. Regular follow-up assessments are

> ### Key Point
> Regularly assessing the performance of your class participants is essential.

also an effective way of motivating your participants to continue attending the program because of the improvement they have made in one or more areas of balance. Because you are continually increasing the difficulty of most exercises, it is often hard for a participant to see the positive changes resulting from each class. Thus, these tests become a means of objectively demonstrating positive change.

All of the tests that make up the FallProof program assessment were selected based on their reliability, their validity, and their ability to detect changes in performance over time. As long as you conduct each follow-up test using the same care you exercised during the initial assessment, you are sure to see positive and meaningful changes in one or more of the dimensions of balance and mobility you are reevaluating. Because you probably have not conducted the tests within the previous 2 months (the recommended minimum time between follow-up assessments), you will need to review the test instructions for each test so you can readminister them reliably. You should also review the participant's file just before conducting each follow-up test to see whether certain tests were modified during the initial

> **Key Point**
>
> To ensure that your follow-up test results are valid, have your participants perform each test in exactly the same way they performed it on the previous assessment. Also ensure that they use the same assistive device.

assessment. For example, some older adults may have needed to use an assistive device while performing mobility tests such as the 8-foot (2.4 m) up-and-go test and the 30-foot (9 m) walk test, or they may have required additional support while performing other tests (e.g., used their hands to rise from the chair during the chair stand). To ensure that your follow-up test results are valid, have the participants perform each test in exactly the same way they performed the test in the previous assessment. If time permits, you can also allow your participants to perform the test without the assistive device or additional support, but that should not occur during the first readministration of the test.

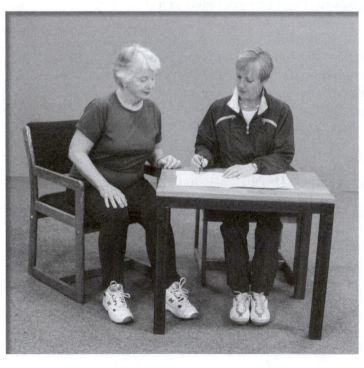

Figure 11.6 Share test results with clients in a timely fashion.

Once you have reevaluated each participant, share the results with the participant in a timely fashion (figure 11.6). You can share results via a short interview or by giving a report card that indicates the actual changes (if any) that occurred in test scores, what the changes mean in terms your clients can understand, and any areas that may require more attention during and between future class sessions. Form 3.3 on pages 93-94 is a sample report card.

The improvement in performance you observe on reassessment is likely to vary among your class participants due to differences in their initial functional level and the type of balance and mobility problems (e.g., temporary versus permanent) they are experiencing. Thus, participants should be discouraged from comparing their test scores with each other and should focus only on their own individual improvements. In this regard, you should show participants how the changes you are seeing in their balance and mobility are likely to influence their performance of daily activities. Ask participants whether they think the program has positively influenced their performance of daily tasks, and in what ways, before sharing the test results with them. Also spend time reviewing each participants' program goals and how they feel about their progress toward meeting those goals. This conversation not only will help you form a personal connection with your clients but also will provide you with information for selecting the next set of progressive exercises for them.

COMMUNICATING WITH CLASS PARTICIPANTS

Although it is beyond the scope of this instructor guide to discuss the many techniques associated with good leadership, one area in particular is important to a successful class: the way in which you communicate with your program participants, both verbally and nonverbally. Good communication skills are essential to the success of any program in which you are trying to motivate individuals to change their behavior. In fact, how well you deliver feedback to your class participants about their performance will often determine how well they perform on subsequent attempts.

> ## Key Point
>
> How well you deliver feedback to your class participants will often determine how well they perform on subsequent practice attempts.

Among the many leadership skills that are desirable if you are going to be an effective and successful instructor of older adults is the ability to express a genuine professional interest in and concern for each individual who attends your classes. You demonstrate interest and concern not only by what you say to individual clients before, during, and after each class but also by what you convey through body language. Tailor your communication to the individual personalities within your class. Whereas some class participants need lots of reassuring and motivating words, others prefer less positive reinforcement and more corrective feedback on their performance. When in doubt, ask your class participants if they feel they are receiving sufficient and meaningful feedback.

Addressing class participants respectfully is essential for effective communication. Substitute slang terms such as *you guys* with more appropriate ones such as *ladies and gentlemen* or *class* when addressing the group as a whole. Also learn the names of your participants as soon as possible. A good way to do this during the early classes is to provide participants with name tags to help you and other class members learn each other's names. Knowing the names of your class participants not only facilitates good communication but also makes participants feel just that little bit more special.

As important as it is to communicate effectively, it is equally important to listen well. Never interrupt class participants when they are speaking, and always maintain good eye contact. If you need to end a conversation in order to start the class or change activities, indicate your need to curtail the conversation but also let the participant know that you would be happy to continue the conversation at the end of class or before the next class.

If possible, allow time after class to talk with participants and answer any questions. This is also a good time to provide positive feedback to participants so that they leave the class feeling successful and optimistic about their progress. In addition, be sure to thank each of them for coming to class and tell them how much you are looking forward to seeing them the next time. For participants

> **Key Point**
>
> Allow time after class to talk with participants and answer any questions.

with more severe balance problems, a change in performance will not come quickly; you need to provide these participants with feedback that acknowledges their efforts and motivates them to attend regularly.

Evaluate your communication skills periodically. Consider videotaping yourself instructing a class so you can evaluate your communication skills in that setting. During your review, focus on what you are saying, when and how often you are saying it, and what tone you are using. In addition, consider soliciting occasional feedback from class members, particularly those who appear to have difficulty understanding what you are asking them to do. It is helpful to know if they have any areas of concern or confusion about the exercise progressions you have taught them and if they understand how the various types of activities they have learned relate to their daily lives. Because some activities may not seem immediately meaningful to your class participants, you must explain how these activities might be related to certain daily activities, how they might influence how well a certain task is performed, or how they may help participants cope with different sensory environments.

> **Key Point**
>
> It is important to explain to participants how the balance activities presented in class relate to the performance of daily activities.

SUMMARY

The success of the program you design using this instructor guide will be determined not only by how well you plan each individual class session but also by how effectively you present the content you have selected. Good organization skills are essential if you are going to be an effective balance and mobility instructor. Just as it takes time to learn how to interpret assessment results and then match the appropriate exercise progressions to the capabilities of your participants, it takes time and effort to develop your class organization skills. Individualizing a program used in a group setting is not an easy task, but it is a necessary skill to master in order to optimize the progress of each participant in your program. Programming for older adults with balance and mobility disorders can also be challenging because many of them will have developed elaborate ways of compensating for their problems that are often inappropriate or difficult to change. Careful planning, good communication skills, and patience are the keys to your success as a balance and mobility instructor. The success of the FallProof program over the years has been due not only to the quality of the exercise progressions developed but also to the many instructors who have become certified to teach the program and systematically deliver the program components after becoming familiar with the content in this instructor guide.

Test Your Understanding

1. After completing the preprogram assessment, the first task is to
    a. begin selecting appropriate exercises based on the results obtained
    b. identify and list the types of balance and mobility problems observed
    c. determine which clients should use a Dyna-Disc as opposed to a balance ball during the seated COG balance activities

    d. develop a list of the balance problems observed that are permanent and a list of the impairments that are more temporary

    e. assign certain exercises for homework

2. Which of the following will *not* determine the starting point for each participant in the program?

    a. previous motor skill experience

    b. current level of physical activity

    c. type of impairments identified during the initial assessment

    d. age and gender of the participant

    e. level of balance-related self-confidence

3. It is suggested that each class include the following components:

    a. 10-minute warm-up, 40-minute skills section, and 10-minute cool-down

    b. 15-minute warm-up, 35-minute skills section, and 10-minute cool-down

    c. 20-minute warm-up, 40-minute skills section, and no cool-down

    d. a warm-up, skills section, and cool-down of any length the instructor chooses

    e. 40-minute skills section and 20-minute cool-down

4. The major advantage of presenting certain activities to the whole class is that

    a. the social atmosphere of the class is enhanced

    b. you do not have to repeat your verbal instructions to multiple groups

    c. you are able to monitor each client's progress more directly

    d. the class participants do not have to move between groups so their risk of falling is decreased

    e. transition time between groups is eliminated

5. The primary reason for incorporating small-group station activities into a class is so the instructor can

    a. take a well-earned rest from teaching the class

    b. individualize the program a little more for each participant

    c. group participants according to ability

    d. use more of the space available

    e. better distribute attention among the groups

6. The primary reason for including a cool-down at the end of each class is to

    a. elevate the heart rate following the skills section

    b. solicit feedback from participants about the class

    c. assign homework to be completed before the next class

    d. lower the heart rate and anxiety level of class participants

    e. recognize the efforts of individual participants

7. When working with class participants who have very low balance-related self-confidence,

    a. make sure that the exercises performed are easy enough that the participant will always be successful

    b. always provide close supervision and additional manual support

    c. have them perform all exercises in a seated position so their risk for falling is decreased

    d. present challenging balance activities that will help them forget they have a confidence problem

    e. select exercises that will challenge their balance abilities but also ensure that they are successful on a large percentage of practice attempts

8. The best way to evaluate your class management skills is to
   a. determine how quickly class participants move from one activity to the next
   b. ask the participants for feedback during the cool-down
   c. estimate the amount of time the class participants spend exercising during the time allocated for the class
   d. check whether your class ends at the designated time
   e. determine how long it requires you or your assistants to get all the necessary equipment needed for the class

9. Which of the following is *not* a good reason for conducting regular balance and mobility assessments?
   a. to identify which dimensions of balance are beginning to show improvement in each client
   b. to identify which dimensions of balance still need improving in each client
   c. to evaluate your effectiveness as an instructor
   d. to practice your test administration skills
   e. to motivate participants to continue attending classes

10. The following are all examples of effective communication skills *except*
    a. addressing class participants in a respectful manner
    b. taking the time to point out each individual class member's errors during the cool-down
    c. knowing the names of class participants
    d. not interrupting when a client is speaking
    e. allowing time to talk with clients individually after class

Practical Problems

1. Review the sample lesson plan presented in figure 11.2. Develop a similar lesson plan for a 60-minute class that includes Phoebe and Larry. Indicate whether the lesson plan you develop is one that will be presented early or later in the program.

2. Videotape yourself leading an activity class for a group of older adults. Review the tape and evaluate the following components, listing all the things you feel you did well in addition to the things you feel need improvement:
   a. Classroom management skills (e.g., record the amount of time participants were engaged in activity, note the efficiency of the classroom setup)
   b. Communication skills
   c. Positioning during class and quality of verbal cuing and feedback provided to participants

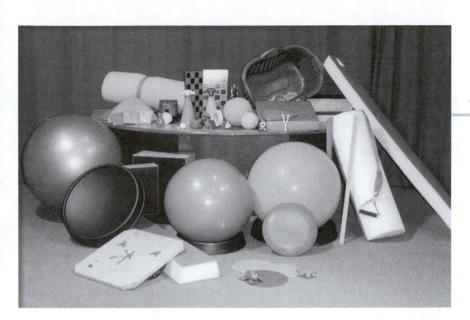

Balance Kit Inventory

- Lightweight balls (6)
  - 3 small
  - 3 large
- Balance balls (5)
  - One 55 cm ball
  - Two 65 cm balls
  - One 75 cm ball
  - One 80 cm ball
- Large ball holders (5)
- Weighted balls (3)
  - One 1 kg ball
  - One 2 kg ball
  - One 3 kg ball
- Dyna-Discs (4)
- Stacking cones, small (set of 30)
- Stacking cones, large (set of 10)
- Large rocker boards (2)
- Nested benches (2 sets of 2-, 4-, and 6-inch benches)
- Airex balance pads (6)

- Thin foam mats (floor, Yoga) (4)
- Large Airex pad
- Half foam roller (2 mats, 6 × 36 inches)
- Half foam roller (2 mats, 12 × 36 × 0.5 inches)
- Spots (3 sets of 10)
- Resistance band (1 box of light, medium, heavy)
- Laundry baskets (2)
- Small parachute with handles
- Large parachute with handles
- Bean bags (20)
- Soft critters (frogs, turtles, etc.)
- Stepping stones (1 set of small, 1 set of large)
- Plastic trays (4)
- Plastic cups, plates, bowls

Answer Key for Test Your Understanding Questions

Chapter 1

1. b
2. e
3. b
4. b
5. a
6. d
7. c
8. c
9. b
10. c

Chapter 2

1. d
2. b
3. e
4. d
5. a
6. b
7. b
8. d
9. a
10. c

Chapter 3

1. c
2. c
3. d
4. b
5. a
6. a
7. e
8. c
9. d
10. a

Chapter 4

1. b
2. e
3. d
4. e
5. b
6. a
7. c
8. b
9. e

Chapter 5

1. d
2. e
3. c
4. b
5. a
6. c
7. b
8. a
9. b
10. b

Chapter 6

1. a
2. c
3. c
4. b
5. c
6. b
7. a
8. a
9. d

Chapter 7

1. d
2. c
3. d
4. d
5. b
6. a
7. a
8. d
9. e
10. c

Chapter 8

1. c
2. c
3. b
4. d
5. b
6. a
7. e
8. b
9. a
10. c

Chapter 9

1. b
2. d
3. c
4. c
5. c
6. d
7. c
8. a
9. b
10. b

Chapter 10

1. b
2. c
3. b
4. a
5. d
6. e
7. b
8. d
9. c
10. b

Chapter 11

1. b
2. d
3. a
4. c
5. b
6. d
7. e
8. c
9. d
10. b

Bibliography

Adams, P.F., Dey, A.N., & Vickerie, J.L. (2007). Summary health statistics for the U.S. population: National health interview survey, 2005. *Vital and Health Statistics. Series 10, Data from the National Health Survey, 233,* 1-104.

Akima, H., Kano, Y., Enomoto, Y., Ishizu, M., Okada, M., Oishi, Y., Katsuta, S., & Kuno, S.Y. (2001). Muscle function in 164 men and women aged 20-84 yr. *Medicine and Science in Sports and Exercise, 33,* 220-226.

Alexander, N. (1994). Postural control in older adults. *Journal of the American Geriatrics Society, 42,* 93-108.

Allison, L., & Rose, D.J. (1998). The relationship between postural control system impairments and disabilities in older adults. *Physical Therapy, 78*(5), S69-70.

Aloia, J.F., McGowan, D.M., Vaswani, A.N., Ross, P., Cohn, S.H. (1991). Relationship of menopause to skeletal and muscle mass. *American Journal of Clinical Nutrition, 53,* 1378-1383.

American College of Sports Medicine. (1998). Position stand on exercise and physical activity for older adults. *Medicine and Science in Sports and Exercise, 30,* 992-1008.

American College of Sports Medicine. (2002). Progression models in resistance training for healthy adults. *Medicine and Science in Sports and Exercise, 34,* 364-380.

American Heart Association. (2002). *Heart facts 2002: All Americans.* Dallas, TX: American Heart Association.

Asp, K. (2000). The role of stretching exercises: From warm-ups to cool-downs. *IDEA Fitness Edge, November-December,* 7-10.

Bandy, W.D., & Sanders, B. (2001). *Therapeutic exercise.* Baltimore: Lippincott Williams & Wilkins.

Barak, Y., Wagenaar, R.C., & Holt, K.G. (2006). Gait characteristics of elderly people with a history of falls: a dynamic approach. *Physical Therapy, 86,* 1501-1510.

Basmajian, J.V., & De Luca, C.J. (1985). *Muscles alive: Their functions revealed by electromyography* (5th ed.). Baltimore: Williams & Wilkins.

Bell, R., & Hoshizaki, T. (1981). Relationships of age and sex with joint range of motion of seventeen joint actions in humans. *Canadian Journal of Applied Sport Sciences, 6,* 202-206.

Berg, K., Wood-Dauphinee, S., & Williams, J.I. (1995). The balance scale: Reliability assessment with elderly residents and patients with acute stroke. *Scandinavian Journal of Rehabilitation Medicine, 27,* 27-36.

Berg, K., Wood-Dauphinee, S.L., Williams, J.I., & Gayton, D. (1989). Measuring balance in the elderly: Preliminary development of an instrument. *Physiotherapy Canada, 41,* 304-311.

Berg, K.O., Wood-Dauphinee, S.L., Williams, J.I., & Maki, B. (1992). Measuring balance in the elderly: Validation of an instrument. *Canadian Journal of Public Health, 2,* S7-S11.

Berthoz, A., & Pozzo, T. (1994). Head and body coordination during locomotion and complex movements. In S.P. Swinnen, H. Heuer, J. Massion, & P. Casaer (Eds.), *Interlimb coordination: Neural, dynamical and cognitive constraints* (pp. 147-165). San Diego: Academic Press.

Blaszczyk, J.W., Hansen, P.D., Lowe, DL. (1993). Postural sway and perception of the upright stance stability borders. *Perception, 22,* 56-62.

Brady, T.J., Kruger, J.M., Helmick, C.G., Callahan, L.F., Boutaugh, M.L. (2003). Intervention programs for arthritis and other rheumatic diseases. *Health Education & Behavior, 30*(1), 44-63.

Brandt, K.D., & Slemenda, C.W. (1993). Osteoarthritis epidemiology, pathology, and pathogenesis. In H.R. Schumacher, Jr. (Ed.), *Primer on the rheumatic disease* (10th ed., pp. 184-187). Atlanta: Arthritis Foundation.

Brauer, S.G., Woollacott, M., & Shumway-Cook, A. (2002). The influence of a concurrent cognitive task on the compensatory stepping response to a perturbation in balance-impaired and healthy elders. *Gait and Posture, 15,* 83-93.

Brown, L.A., Shumway-Cook, A., & Woollacott, M.H. (1999). Attentional demands and postural recovery: The effects of aging. *Journal of Gerontology, 54A,* M165-171.

Buchner, D.M., Cress, M.E., de Lateur, B.J., Esselman, P.C., Margherita, A.J., Price, R., & Wagner, E.H. (1997). The effect of strength and endurance training on gait, balance, fall risk, and health services use in community-living older adults. *Journal of Gerontology, 52,* M218-M224.

Campbell, A., Borrie, M.J., & Spears, G.F. (1989). Risk factors for falls in a community-based prospective study of people 70 years and older. *Journal of Gerontology, 44,* 112-117.

Campbell, Robertson, Gardner, Norton, & Buchner. (1999) Economic evaluation of a community based exercise programme to prevent falls. *Journal of Epidemiological Community Health.* 2001 August; 55(8): 600–606.

Centers for Disease Control and Prevention. (2008). Stroke Facts and Statistics. http://www.cdc.gov/Stroke/stroke_facts.htm

Centers for Disease Control and Prevention. *Stay Independent Self-Risk Assessment Guide.* Currently being evaluated at the Fall Prevention Center of Excellence.

Chandler, J.M. (1996). Invited commentary. *Physical Therapy, 76,* 584-585.

Chandler, J.M., & Hadley, E.C. (1996). Exercise to improve physiologic and functional performance in old age. *Clinics in Geriatric Medicine, 12,* 761-784.

Chang, J. T., Morton, S. C., Rubenstein, L. Z., Mojica, W. A., Maglione, M., Suttorp, M. J., Roth, E. A., Shekelle, P. G. (2004). Interventions for the prevention of falls in older adults: Systematic review and meta-analysis of randomised clinical trials. *British Medical Journal, 328,* 680.

Chen, H.-C., Ashton-Miller, J.A., Alexander, N.B., & Schultz, A.B. (1991). Stepping over obstacles: Gait patterns of healthy young and old adults. *Journal of Gerontology, 46,* M196-203.

Chou, C., Chien, C., Hsueh, I., Sheu, C., Wang, C. & Hsieh, C. (2006). Developing a Short Form of the Berg Balance Scale for People With Stroke. *Physical Therapy,* 86(2),195-204.

Clemson, L, Cumming, R.G., Kendig, H., Swann, M., Heard, R., & Taylor, K. (2004). The effectiveness of a community-based program for reducing the incidence of falls in the elderly: a randomized trial. *Journal of the American Geriatric Society, 9,* 1487-94.

Cromwell, R.L., & Newton, R.A. (2004). Relationship between balance and gait stability in healthy older adults. *Journal of Aging and Physical Activity, 11,* 90-100.

Danion, F., Varraine, E., Bonnard, M., Pailhous, J. (2003). Stride variability in human gait: the effect of frequency, amplitude and walking speed. *Gait and Posture, 18,* 69-77.

Deyle, G.D., Henderson, N.E., Matekel, R.L., Ryder, M.G., Garber, M.B., & Allison, S.C. (2000). Effectiveness of manual physical therapy and exercise in osteoarthritis of the knee. *Annals of Internal Medicine, 132,* 129-133.

Dickin, D.C., & Rose, D.J. (2004). Sensory organization abilities during upright stance in late-onset Alzheimer's-type dementia. *Experimental Aging Research, 30*(4), 373-90.

Diener, H.C., & Nutt, J.G. (1997). Vestibular and cerebellar disorders of equilibrium and gait. In J.C. Masdeu, L. Sudarsky, & L. Wolfson (Eds.), *Gait disorders of aging. Falls and therapeutic strategies* (pp. 261-272). Philadelphia: Lippincott-Raven.

Di Pietro, L. (1996). The epidemiology of physical activity and physical function in older people. *Medicine and Science in Sports and Exercise, 28,* 596-600.

Eisenberg, D.M., Davis, R.B., Ettner, S.L., Appel, S., Wilkey, S., Van Rompay, M., & Kessler, R.C. (1998). Trends in alternative medicine use in the United States, 1990-1997. Results of a follow-up national survey. *Journal of the American Medical Association, 280,* 1569-1575.

Eisenberg, D.M., Kessler, R.C., Foster, C., Norlock, F.E., Calkins, D.R., & Delbanco, T.L. (1993). Unconventional medicine in the United States: Prevalence, costs, and patterns of use. *New England Journal of Medicine, 328,* 246-252.

Elble, R.J. (1997). Changes in gait with normal aging. In J.C. Masdeu, L. Sudarsky, & L. Wolfson (Eds.), *Gait disorders of aging. Falls and therapeutic strategies* (pp. 93-106). Philadelphia: Lippincott-Raven.

Elble, R.J., Thomas, S.S., Higgins, C., & Colliver, J. (1991). Stride-dependent changes in gait of older people. *Journal of Neurology, 238,* 1-5.

Erim, Z., Beg, M.F., Burke, D.T., & De Luca, C.J. (1999). Effects of aging on motor-unit control properties. *Journal of Neurophysiology, 82,* 2081-2091.

Ettinger, W.H., Burns, R., & Messier, S.P. (1999). A randomized trial comparing aerobic exercise and resistance exercise with a health education program in older adults with knee osteoarthritis. The Fitness Arthritis and Seniors Trial (FAST). *Journal of the American Medical Association, 277,* 1361-1369.

Farrar, K., & Rose, D.J. (2007). The Association between Sensory Impairment and Functional Limitations in Balance in Community-Dwelling Older Adults. *The Gerontologist, 47,* 2, 78.

Fitts, P.M., & Posner, M.I. (1967). *Human performance.* Belmont, CA: Brooks/Cole.

Foldvari, M., Clark, M., Laviolette, L.A., Bernstein, M.A., Kaliton, D., Castaneda, C., Pu, C.T., Hausdorff, J.M., Fielding, R.A., & Fiatarone-Singh, M.A. (2000). Association of muscle power with functional status in community-dwelling elderly women. *Journal of Gerontology, 55A*, M192-M199.

Foley, A., Halbert, J., Hewill, T., & Crotty, M. (2003). Does hydrotherapy improve strength and physical function in patients with osteoarthritis—a randomised controlled trial comparing a gym based and a hydrotherapy based strengthening programme. *Annals of the Rheumatic Diseases, 2*(12), 1162-1167.

Fransen, M., Nairn L., Winstanley J., Lam P., Edmonds J. (2007). Physical activity for osteoarthritis management: a randomized controlled clinical trial evaluating hydrotherapy or Tai Chi classes. *Arthritis Care & Research, 57*(3), 407-414.

Gehlson GM, Whaley MH. (1990). Falls in the elderly: part II, balance, strength, and flexibility. *Archives of Physical Medicine and Rehabilitation, 71*, 739-741.

Gentile, A.M. (1972). A working model of skill acquisition with application to teaching. *Quest, Monograph XVII*, 3-23.

Gentile, A.M. (1987). Skill acquisition: Action, movement, and neuromotor processes. In J.H. Carr, R.B. Shephard, J. Gordon, A.M. Gentile, & J.M. Held (Eds.), *Movement science. Foundations for physical therapy in rehabilitation* (pp. 93-154). Rockville, MD: Aspen.

Gentile, A.M. (2000). Skill acquisition: Action, movement, and neuromotor processes. In J.H. Carr & R.B. Shephard (Eds.), *Movement science. Foundations for physical therapy in rehabilitation* (2nd ed., pp. 111-187). Rockville, MD: Aspen.

Gillespie, L.D., Gillespie, W.J., Robertson, M.C., Lamb S.E., Cumming, R.G., & Rowe, B.H. (2009). Interventions for preventing falls in older people living in the community. Cochrane Database of Systematic Reviews (online). 2009 Apr 15; (2): CD007146.

Goode, S.L., & Magill, R.A. (1986). The contextual interference effect in learning three badminton serves. *Research Quarterly for Exercise and Sport, 57*, 308-314.

Gunter, K., DeCosta, J., White, K., Hooker, K., Hayes, W.T., Snow, C. (2003). Balance self-efficacy predicts risk factors for side falls and frequent falls in community-dwelling elderly. *Journal of Aging and Physical Activity, 11*, 28-39.

Hall, K.G., Domingues, D.A., & Cavazos, R. (1994). Contextual interference effects with skilled baseball players. *Perceptual and Motor Skills, 78*, 835-841.

Harada, N., Chiu, V., Fowler, E., Lee, M., & Reuben, D.B. (1995). Physical therapy to improve functioning of older people in residential care facilities. *Physical Therapy, 75*, 830-838.

Helmick et al. (2008). Estimates of the Prevalence of Arthritis and Other Rheumatic Conditions in the United States, Part I. *Arthritis and Rheumatism, 58*(1), 15-25.

Herdman, S.J. (2007). *Vestibular rehabilitation* (3rd ed.). Philadelphia: Davis.

Hernandez, D., & Rose, D.J. (2008). Predicting which older adults will and will not fall using the Fullerton Advanced Balance Scale. *Archives of Physical Medicine and Rehabilitation, 89*(12), 2309-2315.

Hernandez, D., Rose, D.J., & Theou, O. (2008). Can gait velocity predict which older adults will or will not fall? *Journal of Physical Activity and Aging, 16*, S209.

Holland, G.J., Tanaka, K., Shigematsu, R., & Nakagaichi, M. (2002). Flexibility and physical functions of older adults: A review. *Journal of Aging and Physical Activity, 10*, 169-206.

Horak, F.B., & Nashner, L.M. (1986). Central programming of postural movements: Adaptations to altered support surface configurations. *Journal of Neurophysiology, 55*, 1369-1381.

Howland, J., Peterson, E., & Ohayon, H. (2000). Fear of falling: a primer for cargivers. *Stride*, February/March, 4-6.

Hu, M.H., & Woollacott, M. (1994a). Multisensory training of standing balance in older adults: I. Postural stability and one-leg stance balance. *Journal of Gerontology, 49*, M52-M61.

Hu, M.H., & Woollacott, M. (1994b). Multisensory training of standing balance in older adults: II. Kinetic and electromyographic postural responses. *Journal of Gerontology, 49*, M62-M71.

Ivers, R.Q., Cumming, R.G., Mitchell, P., & Attebo, K. (1998). Visual impairment and falls in older adults: the Blue Mountains Eye Study. *Journal of the American Geriatrics Society, 46*(1), 58–64.

Jensen, J.L., Bothner, K.E., & Woollacott, M.H. (1996). Balance control: the scaling of the kinetic response to accommodate increasing perturbation magnitudes. *Journal of Sport and Exercise Psychology, 18*. S45.

Jette, A.M., Branch, L.G., & Berlin, J. (1990). Musculoskeletal impairments and physical disablement among the elderly. *Journal of Gerontology, 45*, M203-M208.

Johnell O, Melton LJ, 3rd, Atkinson EJ, O'Fallon WM, Kurland LT. (1992). Fracture risk in patients with parkinsonism: a population-based study in Olmsted County, Minnesota. *Age and Ageing*, 21(1), 32–38.

Kenshalo, D.R. (1986). Somesthetic sensitivity in young and elderly humans. *Journal of Gerontology*, 41, 732-742.

Kisner, C., & Colby, L.A. (1990). *Therapeutic exercise foundations and techniques* (2nd ed.). Philadelphia: Davis.

Lach H.W. Incidence and risk factors for developing fear of falling in older adults. (2005). *Public Health Nursing*, 22, 45–52.

Landers, K.A., Hunter, G.R., Wetzstein, C.J., Bamman, M.M., & Wiensier, R.L. (2001). The interrelationship among muscle mass, strength, and the ability to perform physical tasks of daily living in younger and older women. *Journal of Gerontology*, 56A, B443-B448.

Leape, L.L. (2000). Preventable medical injuries in older patients. *Archives of Internal Medicine*, 160, 2717-2728.

Leipzig, R.M., Cumming, R.G., & Tinetti, M.E. (1999a). Drugs and falls: A systematic review and meta-analysis: I. Psychotropic drugs. *Journal of the American Geriatrics Society*, 47, 30-39.

Leipzig, R.M., Cumming, R.G., & Tinetti M.E. (1999b). Drugs and falls: A systematic review and meta-analysis: II. Cardiac and analgesic drugs. *Journal of the American Geriatrics Society*, 47, 40-50.

Lindle, R.S., Metter, E.J., Lynch, N.A., Fleg, J.L., Fozard, J.L., Tobin, J., Roy, T.A., & Hurley, B.F. (1997). Age and gender comparisons of muscle strength in 654 women and men aged 20-93 yr. *Journal of Applied Physiology*, 83, 1581-1587.

Lipsitz, L.A., Jonsson, P.V., Kelley, M.M., & Koestner, J.S. (1991). Causes and correlates of recurrent falls in ambulatory frail elderly. *Journal of Gerontology*, 46, M114-M122.

Lord, S.R., Clark, R.D., & Webster, I.W. (1991). Visual acuity and contrast sensitivity in relation to falls in an elderly population. *Age and Ageing*, 20(3), 175-181.

Lord, S.R., McLean, D., & Stathers, G. (1992). Physiological Factors Associated with Injurious Falls in Older People Living in the Community. *Gerontology*, 3, 338-346.

Lord, S.R., Castell, S.L., Corcoran, J., Dayhew, J., Matters, B., & Shan, A. (2003). The effect of group exercise on physical functioning and falls in frail older people living in retirement villages: A randomized, controlled trial. *Journal of the American Geriatrics Society*, 51, 1685-1692.

Lord, S.R., Sherrington, C., Menz, H.B., & Close, J.C. (2007). *Falls in older people: risk factors and strategies for prevention* (2nd ed). Cambridge: Cambridge University Press.

Luff, A.R. (1998). Age-associated changes in the innervation muscle fibers and changes in the mechanical properties of motor units. *Annals of the New York Academy of Science*, 854, 92-101.

Lui, J., & Wrisberg, C.A. (1997). The effect of knowledge of results delay and the subjective estimation of movement form on the acquisition and retention of a motor skill. *Research Quarterly for Exercise and Sport*, 68, 145-151.

Lundin-Olsson, L., Nyberg, L., & Gustafson, Y. (1997). "Stops walking when talking" as a predictor of falls in elderly people. *Lancet*, 349, 617.

Lung, M.W., Hartsell, H.D., & Vandervoort, A.A. (1996). Effects of aging on joint stiffness: Implications for exercise. *Physiotherapy Canada*, 48, 96-106.

Magill, R.A. (2007). *Motor learning. Concepts and applications* (8th ed.). Boston: McGraw-Hill.

Magill, R.A., & Hall, K.G. (1990). A review of the contextual interference effect in motor skill acquisition. *Human Movement Science*, 9, 241-289.

McCarthy, B. (1987). *The 4MAT System: Teaching to Learning Styles with Right/Left Mode Techniques*. Barrington, IL: Excel, Inc.

McCullagh, P., & Meyer, K.N. (1997). Learning versus correct models: Influence of model type on the learning of a free-weight squat lift. *Research Quarterly for Exercise and Sport*, 68, 56-61.

McGibbon, C., & Krebs, D.E. (1999). The effects of age and functional limitations on leg joint power and work during stance phase of gait. *Journal of Rehabilitation Research and Development*, 36, 173–182.

McGibbon, C., Krebs, D.E., & Puniello, M.S. (2001). Mechanical energy analysis identifies compensatory strategies in disabled elders gait. *Journal of Biomechanics*, 34, 481–490.

Metter, E.J., Conwitt, R., Tobin, J., & Fozard, J.L. (1997). Age-associated loss of power and strength in the upper extremities in woman and men. *Journal of Gerontology: Biological Sciences*, 52A(5), B267-B276.

Morey, M.C., Pieper, C.F., & Cornoni-Huntley, J.C. (1998). Physical fitness and functional limitations in community dwelling older adults. *Medicine and Science in Sports and Exercise*, 30, 715-723.

Morris, M.E (2006). Locomotor Training in People With Parkinson Disease. *Physical Therapy Journal* 86, 1426-1435.

Muir, S.W., Berg, K., Chesworth, B., & Speechley, M. (2008). Use of the Berg Balance Scale for Predicting Multiple Falls in Community-Dwelling Elderly People: A Prospective Study. *Physical Therapy*, 88(4), 449-459.

Murphy, J., & Isaacs, B. (1982). The post-fall syndrome. *Gerontology*, 28, 265-270.

Nashner, L.M. (1989). Sensory, neuromuscular, and biomechanical contributions to human balance. In P.W. Duncan (Ed.), *Balance: Proceedings of the APTA Forum*. Alexandria, Virginia: American Physical Therapy Association, 5-12.

Nelson, M.E., Rejeski, W.J., Blair, S.N., Duncan, P.W., Judge, J.O., King, A.C., Macera, C.A., and Castane-dasceppa, C. (2007). Physical Activity and Public Health in Older Adults: Recommendation from the American College of Sports Medicine and the American Heart Association. *Medicine and Science in Sports and Exercise*, 39(8), 1435-1445.

Neutel, S.W., Perry, S., & Maxwell, C. (2002). Medication use and risk of falls. *Pharmacoepidemiology and Drug Safety*, 11(2), 97-104.

Nevitt, M.C. (1997). Falls in the elderly: Risk factors and prevention. In J.C. Masdeu, L. Sudarsky, & L. Wolfson (Eds.), *Gait disorders of aging. Falls and therapeutic strategies* (pp. 13-36). Philadelphia: Lippincott-Raven.

Office of the Surgeon General. (2004). *Bone health & osteoporosis: A report of the surgeon general*. U.S. Department of Health and Human Services, Issued October 14, 2004.

Patla, A.E. (1997). Understanding the roles of vision in the control of human locomotion. *Gait and Posture*, 5, 54-69.

Perret, E., & Reglis, F. (1970). Age and the perceptual threshold for vibratory stimuli. *European Neurology*, 4, 65-76.

Pollock, B.J., & Lee, T.D. (1992). Effects of the model's skill level on observational learning. *Research Quarterly for Exercise and Sport*, 63, 25-29.

Ray, W.A., & Griffin, M.R. (1990). Prescribed medications and the risk of falling. *Topics in Geriatric Rehabilitation*, 5, 12-20.

Rhodes, E.C., Martin, A.D., Taunton, J.E., Donnelly, M., Warren, J., & Elliot, J. (2000). Effects of one year of resistance training on the relation between muscular strength and bone density in elderly women. *British Journal of Sports Medicine*, 34, 18-22.

Riddle, D.L., Stratford, P.W. (1999). Interpreting validity indexes for diagnostic tests: An illustration using the Berg Balance Test. *Physical Therapy*, 79(10): 939-948.

Rikli, R.E., & Jones, C.J. (1997). Assessing physical performance in independent older adults: Issues and guidelines. *Journal of Aging and Physical Activity, 5*, 244-261.

Rikli, R.E., & Jones, C.J. (1998). The reliability and validity of a 6-minute walk test as a measure of physical endurance in older adults. *Journal of Aging and Physical Activity, 6*, 363-375.

Rikli, R.E., & Jones, C.J. (1999a). The development and validation of a functional fitness test for community-residing older adults. *Journal of Aging and Physical Activity, 7*, 129-161.

Rikli, R.E., & Jones, C.J. (1999b). Functional fitness normative scores for community-residing adults, ages 60-94. *Journal of Aging and Physical Activity, 7*, 162-181.

Rikli, R.E., & Jones, C.J. (2001). *Senior Fitness Test manual*. Champaign, IL: Human Kinetics.

Rimmer, J.H. (2005). Exercise and physical activity in persons aging with a physical disability. *Physical Medicine and Rehabilitation Clinics of North America*,16(1), 41-56.

Rose, D.J. (2003). FallProof. A comprehensive balance and mobility program. Champaign, IL: Human Kinetics.

Rose, D.J. (2005). Posture, Balance, and Locomotion. In Spirduso, W., MacCrae, P., & Francis, K., *Physical Dimensions of Aging*, Champaign, IL: Human Kinetics, 131-155.

Rose, D.J., & Christina, R.W. (2007). *A multilevel approach to the study of motor control and learning* (2nd ed.). San Francisco: Benjamin-Cummings.

Rose, D.J., & Clark, S. (2000). Can the control of bodily orientation be improved in a group of older adults with a history of falls? *Journal of the American Geriatrics Society*, 48, 275-282.

Rose, D.J., Jones, C.J., & Lucchese, N. (2002). Predicting the probability of falls in community-residing older adults using the 8 foot up and go: A new measure of functional mobility. *Journal of Aging and Physical Activity*, 10, 466-475.

Rose, D.J., Lucchese, N., & Wiersma, L.D. (2006). Development of a multidimensional balance scale for use with functionally independent older adults. *Archives of Physical Medicine and Rehabilitation*, 87(11), 1478-85.

Roubenoff, R. (2001). Origins and Clinical Relevance of Sarcopenia. *Canadian Journal of Applied Physiology*, 26(1), 78-89.

Rubenstein, L.Z., & Josephson, K.R. (1992). Causes and prevention of falls in elderly people. In B. Vellas et al. (Eds.), *Falls, balance and gait disorders in the elderly* (pp. 21-38). Paris: Elsevier.

Schiller, J.S., Kramarow, E., & Dey A.N. (2007). *Fall injury episodes among noninstitutionalized older adults: United States, 2001-2003*. Hyattsville, MD: National Center for Health Statistics.

Schmidt, R.A., & Wrisberg, C.A. (2008). *Motor learning and performance* (4th ed.). Champaign, IL: Human Kinetics.

Scott, V., Dukeshire, S., Gallagher, E. & Scanlan, A. (2001). A best practices guide for the prevention of falls among seniors living in the community. Prepared for the Federal/Provincial/Territorial Ministers of Health and Ministers Responsible for Seniors.

Shea, J.B., & Morgan, R.L. (1979). Contextual interference effects on the acquisition, retention, and transfer of a motor skill. *Journal of Experimental Psychology: Human Learning and Memory, 5*, 179-187.

Shumway-Cook, A., Baldwin, M., Polissar, N.L., & Gruber, W. (1997). Predicting the probability for falls in community-dwelling older adults. *Physical Therapy, 77*(8), 812-819.

Shumway-Cook, A., Gruber, W., Baldwin, M., & Liao, S. (1997). The effect of multidimensional exercises on balance, mobility, and fall risk in community-dwelling older adults. *Physical Therapy, 77*(1), 46-56.

Shumway-Cook, A., & Woollacott, M. (2000). Attentional demands and postural control: The effect of sensory context. *Journal of Gerontology, 55A*, M10-M16.

Shumway-Cook, A., & Woollacott, M.H. (2005). *Motor control. Theory and practical applications* (3rd ed.). Philadelphia: Lippincott Williams & Wilkins.

Shumway-Cook, A., & Woollacott, M.H. (2007). Attentional demands and postural control: the effect of sensory context. *Journals of Gerontology Series A: Biological Sciences and Medical Sciences, 55*(1), M10-M16.

Shumway-Cook, A., Woollacott, M., Baldwin, M., & Kerns, K. (1997). The effects of cognitive demands on postural sway in elderly fallers and non-fallers. *Journal of Gerontology: Medical Sciences, 52A*, M232-M240.

Skelton, D.A., Greig, C.A., Davies, J.M., & Young, A. (1994). Strength, power and related functional ability of healthy people aged 65-89 years. *Age and Ageing, 23*(5), 371-377.

Spirduso, W.W., Francis, K.L., & MacRae, P.G. (2005). *Physical dimensions of aging* (2nd ed.). Champaign, IL: Human Kinetics.

Stelmach, G.E., Phillips, J., DiFabio, R.P., & Teasdale, N. (1989). Age, functional postural reflexes, and voluntary sway. *Journal of Gerontology: Biological Sciences, 44*, B100-B106.

Studenski, S., Duncan, P.W., Chandler, J., Samsa, G., Prescoh, B., et al. (1994). Predicting falls: The role of mobility and nonphysical factors. *Journal of the American Geriatrics Society, 42*, 297-302.

Swinnen, S.P. (1990). Interpolated activities during the knowledge of results and post knowledge of results interval: Effects of performance and learning. *Journal of Experimental Psychology: Learning, Memory, and Cognition, 19*, 1321-1344.

Tennstedt S., Howland J., Lachman E.P., Peterson E., Kasten L., & Jette A. (1998). A randomized, controlled trial of a group intervention to reduce fear of falling and associated activity restriction in older adults. *Journal of Gerontology: Psychological Sciences, 53B*, P384-P392.

Thapa, P.B., Gideon, P., Cost, T.W., Milam, A.B., & Ray, W.A. (1998). Antidepressants and the risk of falls among nursing home residents. *New England Journal of Medicine, 339*, 875-882.

Thelen, D.G., Brockmiller, C., Ashton-Miller, J.A., Schultz, A.B., & Alexander, N.B. (1998). Thresholds for sensing ankle dorsi- and/or plantarflexor rotation during upright stance: Effects of age and velocity. *Journal of Gerontology: Medical Sciences, 53A*, M33-M38. 1998.

Theou, 0., French, J., Hernandez, D., & Rose, D.J. (2006). Measuring older adult gait speed in community settings using the 30 foot-walk at preferred and maximum speed. *Medicine and Science in Sports and Exercise, 38*(5), S330.

Thorbahn, L., & Newton, R. (1996). Use of the Berg Balance Test to predict falls in elderly persons. *Physical Therapy, 76*, 576-585.

Tinetti, M.E. (2003). Clinical practice. Preventing falls in elderly persons. *New England Journal of Medicine, 348*(1), 42-49.

Tinetti, M.E., Mendes de Leon, C.F., Doucette, J.T., & Baker, D.I. (1994). Fear-of-falling and fall-related efficacy in relationship to functioning among community-living elders. *Journal of Gerontology, 49*, M140-M147.

Tinetti, M.E., Richman, D., & Powell, L. (1990). Falls efficacy as a measure of fear of falling. *Journal of Gerontology: Psychological Sciences, 45*(6), P239-243.

Tinetti, M.E., Speechley, M., & Ginter, S.F. (1988). Risk factors for falls among elderly people living in the community. *New England Journal of Medicine, 319*, 1701-1707.

Van den Ende, C.H.M., Vliet Vlieland, T.P.M., Munneke, M., & Hazes, J.M.W. (1998). Dynamic exercise therapy in rheumatoid arthritis: A systematic review of randomized clinical trials. *British Journal of Rheumatology, 42,* 677-687.

van Dijk, P.T., Meulenberg, O.G., van de Sande, H.J., & Habbema, J.D. (1993). Falls in dementia patients. *Gerontologist, 33,* 200-204.

Vereijken, B. (1991). *The dynamics of skill acquisition.* Unpublished doctoral dissertation, Free University, Netherlands.

Wagenaar, R.C., Holt, K.G., Kubo, M., & Ho, C. (2002). Gait risk factor for falls in older adults: a dynamic prospective. *Generation, 26,* 28-32.

Weir, P.L., & Leavitt, J.L. (1990). The effects of model's skill level and model's knowledge of results on the acquisition of an aiming task. *Human Movement Science, 9,* 369-383.

WHO Study Group. (1994). Assessment of fracture risk and its application to screening for postmenopausal osteoporosis. *WHO Technical Report Series, 843,* 1-129.

Wolfson, L. (1997). Balance decrements in older persons: Effects of age and disease. In J.C. Masdeau, L. Sudarsky, & L. Wolfson (Eds.), *Gait disorders of aging. Falls and therapeutic strategies* (pp. 79-92). Philadelphia: Lippincott-Raven.

Wolfson, L., Whipple, R., Derby, C., Judge, J., King, M., Amerman, P., Schmidt, L., & Smyers, D. (1996). Balance and strength training in older adults: Intervention gains and t'ai chi maintenance. *Journal of the American Geriatrics Society, 44,* 498-506.

Wood, B. H., Bilclough, J. A., Bowron, A., & Walker, R. W. (2002). Incidence and prediction of falls in Parkinson's disease: A prospective multidisciplinary study. *Journal of Neurology, Neurosurgery and Psychiatry, 72,* 721–725.

WHO Falls Global Report Working Party (Kalache, A., (Chair) Al-Faisal, W., Beattie, B., Belton, K,, Chodzko-Zajko, W., Fu, D., Fu, H., Gnanasambandam, U., Graham, T., Herman, M., James, K., Kalula, S., Kronfol, N., Marin, P.P., Perracini, M., Pike, I., Rose, D., Sachiyo, Y., Scott, V., Stevens, J., Todd, C., Yu, W.,). (2007). Global Report on Falls Prevention in Older Age. Geneva: World Health Organization. http://www.who.int/ageing/publications/Falls_prevention7March.pdf

Wrisberg, C.A., & Lui, Z. (1991). The effect of contextual variety on the practice, retention, and transfer of an applied motor skill. *Research Quarterly for Exercise and Sport, 62,* 406-412.

Yaffe, K., Barnes, D., Nevitt, M., Lui, L.Y., & Covinski, K. (2001). A prospective study of physical activity and cognitive decline in elderly women: Women who walk. *Archives of Internal Medicine, 161,* 1703-1708.

Index

Note: The italicized *f* and *t* following page numbers refer to figures and tables, respectively.

About the Author

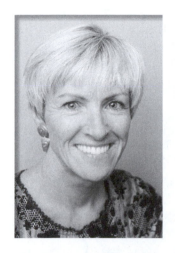

Debra Rose, PhD, is a professor in the division of kinesiology and health science and director of the Center for Successful Aging at California State University at Fullerton. She also serves as co-director of the Fall Prevention Center of Excellence at the University of Southern California. Her primary research focus is on the enhancement of mobility and the prevention of falls in later years.

Dr. Rose is nationally and internationally recognized for her work in assessment and programming for fall risk reduction. Her research in fall risk reduction in the elderly has been published in numerous peer-reviewed publications, including the *Journal of the American Geriatric Society, Archives of Physical Medicine and Rehabilitation, Neurology Report*, and the *Journal of Aging and Physical Activity*. She was an expert contributor to the *Global Report on Falls Prevention in Older Age* published by the World Health Organization in 2007.

The innovative fall risk reduction program she developed and describes in this manual was recognized by the Health Promotion Institute of the National Council on Aging (NCOA) in 2006 as a "Best Practice" program in health promotion. This program is currently being implemented in numerous community-based settings and retirement communities throughout the United States. The NCOA also awarded Debra the Molly Mettler Award for Leadership in Health Promotion for her work in the area of fall risk reduction in 2007.

Debra is a fellow of the Research Consortium of AAHPERD, a fellow of the American Academy of Kinesiology and Physical Education, former executive board member of the North American Society for the Psychology of Sport and Physical Activity, and past editor in chief of the *Journal of Aging and Physical Activity*.

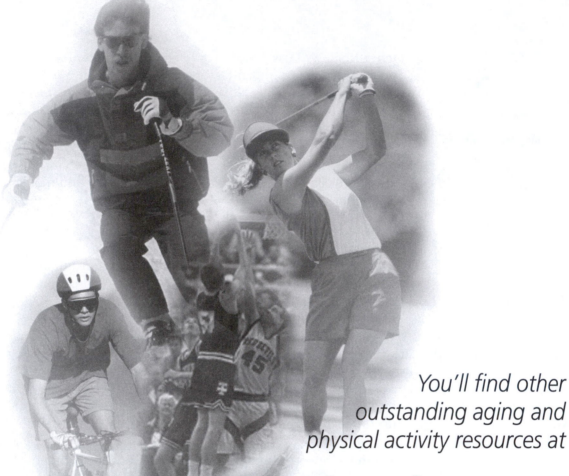

You'll find other outstanding aging and physical activity resources at

www.HumanKinetics.com

In the U.S. call

1-800-747-4457

Australia...08 8372 0999
Canada 1-800-465-7301
Europe...+44 (0) 113 255 5665
New Zealand..0800 222 062

HUMAN KINETICS
The Information Leader in Physical Activity
P.O. Box 5076 • Champaign, IL 61825-5076 USA

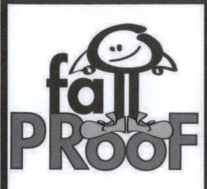

Instructor Certification

Become a Certified FallProof™ Instructor

Get the specialized knowledge and skills needed to lead effective balance and mobility programs. The FallProof™ Balance and Mobility Specialist Instructor Certificate Program is designed to provide physical activity instructors and health care professionals with the knowledge and practical skills necessary to implement an evidence-based balance and mobility training program for older adults at moderate-to-high risk for falls in community and residential care settings.

First of its Kind Certification
The FallProof™ Balance and Mobility Specialist Instructor Certificate Program is the first and only program of its kind to be offered in the U.S. The program has been extensively field-tested and shown to reduce the risk factors associated with falls among older adults.

Students will complete online theoretical coursework and onsite practical competency exams.

Here's a sample of what you'll learn:

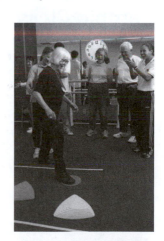

- Theoretical basis for balance and mobility training

- Rationale for the development of multi-dimensional fall risk reduction programs

- The role of intrinsic and extrinsic risk factors in falls

- Multi-dimensional screening and assessment of balance and mobility

- Core components of the FallProof™ program:

  - Center of Gravity Control Training
  - Multi-sensory Training
  - Postural Strategy Training
  - Gait Pattern Enhancement & Variation Training
  - Strength & Flexibility Training

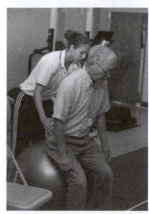

ENROLL on-line at http://hhd.fullerton.edu/csa/
or call 657-278-7994

DVD Menu and User Instructions

DVD MENU

FallProof! Assessments

Fullerton Advanced Balance Scale
30-Foot Walk

Case Study

FallProof! Program Components

Center-of-Gravity Control Training
Multisensory Training
Postural Strategy Training
Gait Pattern Enhancement and Variation Training

Sample Class

Printable Documents

Form 3.1 The FallProof Health and Activity
   Questionnaire
Form 3.2 FallProof Health and Activity Ques-
   tionnaire Short Form
Form 3.3 FallProof Program Report Card
Form 3.4 Score Sheet for Allerton Advanced
   Balance Scale
Form 3.5 Score Sheet for Berg Balance Scale
Form 3.6 Score Sheet for 30-Foot (9 m) Walk
Form 3.7 Score Sheet for Walkie-Talkie Test
Form 3.8 Balance Efficacy Scale
Figure 11.2 Sample Lesson Plan

DVD USER INSTRUCTIONS

The reproducible forms on this DVD-ROM can only be accessed using a DVD-ROM drive in a computer (not a DVD player on a television). To access the reproducible forms, follow these instructions:

Microsoft Windows

1. Place DVD in the DVD-ROM drive of your computer.
2. Double-click on the "My Computer" icon from your desktop.
3. Right-click on the DVD-ROM drive and select the "Open" option from the pop-up menu.
4. Double-click on the "Reproducible Forms" folder.
5. Select the reproducible form that you want to view or print.

Macintosh

1. Place DVD in the DVD-ROM drive of your computer.
2. Double-click the DVD icon on your desktop.
3. Double click on the "Reproducible Forms" folder.
4. Select the reproducible form that you want to view or print.

Note: You must have Adobe Acrobat reader to view the reproducible forms.